D0485535

DIY Clinical Examination
for Medical Students

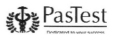

PasTest
Dedicated to your success

 Westminster Publishing Ltd

DIY Clinical Examination
for Medical Students

••••••

a pocket book, incorporating methods of
clinical diagnosis, anatomy, radiology, clinical procedures,
pathology, and a glossary of medical terms

John Lumley MS FRCS

Emeritus Professor of Vascular Surgery
St Bartholomew's and the Royal London
School of Medicine and Dentistry
Honorary Consultant Surgeon
St Bartholomew's Hospital, London
Member of Council, Royal College of Surgeons
England

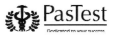

PasTest
Dedicated to your success

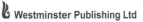
Westminster Publishing Ltd

© 2008 WESTMINSTER PUBLISHING
© 2008 PASTEST LTD
Egerton Court
Parkgate Estate
Knutsford
Cheshire
WA16 8DX

Telephone: 01565 752000

First Published 2008

ISBN: 1 905635 51 6
978 1 905635 51 1
A catalogue record for this book is available from the British Library.

PasTest Revision Books and Intensive Courses

PasTest has been established in the field of postgraduate medical
education since 1972, providing revision books and intensive
study courses for doctors preparing for their professional
examinations.

Books and courses are available for the following specialties:
**MRCGP, MRCP Parts 1 and 2, MRCPCH Parts 1 and 2, MRCS,
MRCOG Parts 1 and 2, DRCOG, DCH, FRCA, Dentistry.**

For further details contact:
PasTest, Freepost, Knutsford, Cheshire WA16 7BR
Tel: 01565 752000   Fax: 01565 650264
www.pastest.co.uk enquiries@pastest.co.uk

Text prepared by Scribe Design
Printed and bound in the UK by Cambridge University Press, Cambridge

Contents

PREFACE

This text provides an illustrated guide to clinical examination. It includes the relevant anatomy to understand these techniques and to undertake routine practical procedures, together with an introduction to basic pathology and its associated radiology. Traditional teaching of anatomy is in excess of the current requirements of most clinical practitioners; even surgeons tend to limit their activities to specific regions of the body. Nevertheless, every clinician examining a patient requires anatomical knowledge, to understand the limits and range of normality, before they can diagnose and manage abnormal states. Thus training in practical anatomy remains essential and relevant.

Most clinicians undertake venepuncture and an increasing number are involved in vascular access; this requires unique knowledge in the choice of vessel and potential complications. Many clinicians have to inject local anesthetic and undertake procedures, such as lumbar puncture, pleural and peritoneal drainage, and organ biopsy, requiring associated anatomical knowledge. Injuries can involve any part of the body, and require knowledge of the structures that may be damaged and need treatment. Some disciplines, including sports medicine, physical medicine and physiotherapy, require knowledge of functional anatomy, with an emphasis on palpable anatomy and movement.

The recent remarkable developments in radiological imaging have increased the need for a comprehensive knowledge of anatomy for their interpretation. This is particularly so for the deeper structures that were only previously accessible to the surgeon and pathologist, e.g., within the head, chest, and abdomen. Multi-media diagnosis requires the use of appropriate techniques for specific areas, and whole body imaging requires knowledge of "joined-up" anatomy and the ability to follow structures across adjacent regions.

Surgeons require more anatomical knowledge of their specialist area than is included in this text, but they also should be skilled clinicians and diagnosticians, and require enough general anatomy to bring this about. All clinicians should know the operation that has probably been undertaken through an observed scar.

An extensive number of clinicians from multiple disciplines treat disease and dysfunction, each discipline requiring its own body of knowledge and expertise. The anatomical requirements of these groups vary, but may be very specialized, as with acupuncture and chiropody.

This book addresses many of the needs of all specialties, but the main audience is the general medical practitioner and those practicing all aspects of physical medicine. This is particularly at the start of clinical studies, but the student continually needs to perfect clinical skills and to demonstrate competence in their final examination. In the latter, students can expect to be observed examining patients and this tests the security of the clinical examination to its fullest extent.

Postgraduate students also need careful reappraisal of their techniques of clinical examination before presenting themselves for work-based appraisal and to higher examining authorities. The aim of this title is to provide a reliable yet flexible method of clinical assessment, appropriate to life-long professional application.

AIMS, ORGANIZATION, and CLINICAL SKILLS

The aims of this book are to:

- Demonstrate a system of examination of the body, including the assessment of function, and the use of common clinical tools
- Display observable and palpable anatomy of relevance to clinical practice
- Examine radiological images and their associated anatomy
- Illustrate points for vascular access and injection of local anesthetic
- Consider the anatomy of common clinical procedures, tendon and joint injections, surgical incisions, and access points for minimally invasive surgery
- Highlight and selectively illustrate common disease entities
- Include tables and appendices on practical areas of clinical management
- Provide a glossary of common medical terms

There is no single right way to examine a patient, as this is adapted to the patient's condition, and each specialty has its own preferred approach. Whereas anatomy is most easily worked out and understood through a regional approach, medicine is taught primarily by system, and systemic examination crosses regional boundaries, requiring joined up anatomy. In this text, a **regional** order is followed but it is linked to a **systemic approach**. The chest includes the cardiovascular and respiratory systems; the abdomen, the alimentary and urogenital systems. The musculoskeletal system includes the muscles of the back and limbs, and the nervous and vascular systems are considered as separate entities.

The text for each system is brief, to make it easier to read, understand and remember. Sections start with essential anatomy and the muscle details are tabulated. There follows a summary of frequently encountered diseases; this has been highlighted in blue; additional information is integrated into the text and tables. The bulk of the book is a fully illustrated method of clinical examination. Further sections consider vascular access and local anesthetic techniques; incisions and practical procedures are placed with the relevant system.

The illustrations are predominantly photographs of clinical examination, emphasizing this important aspect of diagnosis. Clinical examination is linked to its anatomy, considering **observation**, **palpation**, **percussion**, and **auscultation**. With muscles, their **active**, **passive**, and **resisted**

movements are examined, and in joints, the traditional order of **look**, **feel**, **move**, and **measure** is followed by **imaging**.

Radiological images complement the text and indicate the current preferred investigations. These include plain radiographs, computed tomography (CT) and magnetic resonance imaging (MRI); vascular images include duplex ultrasound, spiral CT, and angiography.

The number of anatomical and medical terms is initially daunting to a student. **Appendix 1** considers the terms used for **anatomical description**. An extensive **glossary** is intended to ease your induction; it covers medical terms in the text, but not all those from the tables. It provides a useful bedside aid but use an online medical dictionary to define other terms and the diseases you encounter.

The book lays emphasis on clinical examination, but **Appendix 2** includes **historical notes** for each system. **Appendix 3** considers the tools of examination, the examination of **lumps** and **ulcers**, and includes a **method of diagnosis**. Everyone loves tables, even if it's only to complain of their content or decry their inclusion. The **diagnostic tables** are not for the whingers, but for those who like facts and lists to hang their information on; they include practical useful information to help you sort out common problems.

Although the information presented provides a logical approach to diagnosis, there must be flexibility to adapt this approach, to match the patient's presenting condition. **Clinical examination** generally commences with the hands followed by the head and neck, and then an examination from top to toe. You are encouraged to develop your own method of assessment, based on the guidelines provided in the text. Training in clinical examination should begin with self-examination, and examining peers and models, before approaching a patient.

CLINICAL SKILLS

A patient presents to a doctor because of a problem/complaint/symptom/sign. The consultation may be at home/clinic/hospital, and the patient may be walking/supported/transported. The doctor communicates with the patient to determine what is/is not the cause (diagnosis). This is through a history, examination, and investigations – a pattern emerges of a possible diagnosis, together with its severity.

This is followed by frank discussion, with explanation and advice, initiating treatment to make the patient better (and to do no harm). This treatment may have to be started before completing a diagnosis (e.g., trauma, hemorrhage), and may be just reassurance – for self-limiting or trivial diseases, and addressing any fears or anxiety about potential disease. The problem may be social or psychological. When discussing follow-up, consider whether the patient is likely to come back.

HISTORY

The history is the single most important aspect of diagnosis – let the patient talk and listen without interruption.

Communication depends on the patient's understanding, intelligence, education, background, and personality, and is based on the mutual confidence and comfort of the patient/doctor relationship, and the environment.

If the patient is unable to give a history, e.g., a child, a poor historian, because of physical or mental handicap, an unreliable witness or linguistic problems, a third party is used, but the responses are more difficulty to interpret (make a note of the informant).

Although there may be physical (organic/pathological) disease, the primary or secondary features may be due to socio-psychological effects.

The initial questions concern identity: **date**, **name**, **age**, **occupation** (present/previous), **marital status**, and **children**.

Presenting Problem (see also *Appendix 2*)

Use simple, single and understandable questions; wait for and listen carefully to the answers; never be confrontational

Don't suggest, direct, shape, flavour or elaborate answers

If asking leading questions (as with the review of the systems), allow free choice of answers

Avoid fitting questions and answers to a classical picture, as this can lead to a misdiagnosis

Enquire of recent illness, trauma, weight loss, medication, contacts, and overseas visits

Note previous bouts of the same problem, the diagnosis, investigations, treatment, and precipitating and associated features

NB: When recording the problem, use the patient's own words and place events chronologically; if there is more than one problem, document these separately (e.g., breathless for two weeks/vomited fresh blood last night).

Pain

Pain is a frequent presenting problem, it is often diagnostic, but it can be subjective, influenced by potential implications and its effect on lifestyle: its presence may also influence history taking and examination.

In its diagnosis, consider the following headings, turning them into a memorable form, such as a flow chart or an anagram.

Site

Focal: can be pinpointed and pointed out (e.g., trauma, superficial infection)

Diffuse: (e.g., from thoracic and abdominal viscera)

Referred: from a viscus to its somatic nerve root (e.g., diaphragm to the tip of the shoulder)

Radiating: along a nerve root (e.g., down the leg, due to pressure from an intervertebral disc)

Timing (of current episode)

Onset: when first noticed – sudden (e.g., related to an activity, trauma, vascular ischemic event, perforation of a viscus) – gradual (e.g., inflammatory)

Duration: continuous, fluctuating, intermittent, colic, frequency, progress, changing pattern

Offset: sudden/gradual, modification (see below)

Previous episode: when, frequency, course, differences, diagnosis, management

Quality: sharp, stabbing, aching, burning, throbbing, crushing, bloated, distended

Severity: on a scale of 0 to 10, percentage disability, what do you do, pain tolerance. Anxiety about effect and implication of diagnosis on way of life

Modification

Aggravation: cough, movement, posture, feet up/down, bright light, food

Relief: lying down, staying still, sitting, standing, feet down/up, closing eyes, food, medication, intervention

Effect on systems and lifestyle

Sweating, pyrexia, malaise, photophobia, loss of sleep

Vomiting, diarrhea, focal effects (e.g., paresthesia, muscle wasting)

Inactivity at home, reduction of sport and social activity

Stopping work and socio-economic effect

Past Medical History

Previous non-trivial illnesses, operations, accidents, admissions to hospital; with dates

In children, note illnesses, investigations, and immunizations

In adults, note relevant childhood problems, e.g., chronic respiratory disease, rheumatic fever

Drugs and Allergies

Drugs being taken – doses, duration

Previous drugs – when, what, why?

Allergies/allergic symptoms (describe), precipitating causes

Social and Personal History

Smoking – number per day (number of years), changes

Alcohol – units per day (week), what drunk, ever heavy drinker?

Recreational drugs – which? – current/previous

Difficulties with job, family or finance, recent mental stress or sleeping problems

Social arrangements, spouse, partner, living arrangements

Accommodation, ownership, which floor/lifts?; toilet same floor?

Friends/relatives nearby

Receives or needs meals on wheels/home help

Pets

Able to return to previous residence or employment

Family History

State of health/cause of death: parents, siblings, other close relatives, spouse, children

Members of family suffering from the same or other disorder, or serious illnesses (draw a family tree)

CLINICAL EXAMINATION

Examination of a patient commences from the moment you first meet, observing them carefully from this point onwards; throughout the history, examination, and subsequent discussion.

Observation

When you observe a person sitting in a restaurant or walking down the street, you gain an impression of their general well-being. Although the "first impressions can be deceiving," when they are, you usually look for the reason why this is so. Similarly, when a patient arrives for a consultation, you should carefully observe their **body language** for evidence of disease and discomfort, and how this is affecting them.

From the referral letter, you will know a patient's presenting complaint, and something of their *social* and *cultural* background. You can therefore decide whether their clothing and state of cleanliness are in keeping with these expectations. **Physical** as well as **mental** problems can reflect in a patient's face, showing discomfort, anxiety and cachexia – skin discoloration, weight loss and drawn features. **Posture** may indicate **discomfort** in a part of the body, accompanied by breathlessness and general misery from this condition. **Deformity** may be present and, if the patient is walking, the above factors, together with any weakness or joint problems, influence their **gait**, and whether they require physical or any other form of support.

A **handshake** is an appropriate introduction to most patients, but may not be in some cultures – this should be obvious from a patient's response. Provided there is no discomfort in this limb, the handshake provides a good deal of information on the confidence of the patient, their reluctance or willingness to communicate, together with local power, muscle wasting, coordination, and abnormal limb movement. This is the first **skin** contact and may indicate dryness, moisture or skin abnormality. Many of the above features are also reflected in your **eye contact** with a patient during the initial introduction, and subsequent history and examination. It is essential that your own body language indicates confidence, and offers **understanding** and **support** to every patient under your care.

Palpation

Palpation is undertaken with the fingers and palm of your hand, and between the thumb and finger, or between the hands, exploring and defining normal and abnormal anatomy. It confirms what you have already observed and adds information on the feel of the skin and the structures deep to it. This information includes the **texture**, **temperature**, and **dampness** of the skin, **tenderness** due to injury and infection, **swelling** and **deformity**, abnormalities of **sensation** and in **movement**, and information on the neurological and musculoskeletal systems.

Tactile communication varies in different cultures and societies, but even if an invited handshake is declined, patients realize that palpation is an essential diagnostic tool and may also be a therapeutic measure, as with movement, mobilization, massage, and manipulation.

The confidence with which a patient accepts examination and cooperates with the examiner relates to the relationship developed during history taking, your tact and diplomacy, and your ability to palpate, defining abnormality and avoiding discomfort. The patient is soon fully aware of your skills and whether they can relax and let you proceed. **Palpation is a two-way process**, building up mutual understanding. As you define abnormality, the patient becomes increasingly aware of the nature of their problem.

Discussion is continued during the examination and, as confidence increases, new factors in the history are defined and sometimes other unexpected topics introduced. Be continually on the lookout for information that the patient has previously, intentionally or unintentionally, withheld.

Palpation requires training and practice and a sound knowledge of normal anatomy. This should begin with **self-examination** and extend to supervised, directed examination of peers and models, before you examine patients. Confidence, speed, and quality develop with regular use and experience. Although tactile skills vary in different individuals, they can be acquired, developed, and improved.

When examining, your **hands should be clean** with no grease or sticky material that could act as a barrier to tactile sensation. Your nails should be short, smooth, and clean. Your palmar surface should be as smooth as possible. Special care is required after rope and rock climbing, rowing and car maintenance, but avoid using aggressive soaps and detergents. Before examining, make sure your hands are **warm**; if necessary, soak them in warm water.

Tactile awareness can be improved by feeling coins and other common objects, under direct vision, out of sight, and within plastic and canvas bags. Recognition of surface markings, such as the imprint of a coin, is undertaken with the gentle touch of the fingers. The fingers must be firmer, stronger, and more rigid to identify ill-defined contours, such as through the canvas bag. The top and sides of an object have to be accessible for examination between finger and thumb or bimanually. The effects of compression can be examined by compressing a water-filled balloon or a squeegee ketchup bottle. Joints can be considered by opening a hinged box or a door, particularly when these have stiff hinges, slam shut, or are opened too far.

Examination must always begin gently and you must **watch the patient's face** throughout, to identify discomfort, before applying deeper pressure or extended movement. **Moving structures** are best examined with a still hand, such as the placement of two fingers on the superficial temporal artery or the deep placement of fingers, of one or both hands, over, or on either side of, the abdominal aorta. Stationary flat hands are also used to assess thoracic movement and movement of intra-abdominal organs.

Static and **fixed**, normal and abnormal tissues and organs require exploratory movement of the fingers or hand, depending on their relative size, and whether they can be gripped between the finger and thumb, or between the fingers of both hands. Defining features are considered in **Appendix 3**. The **smoothness**, coarseness or irregularity of surfaces must be defined. Their **size** is frequently related to common objects, such as fruit and vegetables, but measurement in **centimeters** is more reproducible. Know the **size of parts of your own hand**, such as the width of your thumbnail, the distance from the tip of your index finger to the metacarpophalangeal joint and your palmar span.

The hardness of a structure is often difficult to define. Bony **hard** can be likened to tapping your forehead, **firm** as pressing the tip of your nose and **soft** as in squeezing your lip. **Superficial palpation** may be quick and gentle, avoiding any pressure that could obscure inflammation and its interpretation. This may be for superficial, cutaneous, and subcutaneous abnormalities, such as counting thoracic spines, or defining the sternal angle and ribs in a thin individual.

Deeper palpation is with firm, rigid fingers, slowly and gradually searching more deeply, the pressure is applied by one hand or downward pressure of one hand on the other. Remember to keep watching the patient's face for evidence of discomfort. Deeper pressure may be required in the abdomen or to locate the shape of the spines of the twelfth thoracic and lumbar vertebrae.

Palpation also identifies underlying movement, such as the cardiac impulse, the resonance of vocal reverberation through the chest, and the fluid thrill of abnormal heart valves and vascular malformations.

Palpation must be undertaken in an **organized fashion** working from outwards to the center or centrally outwards, defining all aspects of a normal or abnormal structure. It is directed by your knowledge of normal anatomy, e.g., palpating nerves and arteries. The examination of muscles, bones, and joints is considered with the musculoskeletal system (page 71).

A specific aspect of palpation that must be considered in every patient is the examination for enlarged **lymph nodes**. This may be as a general examination, as with a disease of the hematopoietic tissue, or related to focal infection and neoplasia.

Percussion

With the tip of the bent middle finger of your dominant hand, gently tap the top of a table, first in the middle and then over a leg. You will note the more hollow sound from the unsupported area. Now place the palm of the other hand over the same two areas and this time tap the middle phalanx of the second or third finger. The sound is amplified and you can both **hear** and **feel** with the resting hand, the difference in the two areas.

This is the principle of percussion that is used in clinical practice. You can directly tap onto a bone or onto your palmed other hand, as just described. First try this out on yourself in the privacy of your room. **Tap various bones**, such as the skull and patella, and get the feel of the wrist movement, and the force needed to make a noise and feel the impact, without hurting yourself. Next place the palm of your other hand on your **belly** and tap the middle finger as with the table. Move the palm around and you will find a different noise as you pass over the hollow area of your gut, in the center of your belly, and the solid liver, as you move over the ribs on the right side.

Repeat this over your **chest**, and note the difference between the air-filled lung laterally and your heart centrally. By moving slowly from a hollow to a solid area, you have a means of defining the edge of an organ, and therefore its size. Percussion can take a lot of practice, to find the appropriate wrist swing and force required to hear and feel differences, without hurting yourself or a patient, so practice regularly on yourself until you are competent.

Auscultation

The sounds emitted by the body include the movements of the **heart valves**, and **blood flow** and **airflow** through the respiratory tract and gut. The **stethoscope bell** can be applied to most areas of the body and the **diaphragm** is used to listen to higher pitched sounds. A fetal stethoscope is used over the pregnant uterus.

An ultrasound (US) probe emits and receives reflected sound. A moving column of blood changes the frequency of the reflected beam, due to the Doppler effect, and, through this frequency change, the US probe can be used to detect flow, and analyze its waveform. US probes are also used to build up images of deep structures, from the position and nature of the reflected beam (e.g., intra-abdominal aorta, liver, and fluid collections), and to detect movement (e.g., the valves of the heart).

Thus with the techniques of **observation, palpation, percussion**, and **auscultation**, you have a powerful means for assessing the structures of the body. For the examination of joints, as considered in the musculoskeletal system, use the classic checklist of **look, feel, move, measure**, and **X ray**.

On completion of your examination ask the patient to dress, and make himself or herself comfortable, on a bed or chair as appropriate. You must now make a preliminary diagnosis, decide on any necessary investigations and formulate a management plan. Consider carefully what the patient thinks is wrong, as this is based on personal experience, reading available literature, an internet search, and an informed family history. It is a sobering thought that most patients progress as well as they expect to do.

General Examination

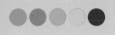

General Examination

In an outpatient consultation, the **pulse**, **blood pressure** (figures 1 & 2), and **urine** should be routinely recorded, together with a patient's **weight** (figure 3). The **height** (figure 4) is usually known, but when growth patterns are being studied, this should be measured, together with span and segments (figure 5a,b). In hospital, examine the **ward chart** for patient details and dates. These commonly record temperature, pulse, respiration, blood pressure, weight, bowel habit, and the results of urine testing. Note all these records carefully, and personally examine all abnormal specimens. The latter include sputum, urine, vomit, feces, the contents of surgical drainage bottles, and any discharges. Discharge may be from ulcers, wounds or other sites, and smaller amounts can be observed on dressings.

In the **physical examination**, keep the patient comfortable, relaxed and reassured. Talk through what is going to happen, if this is not obvious, and ensure minimal discomfort and inconvenience. A **warm environment** is essential and your hands must be warm. The **privacy** of a small room or a curtained area is desirable with optimal, preferably natural, **lighting**. The patient undresses down to underclothes and puts on a dressing gown. They then lie supine on a couch with an adjustable backrest, to provide head support, and are covered with a sheet or blanket. Each area must be **adequately exposed** as required without embarrassment. A **chaperone** may be appropriate when examining members of the opposite sex. Relatives are usually best excluded except when examining children.

Thoroughness of examination is important. Efficiency and speed develop with practice. The examination time should not be prolonged in sick or frail patients; in an emergency it may be appropriate to concentrate on diseased areas, completing a routine examination at a later time.

Stand on the right side of the patient. The **general impression** obtained during the history is expanded during the examination. Note the patient's **physical** and **mental status**, as well as the **severity** of their presenting problems, their **shape**, **posture**, **state of hygiene**, and **mental** and **physical activity**, and **abnormal movements**. In the initial stage, examine particularly the exposed parts, i.e., the **hands**, and the **head and neck**. This provides information of changes of **nutrition** and **hydration**, such as obesity, edema, weight loss, cachexia, loss of skin turgor, and skin laxity. Weight loss with an increased appetite is seen in **diabetes**, **thyrotoxicosis**, and **malabsorption**. Other potent causes of weight loss are **malnutrition** (due to lack of food, inability to eat and lack of desire to eat), **parasitic** disease, particularly of the gut, and progressive **malignancy**.

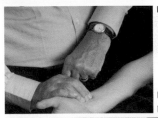

Figure 1 Examination of the pulse.

Figure 2 Measurement of blood pressure.

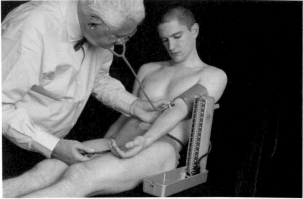

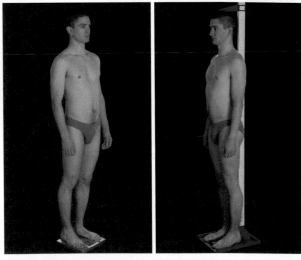

Figure 3 Weight.

Figure 4 Height.

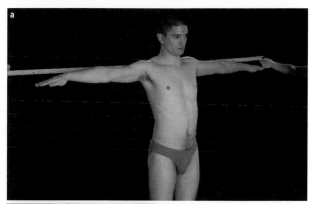

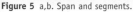

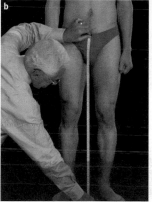

Figure 5 a,b. Span and segments.

In the general examination, the **pulse**, **blood pressure**, **venous** and **arterial pulsation** in the neck, and the **respiratory rate** and **movements**, in the chest and abdomen, are part of the routine. However, they are considered in detail with their respective systems.

MENTAL STATUS

The patient's **behavior** may be influenced by the unaccustomed situation of being a patient, or the effect of their disease, particularly if they are in pain. The latter shows through their **facial expression**, the degree of **eye contact**, **restlessness**, **sweating**, **anxiety**, **apathy**, **depression**, lack of **cooperation** or **aggression**. Stress may be indicated by rapid respiration, but note whether the patient's intelligence and personality equate to what one would expect from the history or whether this could have changed in relation to the disease.

Drugs, head injuries, and other diseases of the central nervous system can effect the **level of consciousness**, varying through alert, slow and confused, lacking concentration, and reduced levels of response to spoken and physical stimuli. The patient's **orientation** in time, place, and person should be noted. The **Glasgow Coma Scale** (**GCS** – page 347) is a valuable way of documenting the level of consciousness for serial measurement. The patient's **speech** may be impaired by disease of the central nervous system, producing dysphasia or dysarthria, and there may be voice changes, such as hoarseness in laryngeal infection or myxedema. Impairment of **motor function** can produce weakness or spasticity and these may affect speech.

The **posture** and **gait** should be noted, and other activities such as undressing. There may be **added movements**, such as the fine tremor of age, thyrotoxicosis, parkinsonism, and alcoholism, the flapping tremor of hepatic, respiratory, renal and cardiac failure, or more specific neurological abnormalities, producing lack of coordination and involuntary movements. If **psychiatric abnormalities** are present, or suspected, note the patient's general behavior, and disturbances of orientation. Record the emotional state, thought processes and content, hallucinations, delusions and compulsive phenomena, and include an assessment of cognitive and intellectual function.

CLINICAL SYNDROMES

A number of **congenital** and **endocrine diseases** have characteristic general features amenable to spot diagnoses; but such changes also occur at the extremes of normality, thus be aware of the danger of jumping to false conclusions. Congenital examples include Down, Turner and Marfan syndromes, achondroplasia, and hereditary telangiectasia. Endocrine abnormalities include acromegaly (figure 6), Cushing's disease, myxedema, and thyrotoxicosis. Other spot diagnoses are Paget disease, Parkinson, and myopathies. General disease states include **weight loss**, **dehydration**, **edema**, and the features of **hepatic** and **renal failure**.

HANDS

The general examination starts with the hands. The initial handshake may identify an **abnormality**, such as the large hand of acromegaly (figure 6) or a deformed hand due to abnormal development or previous injury. There may be excessive **sweating**, due to anxiety, hyperhidrosis or thyrotoxicosis. Skin **color** changes are more easily seen in white skinned individuals, but they are usually visible in all races and must be sought.

The palm gives some indication of the type of work undertaken (figure 7). Note **pallor**, **cyanosis**, and **pigmentation**; stretch the skin of the palm to examine the color in the skin creases, as this provides a better indication than the more exposed areas. **Erythema** of the palmar skin is most marked over the thenar and hypothenar eminences. It is an important finding in liver disease, but may also occur in pregnancy, thyrotoxicosis, polycythemia, leukemia, chronic febrile illnesses and rheumatoid arthritis.

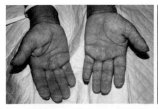
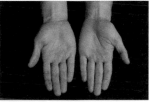

Figure 6 Acromegalic hands. Note the stubby enlarged digits. However, such hands may also be seen in the extremes of normality, and other clinical features and biochemical investigations are required to confirm the diagnosis.

Figure 7 Examination of the palms.

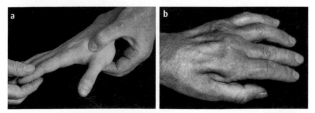

Figure 8 a. Examination for muscle wasting. b. The extreme atrophy of the interossei in this patient is due to a long-standing ulnar nerve lesion.

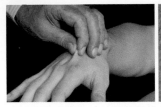

Figure 9 Examination for skin laxity.

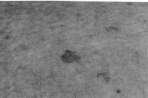

Figure 10 Senile keratosis.

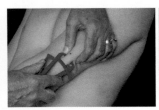

Figure 11 Measurement of skin thickness.

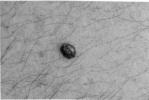

Figure 12 Campbell de Morgan spot.

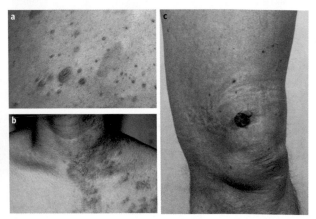

Figure 13 These three classic examples could all be missed unless a complete survey of exposure of the whole body is undertaken as part of your general examination. a. Numerous areas of skin pigmentation and nodular appearance associated with neurofibromatosis. b. Skin changes of a herpes zoster infection c. Malignant melanoma. An early diagnosis is essential if an excision cure is to be obtained in this condition.

Table 1 **SKIN MANIFESTATIONS OF NON-MALIGNANT SYSTEMIC DISEASE**

Erythema	Collagen disease Carcinoid Mitral valve (malar flush) Polycythemia rubra vera Superior vena caval obstruction Liver disease
Erythema multiforme	Fever Inflammatory bowel disease Rheumatoid arthritis Thyrotoxicosis Virus and micoplasma infections
Urticaria	Collagen disorders Xanthomatosis Hereditary angioneurotic edema Urticaria pigmentosa Henoch-Schönlein purpura Cold agglutinins
Scaling	Vitamin deficiencies Hypothyroidism Acromegaly Malabsorption Reiter syndrome
Papules and nodules	Behçet disease Erythema nodusum Erythema induratum Gardner syndrome Necrobiosis lipoidica Neurofibromatosis Polyarteritis nodosum Pseudoxanthoma elasticum Sarcoid Tuberous sclerosis Xanthoma
Blisters	Dermatitis herpetiformis Drugs Glucagonoma Pemphigus Porphyria Vascular disease
Angiomas **Pruritus** (table 11, p.339) **Purpura**	Multiple vascular malformations

Generalized muscle wasting can be detected by examination of the first dorsal interosseous muscles (figure 8a,b).

The back of the hand is best to assess **skin turgidity** and look for generalized pigmentation, bruises, rashes, and **spider nevi**. **Skin laxity** is seen in older subjects, but it may indicate dehydration at all ages (figure 9). Similarly, areas of **bruising** and **senile keratosis** (figure 10) are normal features of aging, but may also indicate non-malignant and malignant disease (tables 1 & 2) and there may be local or generalized skin discoloration (tables 3 & 4). Skin thickness is a useful measure of nutritional status, particularly in children (figure 11). Skin **nodules**, **moles**, and red **Campbell de Morgan spots** (figure 12) are common; skin abnormalities may be encountered anywhere on the body and the general examination must scan all areas (figure 13a–c).

In the **fingers**, note nicotine **staining**, and the **nutrition** of the skin in scleroderma, rheumatoid arthritis, other collagen disorders and ischemic conditions. There may be loss of pulp and small areas of ulceration

Table 2 CUTANEOUS MANIFESTATIONS OF MALIGNANCY

Primary skin malignancy
Gardner syndrome
Secondary malignant invasion (leukemia)
Paget disease of the breast
Pruritis (lymphoreticular disease)
Clubbing (lung)
Hypertrophic pulmonary osteoarthropathy (lung)
Superficial, deep venous thrombosis (occult often lung, gut)
Dermatomyositis (50% associated with malignancy)
Acanthosis nigricans (gut, bronchus)
Ichthyosis (gut)
Alopecia (gastric)
Purpura (thrombocytopenic)
Exfoliative erythroderma (lymphoma)
Erythema gyratum repens (breast, lung)
Erythema nodosum (gut, lung)
Erythema multiforme (gut, lung)
Eczematous dermatitis (gut, lung)
Herpes zoster (lymphoreticular)
Flushing (carcinoid)
Pyoderma gangrenosum (leukemia, multiple myeloma)
Palmar keratosis (bladder, lung)
Disseminating intravascular coagulation (leukemia, lymphoma,
    pancreas, generalized terminal malignant event)
Hypertrichosis lanuginosa (gut)

Table 3 **SKIN DISCOLORATION – LOCAL**

LOCAL SKIN DISCOLORATION	CAUSE
Hemorrhage/ bruising	Trauma Blood dyscrasias Increased capillary fragility Old age Lower limb venous hypertension
Purple	Campbell de Morgan spots Capillary nevus – port wine; strawberry Spider nevi Telangiectasia Pyogenic granuloma Stria – pregnancy, Cushing's, sudden weight loss
Yellow	Xanthelasma Pus
Brown	Freckles – moles, melanoma, basal cell carcinoma Café-au-lait spots – neurofibromatosis Oral spots – Peutz–Jeghers syndrome (with multiple small gut polyps) Erythema ab igne – fires and hot water bottles Pregnancy – areola and midline abdominal Ultraviolet light Radiotherapy Warts, senile keratosis, keratoacanthoma, callosities
Black	Eschar, burns and other scabs Gangrene Anthrax Pyoderma gangrenosum

around the fingertips. Painful **nodules** around the fingertips are seen in infective endocarditis (Osler's nodes) and deformity in rheumatoid arthritis and osteoarthritis (Heberden's nodes). **Warts** (figure 14) are common findings in children. **Thickening** of the palmar fascia (**Dupuytren's contracture** – figure 15) may be idiopathic, hereditary, or associated with cirrhosis, and various gut and pulmonary disorders.

Table 4 **SKIN DISCOLORATION – GENERALIZED**

GENERALIZED SKIN DISCOLORATION	CAUSE
Purpura	Bleeding disorders Vasculitides – collagen diseases, diabetes Septicemia – especially meningococcal Systemic malignancies Cushing disease Ehlers-Danlos syndrome
Yellow	Jaundice Mepacrine
Orange	Carotenemia
Pale brown/yellow	Chronic renal failure Polycythemia
Blue	Methemoglobin Cyanosis Polycythemia
Brown	UV light Acanthosis nigricans Addison disease Nelson syndrome Cushing disease ACTH hypersecretion Hemochromatosis (bronze diabetes) Arsenic and silver poisoning Gardner syndrome Pellagra – nicotinic acid deficiency Rheumatoid arthritis Gaucher syndrome Lichen planus Fixed drug reaction
Pallor	Anemia Hypoalbuminemia
Depigmentation	Albinism (absence of melanocytes) Vitiligo (destruction of melanocytes) Pernicious anemia Gastric cancer Hypo and hyperthyroidism Addison disease Late-onset diabetes Autoimmune disease (Hashimoto) Scleroderma Syphilis Leprosy Idiopathic

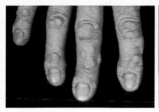

Figure 14 Digital warts

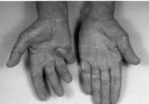

Figure 15 Dupuytren's contracture. This typically involves the ring and little fingers with palmar nodularity.

Skin rashes may be discrete or continuous (confluent) and the lesions may be primary or secondary. **Primary lesions** have specific features:

Macules are flat circumscribed areas of abnormal skin color. They may also have characteristic texture or markings

Papules are circumscribed raised areas of abnormal skin. Larger papules are termed **nodules** or tumors; if greater than 1 cm across, raised abnormal areas may be referred to as **plaques**. They may be due to increased cellular content or edema

Vesicles are raised papules containing clear fluid. Larger collections are termed blisters or bullae

Pustules are raised papules containing pus

Wheals are raised papules with pale centers

Purpura indicates hemorrhage within the skin

Annular lesions may indicate spreading and infiltration or may have a healing center

Secondary lesions develop from the expansion or decline of primary lesions, or may be related to their mechanical effect. Examples are desquamation or crusting, infiltration, ulceration, and scarring. Ichthyosis is thickening of the skin, lichenification is depigmentation and there may be atrophy. Scratching produces specific longitudinal, reddened areas, and there may be some associated skin thickening. Although there are very many and diverse cutaneous lesions, only a few are commonly seen. These include acne, dermatitis, psoriasis, urticaria, warts, skin cancers, and leg ulcers. In your general survey, also examine the hair distribution (table 5).

Table 5 **HAIR CHANGES**

HAIR CHANGES	CAUSE/REACTION
Decrease (alopecia)	Age Genetic-myotonia Damage from chemical treatment Severe illness Malnutrition Immunosuppressive drugs Radiotherapy Lichen planus Psoriasis Systemic lupus erythematosus Fungal

Increase	Racial
	Endocrine (virilizing ovarian tumors)
	    precocious puberty
	    adrenogenital syndrome
	    Cushing syndrome
	    acromegaly
	    drugs
	    steroids (anabolic steroids)
	Anti-epileptic drugs
	Menoxidil; diazoxide
	Anorexia nervosa

NAILS

Nails can be an indicator of local and systemic disease. There can be stunted growth, and they may be brittle and deformed. **Nail biters** (figure 16) can be identified from loss of the projecting nail in any of the digits of either hand. **Whitish spots** under the nail (leukonychia punctata) are associated with minor trauma. **Pallor** of anemia and hypoalbuminemia, **cyanosis** and polycythemia are usually well shown, and **pitting** of the nails is common in psoriasis. **Splinter hemorrhages** are longitudinal brown strips along the length of the middle of the nail; they are found in bacterial endocarditis and vasculitic disorders. Spoon-shaped, central depression of the nail (**koilonychia**) is seen in iron deficiency anemia.

Transverse grooves at a similar level in a number of nails (**Beau's lines**) can denote growth abnormalities related to the onset of a severe

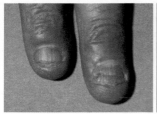

Figure 16 A nail biter.

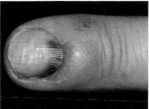

Figure 17 Paronychia. Pus has extended underneath the proximal nail bed with surrounding inflammation.

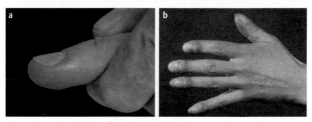

Figure 18 a. Examination for clubbing. b. Clubbing associated with congenital heart disease.

systemic disease. The arch over the base of the nail may become brown (**Mei's lines**) in renal insufficiency, poisoning, and some inflammatory disorders. **Infections** around the nail (**paronychia** – figure 17) are common but always exclude a diabetic etiology.

CLUBBING

In **finger clubbing**, the tissues at the base of the nail are thickened and the angle between the nail base and the adjacent skin on the finger (this should measure approximately 160 degrees – figure 18a,b) becomes obliterated. Application of light pressure at the base of the nail is associated with excessive movement of the nail bed. In clubbing, the nail loses its longitudinal curve and becomes convex from above downwards as well as from side to side. In the late stages, there may be associated swelling of the tips of the fingers. **Hypertrophic pulmonary osteoarthropathy** may be associated with clubbing in bronchial carcinoma; involvement of the wrist joints can be looked for at this stage.

Clubbing may also involve the **toes**, particularly the **congenital** variety. Common causes of clubbing are carcinoma and purulent conditions of the lung (bronchiectasis, lung abscess, empyema), congenital heart disease, and infective endocarditis. Less common conditions are pulmonary fibrosis, fibrosing alveolitis, pulmonary tuberculosis, pleural mesothelioma, cystic fibrosis, celiac and inflammatory bowel disease, cirrhosis, malabsorption, thyrotoxicosis, and bronchial arteriovenous malformations.

FACE

Generalized **weight loss** may be apparent in changing facial and cervical contours. Excess tissue fluid (**edema**) is subject to the effect of gravity and although mostly observed in the lower limbs towards the end of the day, it may also be obvious within the face, particularly the eyelids, after a night's sleep. Regional edema of the head, neck and upper limbs is seen in superior vena caval obstruction and the edema of myxedema may be particularly obvious in the eyelids, associated with skin and hair changes.

Whereas **pallor** and **cyanosis** of the hands may be due to the cold or local arterial disease, these signs in the warm central areas of the lips and tongue have a more generalized significance. The pallor of **anemia** is most noticeable in the mucous membranes, although the sign lacks specificity. The inner surface of the lower eyelid is an important area for demonstration (figure 19), as well as pallor of the mucous membranes and the palmar creases. Other abnormalities around the orbit include xanthelasma and an arcus senilis (figure 20).

Cyanosis is the blue discoloration given to the skin by deoxygenated blood. However, hemoglobin of 5 g/dl is required to produce visible cyanosis; it is thus not detectable in severe anemia. Cyanosis is best observed in areas with a rich blood supply such as the lips and tongue. It may also be noted in the ear lobes and fingernails but these areas can react to cold by vasoconstriction, producing peripheral cyanosis in the presence of normal oxygen saturation.

Cyanosis is usually due to cardiorespiratory abnormalities, but may also occur at high altitudes, with methemoglobinemia and sulfhemoglobinemia. Cardiac conditions include a number of congenital abnormalities with a right-to-left shunt, whilst cyanosis may be related to hypoventilation (head injuries, drug overdose), chronic obstructive airway disease, and mismatched arterial ventilation-perfusion (pulmonary embolism, pulmonary shunts, arteriovenous fistulae). Cyanosis is difficult

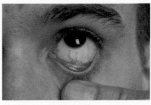

Figure 19 Examining for subconjunctival pallor in anemia beneath the lower lid.

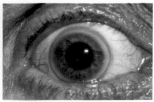

Figure 20 Arcus senilis.The prominent white discoloration around the periphery of the iris commences superiorly and inferiorly but may become circumferential as in this example.

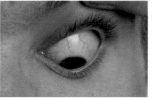

Figure 21 Examining for scleral pigmentation in jaundice.

to elicit in dark skinned people with anemia. **Polycythemia** is an excess of circulating red cells and may produce a purple-blue skin discoloration mimicking cyanosis; however, it is also prominent in the cheeks and the backs of the hands.

Jaundice is yellow discoloration, due to excess circulating bile pigment (table 8, page 315). Mild degrees of jaundice are easily picked up from the staining of the sclera (figure 21). Be careful not to confuse the uniform yellow colour of jaundice with the yellowish peripheral discoloration of the sclera that can be seen in normal individuals. As the jaundice becomes more pronounced, there is yellow skin discoloration, and this may progress to yellow/orange or even dark brown with high levels of plasma pigment.

MOUTH

The mouth is a valuable indicator of systemic disease, as well as local pathology. It has a complex embryological origin, being the site of the junction of ectoderm and endoderm, and receiving contributions from

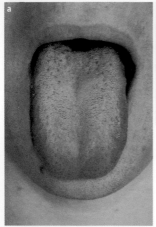

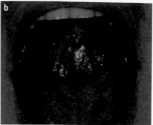

Figure 22 Examination of: a. the tongue and b. oropharynx.

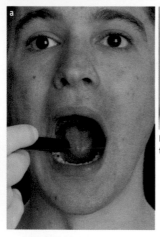

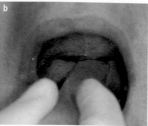

Figure 23 Examining mouth with: a. torch and b. spatula.

pharyngeal arch mesoderm. The tongue muscles are derived from suboccipital somites that have migrated forward around the pharynx, bringing their nerve supply with them. This origin is also reflected in the variety of diseases. These include skin and gut mucosal abnormalities, together with other lesions that encompass a number of medical and surgical disciplines.

The breath must be examined for **halitosis** (offensive or abnormal – fetor oris). This is most commonly due to poor local hygiene, but may be an indicator of respiratory, upper alimentary or systemic disease, and local disease within the oral cavity. Alimentary odors may be related to gastroenteritis, obstruction of the pylorus, and small and large gut, and over-indulgence of food and alcohol; the latter aroma depends on the timing and quantity imbibed.

Systemic disease produces characteristic odors. The sweet smell of ketotic breath may be related to insulin deficiency, but also to an increased metabolic rate, such as with a fever (particularly in childhood disorders) and fasting. There are usually other signs accompanying the fetor of renal and hepatic disease. The ammoniacal smell of hepatic coma has been likened to musty old eggs.

Ask the patient to put out their tongue to assess hydration and to say "ah", to observe the oropharynx (figure 22a,b). A more detailed examination may require a torch and spatula (figure 23a,b), as considered in other sections.

The general examination described is undertaken in all patients; it is followed by examination of one or more systems, depending on the presenting problem, as considered in subsequent sections. On completion of the examination of each region and system, cover the patient and make sure they are comfortable.

Regional Examination

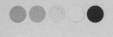

Head and Neck

Examination of the head and neck highlights the overlap between regional and systemic examination. It is part of the general examination (diagnostic features of a number of syndromes, the general mental state, mucous membranes, state of hydration, weight loss, oral hygiene, fetor, and lymphadenopathy), the alimentary system (mouth, pharynx, teeth, tongue, salivary glands), the respiratory system (upper respiratory tract and trachea), the cardiovascular system (the great vessels of the neck), the musculoskeletal system (muscles of mastication and those for head and neck movements), endocrine system (general features and thyroid gland), hematological system (cervical lymph nodes), and the central nervous system (brain and cranial nerve).

As well as incorporating these medical specialties, the head and neck is examined by a number of surgical groups: head and neck surgeons manage predominantly malignancy, but also thyroid and salivary gland pathology; dentists and faciomaxillary surgeons relate to the teeth and jaws; ophthalmic surgeons manage disease of the orbit and eye; neurosurgeons, diseases of the brain and cranial nerves; while the ear, nose and throat (ENT) surgeons overlap the other groups.

In this text, after the initial anatomy, the cranial nerves are used to demonstrate head and neck examination, including the special sensory organs, followed by a general description of the neck, including muscle tables, and the thyroid gland. (The cervical nodes, the mouth, salivary glands, oropharynx, and airway are considered with other systems.)

ANATOMY

The **skull vault** (figure 1a) is formed from the **frontal bone** anteriorly, a **parietal bone**, on each side, and the **occipital bone** posteriorly. At birth there is a diamond-shaped defect between the parietal and frontal bones (**anterior fontanel – bregma** – this closes at 18 months), and a triangular defect between the parietal and occipital bones posteriorly (**posterior fontanel – lambda** – this closes at 6 months).

Figure 1b,c shows the bones and radiograph of the anterior aspect of the skull. The frontal bone contains the **frontal air sinuses** on either side of the midline and, anterior to these, forms the **superciliary arches** (more prominent in the male), before turning backward to form the thin superior orbital roof. A palpable **supraorbital notch**, at the junction of

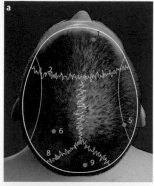

Figure 1
a,b. Bones of skull vault and face, and
c. anteroposterior skull radiograph.

1. Frontal
2. Frontoparietal suture
3. Bregma
4. Sagittal suture
5. Superior temporal line
6. Parietal
7. Lambda
8. Parieto-occipital suture
9. Occipital

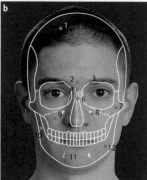

1. Frontal
2. Glabella
3. Supraorbital notch
4. Nasion
5. Zygomatico-frontal suture
6. Nasal bones
7. Zygomatic
8. Infraorbital foramen
9. Maxilla
10. Ramus of mandible
11. Mental foramen
12. Body of mandible

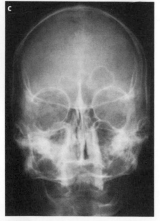

the medial third and lateral two-thirds of the superciliary arch, contains the supraorbital vessels and nerve.

The two **maxillary bones** form the central part of the face. Each contains a **maxillary air sinus**. The thin superior surface of the sinus forms the floor of the orbit, within which lies the infraorbital nerve that emerges through the **infraorbital foramen**. The maxilla forms the medial wall of the nose. This is incomplete and largely covered by the **inferior concha bone**, and the **superior** and **middle conchae** of the **ethmoid bone**. Posteriorly the maxilla overlaps the pterygoid process of the sphenoid bone.

Laterally the maxilla articulates with the **zygomatic bone**. This forms the prominence of the cheek; it extends upwards to meet the frontal bone, at the palpable **zygomatico-frontal suture** in the lateral wall of the orbit. Posteriorly the zygomatic bone articulates with the **zygomatic process** of the **temporal bone** to form the **zygomatic arch**.

The maxilla is thicker and arched inferiorly where its **alveolar process** carries the upper teeth. It has an inferomedial thin horizontal projection, the palatine process; the **palatine processes** from each side form the anterior part of the **hard palate**. The **horizontal process** of the **palatine bone** forms the posterior part of the hard palate on each side; its perpendicular plate completes the back of the lateral wall of the nose. The midline **nasal septum** is formed from the **perpendicular plate** of the ethmoid, posteriorly by the **vomer** and anteriorly by **septal cartilages**; the latter articulate with the **nasal spine** of the frontal bone and the line of union of the **nasal bones**.

The skull is formed laterally by the downward extension of the parietal bone, and the occipital, temporal, and sphenoid bones (figure 2a-d). The **temporal bone** extends medially across the skull base, housing the middle and inner ear. **The body of the sphenoid bone** forms part of the skull base. Laterally it has lesser and greater wings: the **lesser wing** forms the ridge between the anterior and middle cranial fossae. The **greater wing** extends onto the lateral surface of the skull, its union with the frontal, parietal, and temporal bones is known as the **pterion**, which overlies the middle meningeal artery. The skull base is completed posteriorly by the **occipital bone** (figure 2d). This extends anteriorly to the body of the sphenoid, contains the **foramen magnum** and, inferiorly, gives attachment to powerful neck muscles.

The **mandible** is a single bone concerned with mastication. It has a body and a superior ramus on each side. Each **superior ramus** has a **condylar process** (by which the mandible is attached to the skull at the temporomandibular joint) and a **coronoid process** (for attachment of the

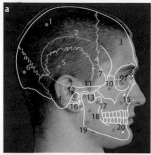

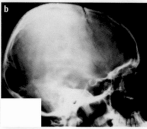

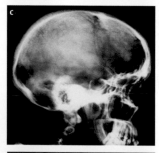

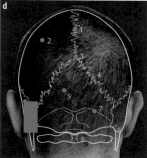

Figure 2

a,b,c,d. Lateral and posterior aspects of head; lateral skull X-rays, note in b. the separation of the frontoparietal sutures associated with trauma and in c. large pituitary fossa associated with pituitary adenoma; compare X-rays with anatomy shown in figures 1 and 2.

a Bones of lateral head

1. Parietal
2. Superior temporal line
3. Frontal
4. Pterion
5. Temporal
6. Occipital
7. Greater wing of sphenoid
8. Nasal
9. Lacrimal
10. Zygomatic
11. Zygomatic arch
12. External acoustic meatus
13. Condylar process
14. Mastoid process
15. Maxilla
16. Styloid process
17. Coronoid process
18. Ramus of mandible
19. Angle of mandible
20. Body of mandible

d Posterior bones of skull

1. Sagittal suture
2. Parietal
3. Lambda
4. Parieto-occipital suture
5. Occipital
6. Temporal
7. Superior nuchal line
8. Mastoid process
9. Atlas
10. Styloid process

temporalis muscle). The upper border of the horseshoe-shaped **body** carries the lower dentition. The inferior alveolar (dental) nerves pass through the bone on each side, and emerge at the **mental foramina**. The mental foramen, the infraorbital foramen, and the supraorbital notch are in line, approximately 1.5 cm from the midline.

CRANIAL NERVES AND SPECIAL SENSES

I Olfactory Nerve; Nose, Olfaction

The **nose** is the first part of the airway, and in it inspired air is humidified, warmed, and smelt. It comprises two arched, narrow cavities situated above the palate and below the anterior and middle cranial fossae, and extends from the **anterior nares** to the **nasopharynx**. The cavities are separated by the **midline septum** and they receive the openings of the **paranasal air sinuses** on each side.

The **olfactory epithelium** is situated at the upper part of each cavity, where 15–20 **olfactory nerves**, surrounded by individual dural sheaths, pass through the cribriform plate of the ethmoid bone to the olfactory bulb.

Defective fusion of the frontonasal and maxillary processes may produce **nasal deformity**, and **medial** and **lateral dermoid cysts** over the bridge of the nose and lateral to the orbit. A number of uncommon inflammatory conditions may produce nasal deformity. These include **Wegener's granulomatosis**, and infection with **syphilis** (congenital and acquired), **tuberculosis**, and **nocardia**. The nose is commonly damaged by direct trauma, and may be enlarged in **acromegaly** and **myxedema**, or become reddened or enlarged in alcoholism. The commonest cause of **nasal obstruction** and **discharge** is infection, such as a cold, but foreign bodies, polyps, and septal deviation are frequently encountered, and occasionally **neoplasms**. **Epistaxis** (bleeding nose) may follow minor trauma; the bleeding point is usually anterior, particularly over the nasal septum (Little's area). High facial **fractures** may extend into the anterior cranial fossa. **Leaking cerebrospinal fluid** may be distinguished from other clear nasal drips by its sugar content, and, when mixed with blood, by a separate diffusion ring on filter paper.

The anterior nares are examined with a nasal speculum (figure 3). This is introduced anteroposteriorly to avoid stimulating the sensitive nasal septum. With the use of a head mirror, light may be directed into the anterior nares to observe the inferior concha, the anterior nasal cavity, and the nasal septum. Bleeding points may be detected and cauterized.

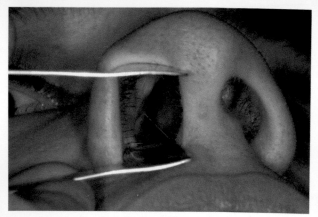

Figure 3 Examination of anterior nares with a speculum.

Nasal endoscopes are used to examine the interior of the nose and the openings of the nasal sinuses.

The posterior nares and adenoids may be observed using a nasal endoscope or head mirror and a small, long-stemmed, angled mirror placed behind the palate.

Apply pressure (gently at first) over the frontal (medial eyebrow) and maxillary (cheek) air sinuses, to look for tenderness due to underlying inflammation.

The olfactory nerves of each side are tested in turn by compressing the contralateral nostril and applying preparations such as cloves, peppermint, and a fetid odor (figure 4a,b). Pungent preparations, such as ammonia, should be avoided, as these also stimulate the fifth nerve and the signs may be misinterpreted. More sophisticated tests require dilution of the odorant to determine threshold levels. Loss of smell (**anosmia**) markedly affects the appreciation of food.

II Optic Nerve; Orbit, Eyeball, Vision

The **orbit** lies beneath the anterior cranial fossa. It is covered anteriorly by the eyelids and contains the eyeball, embedded in fat. Each **eyelid** has a firm, fibrous **tarsal plate**, and the upper and lower tarsal plates are joined by the **medial** and **lateral palpebral ligaments**: only the medial palpebral ligament is attached to bone. The posterior surface of

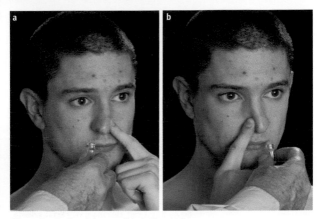

Figure 4 a,b. Examining smell in both nostrils.

the eyelids is covered with conjunctiva and this passes onto the front of the eyeball. When closed, the eyelids form a sealed **conjunctival sac**; tear fluid produced by the **lacrimal gland** (in the superolateral aspect of the orbit) passes through its ducts into the conjunctival sac and lubricates the front of the eyeball. The fluid is drained medially through **lacrimal canaliculi** (figure 5), opening onto the medial end of each lid margin; it passes to the **lacrimal sac** and **duct** to drain into the nose. Because of the medial bony tarsal attachment, when the eyes blink or are screwed up, tears are massaged medially towards the lacrimal apparatus.

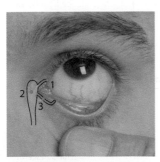

Figure 5 Lacrimal apparatus.

1. Lacrimal puncta
2. Lacrimal sac
3. Lacrimal canaliculi

The **eyeball** is surrounded by orbital fascia and **medial** and **lateral** (**check**) **ligaments** attach it to the lacrimal and zygomatic bones respectively, suspending it within the orbital cavity and allowing it to be moved by the **extraocular muscles**.

The **optic nerve** passes back from the posteromedial aspect of the eyeball, and through the optic canal into the middle cranial fossa. The medial fibers from each side cross (**decussate**) to the opposite side in the **optic chiasm**. Beyond this level, each visual pathway receives impulses from the contralateral field of both eyes.

Diseases of the orbit encompass a large number of conditions, including those of the surrounding skin, the eyelids, and the orbital contents. Internal and external angular **dermoid cysts** represent developmental abnormalities. The skin around the eyelids is a common site for congenital vascular malformations (**capillary hemangiomas/ strawberry nevi**) and skin tumors, particularly **basal cell carcinomas**. **Facial edema**, from myxedema and other general and local causes, usually affects the lax periorbital skin.

The edges of the eyelids and their eyelashes may be turned inwards (**entropion**), causing corneal abrasion, or outwards (**ectropion**), preventing adequate closure of the conjunctival sac and corneal protection. Retention **cysts** occur along the lid margin from the **glands of Moll** and sebaceous glands (**meibomian cysts/chalazion**). These cysts may become infected, and there may be infection of a hair follicle (**stye**), and infection of the conjunctiva (conjunctivitis) or lacrimal apparatus (**dacrocystitis**).

Conjunctivitis may be due to an allergy, foreign bodies, chemicals, trauma, and a number of viral and bacteriological agents. Infection from *Chlamydia trachomatis* is common across the tropics and **trachoma** is one of the commonest causes of blindness in the world. A **red eye** is a common differential diagnosis. It usually is related to inflammatory conditions but an important differential diagnosis is **glaucoma**.

Eye injuries include orbital fractures. A **blow-out fracture** of the orbit (as from the impact of a squash ball) may force the orbital contents through its thin walls into the nose, the anterior cranial fossa or the maxillary air sinus. **Hemorrhage** from the orbit may extend visibly underneath the conjunctiva (an important differential diagnosis is from a spontaneous subconjuntival hemorrhage, where the staining does not go beyond the cornea, and is usually of no clinical significance, although the blood pressure should be checked). **Temporomaxillary fractures** may alter the suspension of the eye and produce diplopia; these fractures may also damage the infraorbital nerve (giving

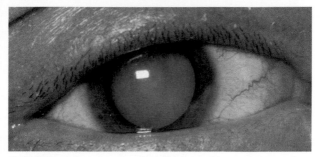

Figure 6 Cataract, note opacity of lens interfering with normal vision and ophthalmoscopy, where there is a reduction of red reflex and difficulty in examination of retina.

anesthesia of the lower eyelid and upper lip) and affect movement of the temporomandibular joint.

Expansion of the orbital contents can produce **proptosis**; this may just affect the eyeball, as with the exophthalmos of thyrotoxicosis, but also includes severe **infection**, **cavernous sinus thrombosis**, and **tumors** of the orbit and its contents.

Visual disorders may be related to corneal disease, opacity of the lens (figure 6), disorders of the eyeball (including **retinal detachment**, **central retinal artery occlusion**, **diabetic retinopathy**, and tumors such as **retinoblastoma** and **malignant melanoma**), and disease of the visual pathway. **Raised intracranial pressure** produces **papilledema**; this swelling of the optic disc is an important physical sign.

Damage to the **optic nerve** produces unilateral visual problems. **Multiple sclerosis** is the commonest cause of optic nerve disease, but it may also occur with trauma and tumors of the orbit. Pressure on the **optic chiasm** is usually due to pituitary tumors, and it produces a **bitemporal hemianopia**; damage beyond this level produces an **homonymous hemianopia**. Damage to the optic tract, optic radiation and the visual cortex are usually due to primary or secondary malignancy: cortical lesions are usually **congruous** (affect the two eyes equally).

When examining the eye, first observe the surrounding skin, the eyelids and their edges (figure 7a,b). Small **foreign bodies** may be detected beneath the lids and the upper may need to be everted for their removal. **Corneal abrasions** and ulcers may need outlining by means of a drop of fluorescein.

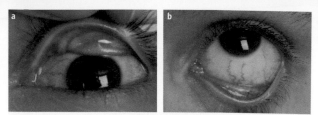

Figure 7 a,b. Examination of under surfaces of eyelids; upper lid may be everted for this purpose.

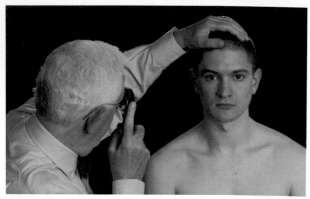

Figure 8 Observation of the retina from a distance to show red retinal reflex.

Observe the **retina** from a distance through an ophthalmoscope (figure 8) to see a red central disc (**red reflex**). This is disturbed by opacities within the lens, or of the aqueous or vitreous humor.

Observation of the retina using an **ophthalmoscope** begins with the subject looking straight ahead and then to each position of gaze (figure 9a-c).

In the normal retina, seen through an ophthalmoscope, the pale optic disc is the site of entry of the optic nerve and vessels that radiate from this point, branching dichotomously (figure 10a,b). The arteries are brighter red and slightly narrower than the veins. The disc is insensitive to light and is termed the "blind spot." The **macula** is the central part of the back of the retina; it is lateral to the disc and is largely devoid of vessels, but has a rich capillary network. The central depression beneath the macula is the **fovea centralis**, where visual resolution is highest.

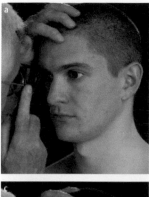
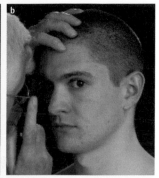

Figure 9
a,b,c. Observation of retinal quadrants with ophthalmoscope.

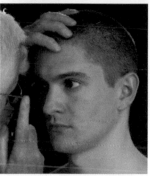

Retinal changes accompany many vascular and neurological abnormalities; these include alteration of the arteriovenous diameter ratio, appearance of hemorrhages and exudates (figure 10c) and swelling of the optic disc in papilledema (figure 10d).

Optic nerve tests encompass visual acuity, color and visual fields, together with the visual component of pupillary reflexes.

Distant vision is assessed with a Snellen chart (figure 11a). Two numbers are reported. The first is the distance of the subject from the chart in meters (usually 6). The chart has 8 rows of letters, which can be seen with the normal eye at respectively 60, 36, 24, 18, 12, 8, 6, and 5 meters away. The second number reported is the distance of the smallest line that can be seen. At 6 meters, this is usually the seventh line and the reported vision is 6/6 for the tested eye. If the acuity is less than 6/60, the subject is moved toward the chart (e.g., 3/60). If the top line

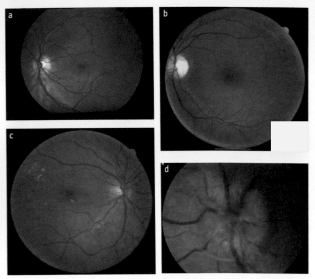

Figure 10 a,b. Normal retina – note color variation commonly observed in the population; c. hard exudates in outer aspect of retina; d. papilledema.

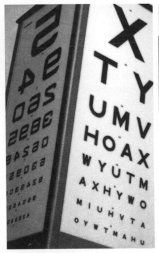

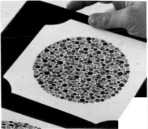

Figure 11 a. Snellen chart; b. Ishihara chart.

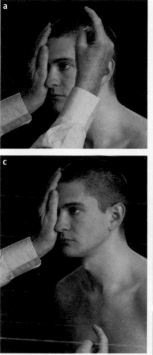
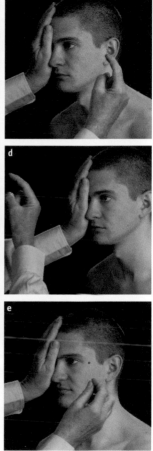

Figure 12 a,b,c,d. Assessment of vision in left eye: upper, middle, and lower field to the left, right mid zone, and e. using red-headed pin as target.

cannot be read at 1 meter (i.e., worse than 1/60) visual acuity is reported as counting fingers (CF), seeing hand movements (HM) or perception of light (PL).

Near vision is assessed with **J charts** of different size prints, each with an assigned code. Color vision is assessed with an **Ishihara chart** (figure 11b). This has the pattern outlined in colors in an otherwise uniform format.

Clinical assessment of the visual field is by confrontation: the observer sits or stands in front of the subject and both cover one opposing eye with a palm (figure 12a-d). The subject fixates on the bridge of the examiner's nose. The examiner then brings a moving finger, or more sensitively a red-headed pin (figure 12e), from outside his/her visual field radially inwards from each quadrant in turn.

A central target is used to identify a **scotoma** (loss of part of the visual field). The subject is asked to say as soon as the finger is noted, or, in the case of the pin, the red color is identified. The examiner compares this with his/her own observation (assuming he/she has normal vision).

Visual **inattention** defects are assessed by the examiner moving fingers of both hands, separately or together; the subject is asked to identify which finger(s) move (figure 13a,b).

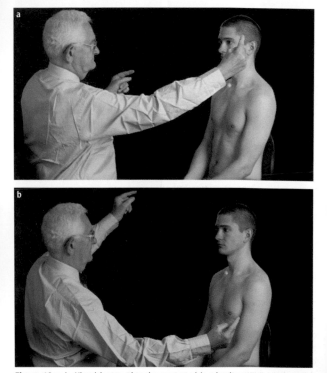

Figure 13 a,b. Visual inattention demonstrated by simultaneous movement in opposing sectors of field.

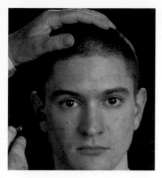

Figure 14 Light reflex; note also consensual response in contralateral eye.

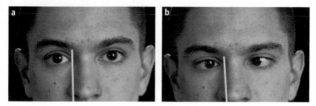

Figure 15 a,b. Accommodation reflex, showing differential size of pupil in far and near vision.

A more precise mapping of the peripheral fields, and of the blind spot, is obtained using **perimetry**. The subject's head is placed, by a chin rest, in the center of the apparatus. This allows a light to be brought in from all directions. Alternatively, the **Bjerrum screen** is used: white and red discs are moved radially inward against a black background. Loss of parts of the visual field and loss of nasal or temporal fields, such as damage to the optic radiation or pituitary tumors pressing on the optic chiasm, can be accurately mapped.

Direct **light reflexes** are tested with a pen torch, examining each eye in turn (figure 14). **Pupillary contraction** is noted in the stimulated and the contralateral eye (**consensual response**).

The **accommodation reflex** is assessed by asking the patient to fixate on a distant object and then on a finger placed close to the bridge of the nose – the pupil constricting on near vision (figure 15a,b). It may be necessary to retract the upper eyelid to better visualize the pupil. The shape of the pupils may be altered by adhesions from local disease, and the pupillary response by neurological disorders.

III Oculomotor; IV Trochlear; VI Abducent Nerves; Eye Movement

Orbital conditions interfere with eye movements, as do a congenital squint, and neurological disorders of the brain and cranial nerves. The oculomotor, trochlea, and abducent nerves are affected by multiple sclerosis and lesions of the midbrain, producing ptosis, squint, and diplopia. The oculomotor nerve may be damaged in **tentorial coning**, the damage to the parasympathetic fibers producing a dilated pupil. **Raised intracranial pressure** may also damage the abducent nerve: this is a non-focal sign, due to the long intracranial course of this fine nerve. **Nystagmus** is particularly associated with disorders of the vestibular apparatus and tumors of the cerebellopontine angle. Muscle weakness interferes with ocular movement, as in **myasthenia gravis**.

When testing eye movements the subject initially is requested to look straight ahead, note being taken of any disconjugate activity (squint), and then into the nine positions of gaze (figure 16).

Normal **eye movements** are demonstrated by asking the subject to follow your finger, moving up and down and then from side to side, the finger following an H shape (figure 17a-d). Note any **nystagmus** (most commonly horizontal flicking of the eye medially from the lateral extreme gaze) to each side, whether there is double vision in any direction of gaze, any squint or any defect in eye movement.

In third nerve palsy, the eye is displaced downward and outward. With **ptosis** (drooping of the upper lid), the only movement is further outward and a little downward. The defect, however, is often only partial and the diagnosis is supported by normal fourth and sixth nerve function. Associated **parasympathetic palsy** produces a dilated pupil.

Although the superior oblique muscle acting independently turns the pupil downward and outward, its most powerful movement is in downward gaze. The oblique end of the muscle is in line with the optical axis, and produces its maximum force when the pupil is turned inward by other optic muscles. The fourth nerve is therefore tested by asking the subject to look downward and inward, noting failure of downward gaze. Sufferers usually keep their head tilted, in an attempt to minimize **diplopia**.

In sixth nerve palsy the eye does not move outward beyond the midline optical axis.

Detecting an abnormality of nerve function can be complicated if the underlying defect is primarily muscular, such as in thyrotoxicosis or myasthenia gravis, as these defects may affect individual muscles selectively.

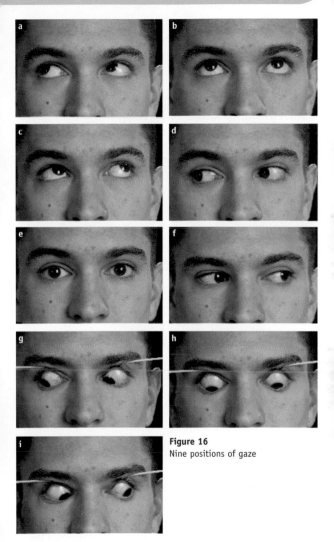

Figure 16
Nine positions of gaze

A **Horner syndrome** (from damage to the cervical sympathetic chain) produces **ptosis**, **miosis** (small pupil), **enophthalmos** (sunken eye), **failure of sweating** on the ipsilateral face and stuffiness of the ipsilateral nasal cavity.

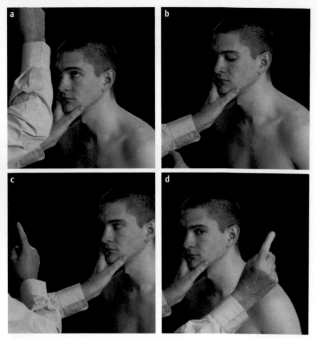

Figure 17 a.b.c.d. Examination of eye movements: up, down, to right, to left.

V Trigeminal nerve

The trigeminal nerve supplies the muscles of mastication and sensation to the face, including the corneal reflex (figure 18). The lingual branch carries taste to the anterior two-thirds of the tongue and parasympathetic fibers to the submandibular ganglion, both derived from the facial nerve. **Herpes zoster** (shingles) infection may cause severe damage to the cornea and may also involve the geniculate and otic ganglia, resulting in deafness, vertigo and facial palsy (**Ramsay Hunt syndrome**). **Trigeminal neuralgia** is a condition of unknown origin; it is characterized by severe intense pain over one or more divisions of the nerve.

Touch, pain, and temperature are tested over the temple, cheek, and jaw, corresponding to the ophthalmic, maxillary, and mandibular divisions of the trigeminal nerve (figure 19a–c).

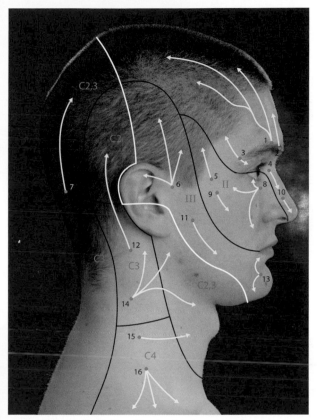

Figure 18 Sensory distribution of head and neck.

1. Supraorbital
2. Supratrochlear
3. Lacrimal
4. Infratrochlear
5. Zygomaticotemporal
6. Auriculotemporal
7. Greater occipital
8. Infraorbital
9. Zygomaticofacial
10. External nasal
11. Buccal

12. Lesser occipital
13. Mental
14. Great auricular
15. Transverse cervical
16. Supraclavicular
C – cervical roots
Trigeminal:
    I ophthalmic
    II maxillary
    III mandibular divisions

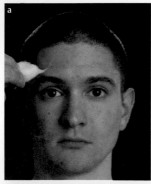
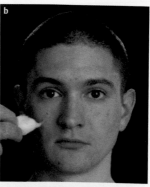
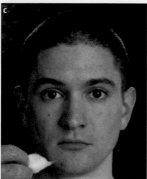
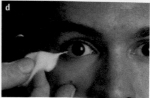
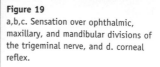

Figure 19
a,b,c. Sensation over ophthalmic, maxillary, and mandibular divisions of the trigeminal nerve, and d. corneal reflex.

To test the **corneal reflex**, twist the corner of a piece of cotton wool into a point (figure 19d). Ask the subject to look toward the other side, and then stroke the cotton wool gently over the exposed cornea. Be sure not to touch the eyelashes and remain out of the line of vision. Note any contact lenses; ask the subject to remove them when testing this reflex. The muscles controlling a blink reflex are innervated by the facial nerve; the trigeminal provides the sensory component.

The motor fibers of the trigeminal nerve supply the **muscles of mastication** (figure 20; table 1). Ask the subject to bite hard and palpate the contracting masseter and temporalis muscles over the angle of the jaw and the temple respectively (figure 21a,b).

Protrusion of the jaw and movements to each side are achieved by the pterygoid muscles and can be assessed against resistance (figure 22a-c).

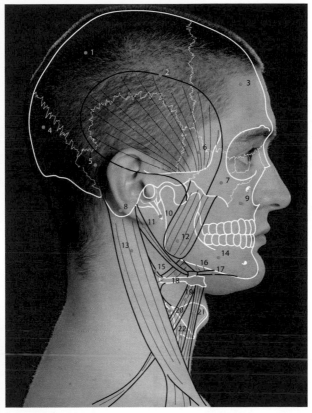

Figure 20
Muscles of mastication.

1. Parietal bone
2. Superior temporal line
3. Frontal bone
4. Occipital bone
5. Temporal bone
6. Temporalis
7. Zygomatic bone
8. Mastoid process
9. Maxillary bone
10. Styloid process
11. Posterior belly of digastric

12. Masseter
13. Sternomastoid
14. Mandible
15. Middle constrictor
16. Mylohyoid
17. Anterior belly of digastric
18. Hyoglossus
19. Omohyoid
20. Inferior constrictor
21. Sternohyoid
22. Sternothyroid

Table 1 MUSCLES OF MASTICATION

MUSCLE	SUPERIOR ATTACHMENT	INFERIOR ATTACHMENT	FUNCTION	NERVE SUPPLY
Masseter	Anterior two-thirds of the inferior border of the zygomatic arch and the zygomatic process of the maxilla	Lower two-thirds of the outer surface of the ramus of the mandible	Elevation, some side to side movement and protrusion of the mandible	Masseter branch of the mandibular
Temporalis	Temporal fossa on the lateral surface of the skull and the temporalis fascia	Superior margin of the coronoid process, extending onto the anterior border of the ramus of the mandible	Elevation, side to side movement and retraction of the mandible	Deep temporal branches of the mandibular
Medial pterygoid	Medial surface of the lateral pterygoid plate, and the adjacent palatine bone and maxillary tuberosity	Lower half of the medial surface of the ramus of the mandible	Elevation, side to side movement and protrusion of the mandible	Medial pterygoid branch of the mandibular
Lateral pterygoid	Upper head: infratemporal surface of the greater wing of the sphenoid bone Lower head: lateral surface of the lateral pterygoid plate	Neck of the mandible and the intra-articular disc of the temporomandibular joint	Side to side movement and protrusion of the mandible: acting together the two heads flatten the disc and open the mouth	Lateral pterygoid branch of the mandibular

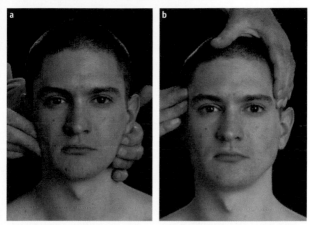

Figure 21 a,b. Palpation of masseter and temporalis muscles on biting.

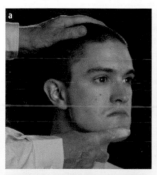

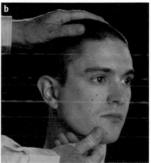

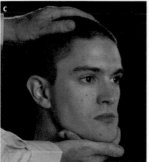

Figure 22 a,b,c. Resisted jaw protrusion, anteriorly, and to right and left.

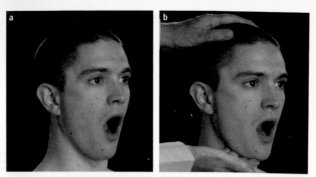

Figure 23 a,b. Active and resisted opening of mouth.

Opening the mouth is partly through the action of the lateral pterygoid muscle drawing the mandibular condyle onto the articular eminence; the muscle pulls the fibrocartilaginous disc forward, flattening it, in this movement (figure 23a,b). The digastric, geniohyoid, and mylohyoid muscles support the movement.

The **temporomandibular joint** is subcutaneous and palpable laterally (figure 24). The condyle can be felt to glide over the articular eminence. The joint may click, and become painful from trauma and arthritic changes. It is very stable in the closed position, but may be **dislocated** by an injury to the open mouth. **Jaw fractures** usually involve the body of the mandible in the region of the first molar: fractures of the angle of the mandible are usually anterior to the attachment of the masseter.

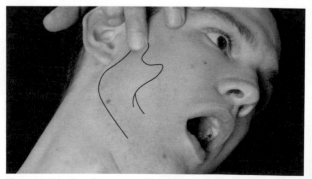

Figure 24 Palpation of temporomandibular joint: feel the condyle move onto the eminence.

VII Facial Nerve

The **motor fibers** of the facial nerve supply predominantly the muscles of facial expression. **Taste** fibers to the anterior two-thirds of the tongue and **parasympathetic** fibers to the submandibular ganglion pass via the chorda tympani, to be distributed with the lingual nerve. The facial nerve has a long course through the skull base, lying adjacent to the inner and middle ear and, on leaving the skull, passes through the parotid gland; it thus may be involved in disease of any of these structures.

The muscles of the upper face are bilaterally innervated and, in **upper motor neuron** lesions, only the lower part of the face is affected (unless there are bilateral lesions that produce a pseudobulbar palsy). Complete paralysis occurs in **lower motor neuron** lesions; the commonest cause is a Bell's palsy. Upper and lower motor neuron lesions may compromise eyelid closure, leaving the cornea exposed and prone to injury. Immediate damage of the facial nerve in a **skull base fracture** is usually permanent, but delayed onset of paralysis is due to edema and undergoes a slow recovery (in spite of the initial severe, usually bilateral, facial paralysis).

Severe **infection** of the middle ear commonly extends to the mastoid air cells and bone involvement may damage the facial nerve, as can surgical drainage of an abscess or other surgical procedures in the region. Malignant **tumors** of the parotid gland may invade the facial nerve and the nerve is easily damaged in any **surgery** of the gland. The mandibular branch on the nerve, supplying the muscles of the lower lip, can be damaged in surgery of the submandibular gland.

Taste in the anterior two-thirds of the tongue (figure 25) is carried to the seventh nerve by the chorda tympani from the mandibular division

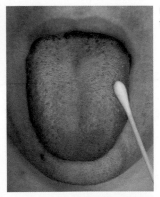

Figure 25 Assessment of taste over the anterior two-thirds of tongue.

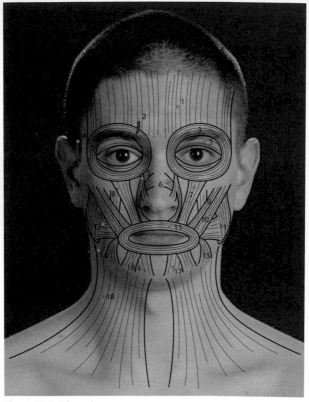

Figure 26 Facial muscles.

1. Frontalis
2. Supraorbital artery
3. Orbicularis oculi
4. Superficial temporal artery
5. Levator labii superioris alaeque nasi
6. Nasalis
7. Levator labii superioris
8. Levator anguli oris (lying deep to zygomatic)
9. Zygomaticus minor
10. Zygomaticus major
11. Masseter
12. Risorius
13. Orbicularis oris
14. Facial artery
15. Depressor anguli oris
16. Depressor labii inferioris
17. Mentalis
18. Platysma

Table 2 **MUSCLES OF THE FACE**

MUSCLE	PROXIMAL ATTACHMENT	DISTAL ATTACHMENT	FUNCTION	NERVE SUPPLY
Occipito-frontalis The two muscles of each side blend with the galea aponeurotica to cover the skull vault	Occipitalis from the lateral two-thirds of the superior nuchal line and mastoid process, passing forward to the dense fibrous galea	Frontalis passes forward from the galea to blend with the orbicularis oculi and other facial muscles	Movement of the scalp and eyebrows	Posterior auricular and temporal branches of the facial
Periorbital: Orbicularis oculi surrounds the orbit and eyelids	Medial margin of the orbit, medial palpebral ligament and the lacrimal sac	Lateral palpebral raphe, with no bony attachment: the thin palpebral portion lies within the eyelids	Orbital sphincter, blink reflex and tear transport	Temporal and zygomatic branches of the facial
Corrugator	Medial supraorbital margin	Medial skin of the forehead	Eyebrow movement and vertical forehead wrinkle	Temporal branch of the facial
Perinasal: procerus and nasalis (dilator and compressor)	Nasal and maxillary bones, around the anterior nasal opening	Nasal skin and cartilages	Wrinkle bridge of the nose and modify nasal aperture	Buccal branch of the facial
Perioral: orbicularis oris	Multilayered circumoral sphincter, partly derived from other facial muscles	No bony attachment, but interlacing nodule (modiolus) on either side	This extensive collection of muscles modifies the position of the mouth and maintains food between the teeth	Buccal and mandibular branches of the facial
Levator labii superioris alaeque nasi	Nasal process of maxilla	Nasal cartilages and skin: upper lip	The facial muscles as a whole are collectively involved in the production of facial expression	Buccal branch of the facial
Levator labii superioris	Maxilla above the infraorbital foramen	Upper lip		Buccal branch of the facial

Table 2 continued **MUSCLES OF THE FACE**

MUSCLE	PROXIMAL ATTACHMENT	DISTAL ATTACHMENT	FUNCTION	NERVE SUPPLY
Levator anguli oris	Maxilla below the infraorbital foramen	Angle of the mouth		Buccal branch of the facial
Zygomaticus major and minor	Zygomatic bone	Upper lip and the angle of the mouth		Buccal branch of the facial
Buccinator	Pterygomandibular raphe, in common with the superior constrictor	Angle of the mouth, and the upper and lower lips		Buccal branches of the facial
Risorius	Parotid fascia	Angle of the mouth		Buccal branch of the facial
Depressor anguli oris	Mandible	Angle of the mouth		Mandibular branch of the facial
Depressor labii inferioris	Mandible, lateral to the mental foramen	Lower lip		Mandibular branch of the facial
Mentalis	Mandible, above the mental foramen	Lower lip		Mandibular branch of the facial
Platysma	Angle of the mouth, lower lip and along the inferior border of the mandible	Broad expansion to the skin of the lateral neck and upper chest		Cervical branch of the facial

of the trigeminal nerve. Dampen three cotton wool buds in tap water and, after dipping them respectively into salt, sugar, and vinegar, assess recognition of each modality on each side of the tongue. Loss of taste is termed **ageusia**.

The facial (seventh) nerve innervates the muscles of **facial expression** (figure 26; table 2). Note facial expression, and any asymmetry at rest, during talking or when smiling. In particular note the symmetry of the nasolabial folds and the angles of the mouth. Ask the subject to close their eyes, show their teeth and to whistle (figure 27a-d).

Assess the power of the facial muscles by trying to open tightly screwed up eyes and the resistance to squashing blown out cheeks (figure 28a,b).

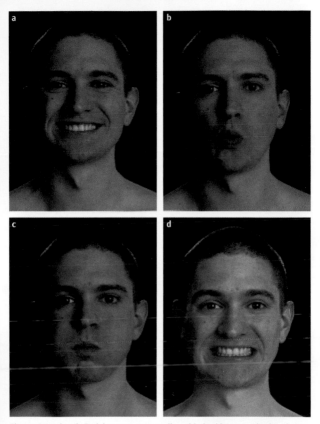

Figure 27 a,b,c,d. Facial movements: smile, whistle, blow out cheeks, show teeth.

Damage to the nerve or its nucleus produces paralysis of the whole face (figure 29).

VIII Vestibulocochlear Nerve; Ear, Hearing, Balance

The ear is the organ of hearing and balance. It comprises external (auricle and external acoustic meatus), middle, and inner parts.

Deformities of the auricle (figure 30), such as bat ears, are common and anomalies may be associated with syndromes such as Down.

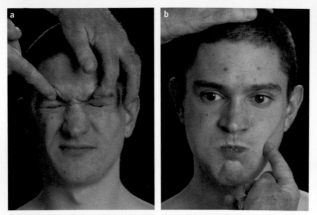

Figure 28 a,b. Resisted facial movements: eye closure and cheek blowing.

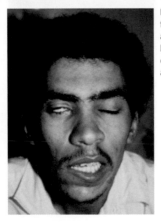

Figure 29 Right lower motor neuron facial palsy. The subject has been asked to close his eyes – this has only been achieved on left side; the face is contorted and eyes elevated, in attempt to close right eye.

Infection of the external acoustic meatus (**otitis externa**) may produce pain and discharge; earache may also be referred from the teeth, temporomandibular joint, laryngopharynx, and cervical spine. Additional symptoms of **middle ear disease** are deafness, tinnitus, and vertigo, although these may also occur in diseases of the central nervous, skeletal, and cardiovascular systems, and with some drugs. Infection of the middle ear (**otitis media**) may produce redness and bulging of the eardrum. Extension of this infection into the mastoid air cells or the

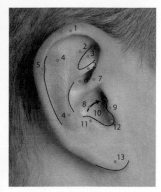

Figure 30 External ear.

1. Helix
2. Crura of antihelix
3. Triangular fossa
4. Antihelix
5. Auricular tubercle
6. Upper and 10. lower parts of concha
7. Crux of helix
8. Arrow leading to external acoustic meatus
9. Tragus
11. Antitragus
12. Intertragic incisura
13. Lobule

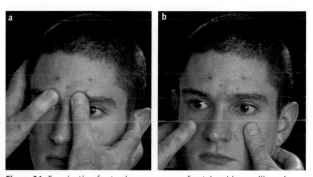

Figure 31 Examination for tenderness over: a. frontal and b. maxillary air sinuses.

paranasal air sinuses may produce tenderness within the ear, or over the cheeks and frontal region (figure 31a,b). Otitis media may be complicated by perforation of the tympanic membrane and damage to the ossicles.

The outer cartilaginous part of the external acoustic meatus can be straightened by gently pulling the auricle upward and backward (figure 32); this facilitates detection of abnormalities within the canal.

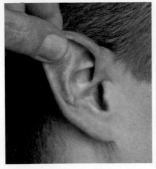

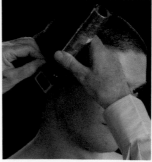

Figure 32 Observe length of external acoustic meatus by pulling ear upward and backward.

Figure 33 In auroscopy, ensure that your hand is resting on the skull, so that there is no uncontrolled advancement of the instrument into the meatus.

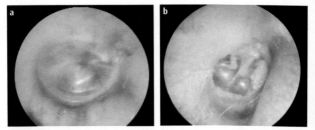

Figure 34 a. Normal right tympanic membrane: membrane faces downward and forward. Prominent lateral process of the malleus bulging into membrane superiorly. Handle of malleus passes downward and forward, attached to center of tympanic membrane at the umbo; this may not be easily seen through pars tensa of membrane. Anterior and posterior folds pass upward from lateral process, bordering pars flaccida of membrane: head of malleus just seen through this part of the tympanic membrane, passing medially. b. **Abnormal left** tympanic membrane has been photographed through the endoscope. There is a large retraction pocket of pars tensa posteriorly, the tympanic membrane is draped over incudo stapedial joint and stapedius muscle tendon. Tympanic membrane has white plaque: this is tympanosclerosis - appearances are sequelae of chronic otitis media.

A detailed view of the drum is provided with an **auroscope**. Ensure that the hand holding the instrument is also resting on the head so that any head movement by the subject carries no risk of the instrument's being forced further into the canal (figure 33). Examination with an auroscope

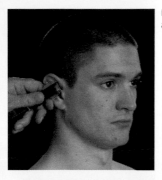

Figure 35 Hearing is initially assessed with whisper or watch.

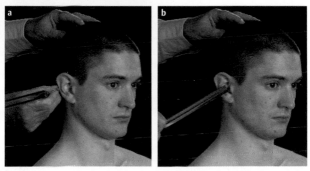

Figure 36 a,b. Bone conduction is normally less than air conduction, and therefore the sound of a tuning fork should reappear when tested through air – Rinne's test.

or endoscope is often diagnostic of middle as well as external ear disease (figure 34a,b).

Assessment of auditory function of the vestibulocochlear nerve is with a whisper or a watch ticking in each ear (figure 35), having checked that there is no wax interfering with air conduction.

Air conduction should be better than bone conduction. Therefore, if the base of a vibrating tuning fork is placed over the mastoid process and the subject is asked to say as soon as the vibration stops, turning the vibrating fork near the ear should be accompanied by return of sound; this is known as **Rinne's test** (figure 36a,b). If the sound does not return, the implication is that bony conduction is better than air and may indicate damage to the tympanic membrane or disease of the middle ear.

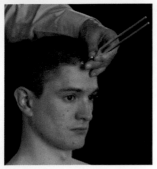

Figure 37 Conduction should be same to both ears – Weber's test.

Comparing the two sides is by **Weber's test** (figure 37) in which the base of a vibrating tuning fork is placed over the middle of the forehead and the subject is asked whether it is heard more distinctly in one ear than the other. The fork is normally heard centrally, but may be lateralized, e.g., in the presence of middle ear disease.

A more precise assessment of hearing is with **audiometry**, applying different noise levels at different frequencies and recording the responses. The balance component of the nerve is assessed by running cold water into each ear in turn. A positive response produces **nystagmus** towards the stimulated side.

IX Glossopharyngeal Nerve

The glossopharyngeal nerve supplies **taste** to the posterior third of the tongue, **parasympathetic** fibers to the parotid gland, and contributes to the pharyngeal plexus. The motor part of the latter, to the stylopharyngeus, cannot be tested, but the sensory component over the tonsil and anterior pillar of the fauces can by examined by the **gag reflex**.

The gag reflex is produced by gently touching the anterior pillar with a wooden spatula (figure 38). Taste over the posterior third of the tongue (figure 39) is assessed as with the facial nerve, but this area is more sensitive to bitter tastes, such as quinine.

X Vagus Nerve

The vagus nerve carries **parasympathetic** fibers to the **heart**, and to **glands** and **smooth muscle**, both in the head and neck, and the

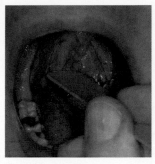

Figure 38 Gag reflex.

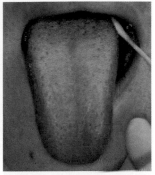

Figure 39 Examining taste over posterior third of tongue.

alimentary tract as far as the splenic flexure. The vagus is involved in **cardiorespiratory reflexes** such as the Valsalva maneuver. Its somatic motor fibers pass to the palate, pharynx, and larynx, and these are most easily examined. In the neck, the nerve can be damaged by **malignant** infiltration, and **surgery** of the thyroid gland, the carotid bifurcation, airway, and pharynx. An auricular branch supplies the posterior aspect of the external acoustic meatus and can provide the afferent pathway of cough and vomiting reflexes.

The motor component of the vagus nerve produces movement of the soft palate and, with the accessory, produces **swallowing** and **speech**. The position of the uvula can be unreliable but ask the patient to say "ah" to assess symmetry (figure 40). Observe or gently palpate the larynx while the patient is swallowing a glass of water (pages 64–5), and note the pitch and power of speech.

Laryngeal and pharyngeal muscles are bilaterally innervated and dysarthria and dysphagia require lower motor neuron or bilateral upper

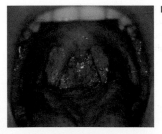

Figure 40 Normal palatal symmetry.

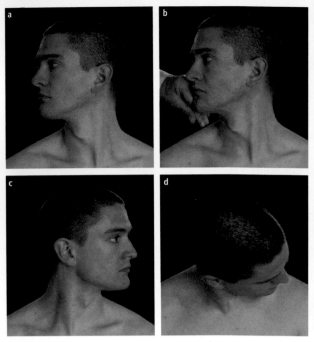

Figure 41
a,b,c,d. Movements of sternomastoid: active and resisted rotation to right, rotation to left with neck flexion.

motor neuron denervation. Unilateral damage to the recurrent laryngeal nerve, which may be produced by neoplasia or surgery of the thyroid gland, interferes with coughing (producing a bovine cough, without the explosive element produced by tight apposition of the vocal cords) and the subject is unable to sing a high pitched "ee".

XI Accessory Nerve

The spinal accessory nerve innervates the sternomastoid and trapezius muscles. Its cranial component contributes to the pharyngeal plexus.

Place the palm of your hand against the right side of the subject's jaw and ask him/her to turn the head to the right against this resistance while observing and feeling the left sternomastoid muscle (figure 41a-d).

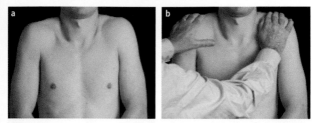

Figure 42 a,b. Shoulder shrugging by trapezius, without and with resistance.

Repeat the procedure for the right. The trapezius is tested by shoulder shrugging (figure 42a,b).

XII Hypoglossal Nerve

The hypoglossal nerve supplies all intrinsic and extrinsic muscles of the **tongue** except the palatopharyngeus (vagus). The nerve may be damaged by infiltrating **malignancies** of the pharynx and **surgery** in the region of the carotid bifurcation. Injury produces paralysis of the ipsilateral side of the tongue, with wasting and fasciculation; the tongue deviates towards the affected side.

Tongue movements are assessed by rapid pointing and withdrawing the tongue (figure 43a,b), and during speech.

Power is assessed by pushing the tongue into the cheek, and against resistance applied to the outside of the cheek (figure 44a,b). In lower

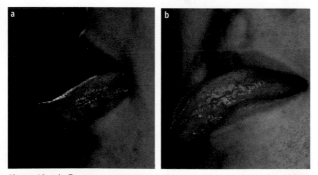

Figure 43 a,b. Tongue movements: repetitive small in and out, and to either side.

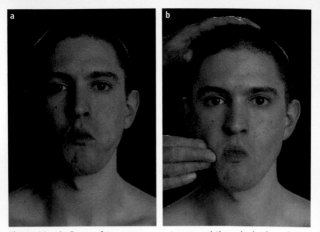

Figure 44 a,b. Power of tongue movements assessed through cheek: active and resisted.

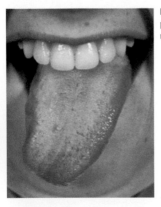

Figure 45 Right-sided twelfth nerve palsy; note deviation to right and right muscle wasting.

motor neuron paralysis, there is muscle wasting and, on putting out the tongue, it deviates to the side of the lesion (figure 45).

The ninth to twelfth cranial nerves can be damaged collectively in the brainstem, producing a **bulbar palsy**, severely affecting swallowing. However, these muscles are bilaterally innervated and require bilateral cortical lesions to produce this effect from upper motor neuron damage (**pseudobulbar palsy**).

Cranial nerve autonomic fibers are carried in III, VII, IX, X. Damage affects lacrimation, salivation, swallowing, and gut motility. Pupillary reflexes may be lost, as are the normal heart rate changes with: respiration (sinus arrhythmia), hyperventilation (30 breaths per minute for 20 seconds should raise the heart rate by 12 beats per minute), Valsalva maneuver (reduction of heart rate), carotid sinus massage (reduction of heart rate), postural change from lying to standing (a rise of 20–30 beats per minute). The latter reflex reduces blood pressure fall, but this may be up to 10 mm of mercury in a normal elderly person.

NECK

The neck provides a powerful, flexible union between the head and the trunk, allowing controlled movement and a wide visual field. The superficial cervical muscles are summarized in table 3 and figure 46, and the cervical spine and deep muscles are considered with the back (page 77).

The neck gives passage to the airway (page 188) and digestive tract (page 285), and the great vessels of the head and brain (page 239), and contains a prominent cervical lymphatic plexus (page 265). This section considers the examination of the thyroid gland and the cervical incisions that provide access to many of the above contents.

Thyroid

The thyroid is an endocrine gland concerned with metabolic activity. It is situated in the anterior neck and its **two lobes** lie on either side of the laryngotracheal junction. The lobes are united across the midline by a short **isthmus** that passes anterior to the second and third tracheal rings. Each lobe is 5 x 3 cm and is related laterally to the carotid sheath. The four parathyroid glands (each 3–6 mm across; endocrine glands concerned with calcium metabolism) are related to the posterior surface of the thyroid (two to each lobe) and are enclosed within its fascial sheath. Due to its fascial attachments, the thyroid gland moves with the larynx on swallowing; it is not usually visible as it is covered anteriorly by the infrahyoid and anterolaterally by the sternomastoid muscles.

Enlargement of the gland (goiter) may be **diffuse**, as with iodine deficiency and the firm gland of Hashimoto disease, or be due to one or more **nodules** The latter are usually **cysts** but may be benign or malignant **neoplasms** (figure 47). Enlargement may compress the trachea, and stretch, invade, and paralyze the recurrent laryngeal nerve: vocal cord paralysis may be observed by direct or indirect laryngoscopy.

Table 3 **MUSCLES OF THE ANTEROLATERAL ASPECT OF THE NECK**

MUSCLE	SUPERIOR ATTACHMENT	INFERIOR ATTACHMENT	FUNCTION	NERVE SUPPLY
Sternomastoid (Divides the neck into anterior and posterior triangles: the small triangular area between its two heads and the clavicle overlies the internal jugular vein)	Lateral surface of the mastoid process and the lateral half of the superior nuchal line	Sternal head: round tendon to the anterior surface of the upper part of the manubrium Clavicular head: from the deep surface of the muscle, passes to the upper medial third of the clavicle	Laterally flexes and rotates the head, as in looking under a table: together, the muscles raise the head from the horizontal and protrude the chin	Accessory and C2,3,4 branches from the cervical plexus
Digastric	Posterior belly from the medial aspect of the mastoid process to the intermediate tendon that is fixed by a fibrous sling to the greater horn of the hyoid bone	Anterior belly passes to the digastric fossa on the back of the mandible close to the midline		Posterior belly by the facial and the anterior belly by the mylohyoid branch of the inferior alveolar
Stylohyoid	Styloid process	Around the intermediate tendon of the digastric to the hyoid bone	The supra- and infra- hyoid muscles act on the hyoid bone (and thus the floor of the mouth) and the larynx: these move- ments of elevation and lowering are concerned	Facial
Mylohyoid	Mylohyoid line on the mandible	The two muscles meet in a midline raphe and also pass to the body of the hyoid bone		Mylohyoid branch of the inferior alveolar
Geniohyoid	Back of the mandible near the midline	Body of the hyoid bone		C1, carried in the hypoglossal

Table 3 continued

MUSCLE	SUPERIOR ATTACHMENT	INFERIOR ATTACHMENT	FUNCTION	NERVE SUPPLY
Thyrohyoid	Greater horn of the hyoid bone	Oblique line of the thyroid cartilage	with chewing, swallowing and speech	C1, carried in the hypoglossal
Sternohyoid	Inferior body of hyoid bone	Posterior aspect of the medial end of the clavicle		Ansa cervicalis (C1,2,3)
Omohyoid	Superior belly from the body of the hyoid bone: intermediate tendon fixed by a fascial sling to the clavicle	Inferior belly to the upper border of the scapula		Ansa cervicalis (C1,2,3)
Sternothyroid	Oblique line on the thyroid cartilage	Posterior aspect of the manubrium		Ansa cervicalis (C1,2,3)
Scalene and prevertebral muscles			Fixation of the rib cage and flexion of the head and neck	Cervical ventral rami

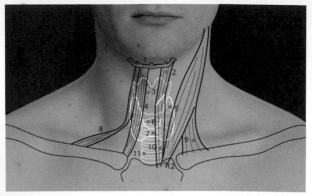

Figure 46
Anatomy of the neck.

Neck

1. Hyoid bone
2. Thyrohyoid
3. Thyroid cartilage
4. Sternohyoid
5. Thyroid gland
6. Cricoid cartilage
7. Isthmus of thyroid
8. Omohyoid
9. Sternomastoid, clavicular head
10. Sternothyroid
11. Tracheal ring
12. Sternomastoid, sternal head

Thyroid over-activity (**thyrotoxicosis**) is accompanied by hyperactivity, anxiety, weight loss, weakness, tremor, and abnormal eye signs (see pages 67, 68). There is tachycardia, and this may be accompanied by auricular fibrillation and cardiac failure. Under-activity (**myxedema**) is characterized by slow mental activity, fatigue, lethargy, weakness, dry skin and hair, facial edema, loss of the lateral eyebrows, slow reacting reflexes, and, more rarely, galactorrhea, pericardial effusion, heart failure, myxedema madness, coma, and hypothermia.

The developing thyroid descends from the back of the tongue, and remnants of this tract may persist as a **thyroglossal cyst**.

Examination of the thyroid commences with observation from the front and the side, looking for enlargement and asymmetry of the lower neck. Observe the thyroid during swallowing. The subject takes a mouthful of water, holds it, extends the neck and then, when requested, swallows; enlargement is more obvious as the gland moves upward on swallowing. Although the female larynx does not have a laryngeal prominence (Adam's apple), enlargement is equally visible on swallowing (figure 48a–d).

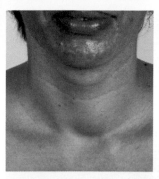

Figure 47 Circular thyroid nodule of approximately 3cm diameter in left lobe.

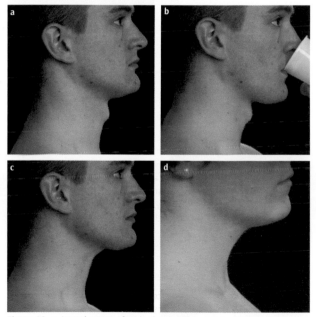

Figure 48 a. Lateral aspect of neck, showing the normal position of the Adam's apple in the male. b,c. When a mouthful of water is swallowed, the larynx rises; d. laryngeal prominance is less obvious in the female, but an enlarged thyroid is more visible in swallowing in both sexes.

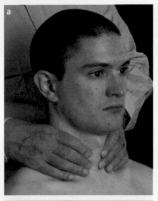

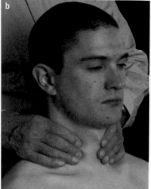

Figure 49 a. Thyroid palpation initially from behind. b,c. Pushing larynx to one side facilitates examination of the thyroid lobe of that side, from behind or in front.

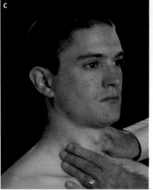

Figure 50 Position of trachea to exclude deviation.

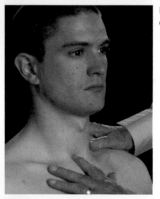

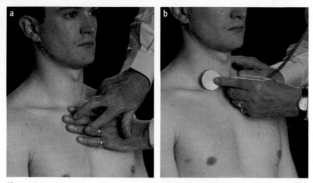

Figure 51 a. Retrosternal extension of enlarged thyroid checked by percussion and b. listening for bruits.

The gland is more easily palpable from behind with the chin slightly down and the neck muscles relaxed (figure 49a). First palpate the isthmus in the midline over the upper tracheal rings, then each lobe in turn. Pushing the larynx to one side makes it easier to palpate the opposite lobe (figure 49b). When examining from the front, the same laryngeal deviation makes the opposite lobe more prominent and palpable (figure 49c).

Check the position of the trachea, as it may be deviated to one side as well as compressed (figure 50).

Enlargement of the thyroid may be into the superior mediastinum. It rises on swallowing, and may also be detected by percussion across the manubrium (figure 51a). A hyperactive gland may have an audible bruit (figure 51b). The bell or the diaphragm of the stethoscope is lightly applied to avoid compression and artifactual production of murmurs from a carotid artery.

Examine the neck for enlarged lymph nodes (page 265) that may be thyroid metastases.

The **exophthalmos** of thyrotoxicosis may produce **lid retraction** with increased visibility of the sclera above (and less commonly below) the iris; the protrusion may be more obvious when observed from the side or from above. There may be **lid lag**: this is demonstrated by asking the subject to follow a finger that is slowly lowered from above downward; noting delay in dropping of the upper lid (figure 52a,b). Also pass your finger laterally to note any **abnormalities of gaze** or differences between the two sides and any **nystagmus** in the lateral extreme (figure 52c).

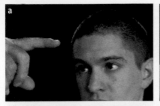

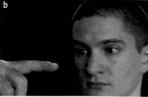

Figure 52 a,b. Abnormal eye movements assessed by gradually dropping finger in front of the eyes, looking for lid lag and c. in lateral extreme, for nystagmus.

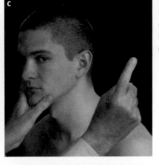

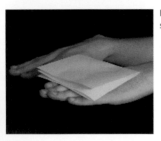

Figure 53 Tremor accentuated by sheet of paper on outstretched hands.

Examine the hands and note any excess sweating, tachycardia or tremor. Ask the subject to hold their hands out straight to observe tremor; this can be accentuated by placing a sheet of paper on the dorsum of the outstretched hands (figure 53).

When examining a thyroglossal cyst, ask the subject to put out their tongue to demonstrate the upward pull from its primary developmental attachment.

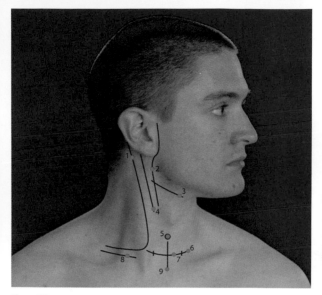

Figure 54
Cervical incisions.

Neck incisions

1. Block dissection of neck
2. Parotid gland
3. Submandibular gland
4. Cervical node sampling/carotid endarterectomy
5. Cricothyroid puncture
6. Thyroidectomy
7. Tracheostomy (transverse)
8. Cervical sympathectomy/ subclavian artery
9. Tracheostomy (vertical)

Neck Incision (figure 54)

The thyroid gland is approached through a transverse (collar) incision, 2 cm above the clavicle; this passes over part of each sternomastoid muscle. A narrower transverse or vertical incision provides access to the upper trachea for **tracheostomy**, separating the infrahyoid muscles. The tracheostomy tube is passed into a circular hole or a flap made in the upper trachea. This is usually through the third and fourth rings, taking care to retract or divide the isthmus of the thyroid and control any bleeding from its associated vessels. An incision through the cricothyroid membrane (**cricoidotomy**) enters the trachea below the vocal cords and is an alternative approach in children. In an emergency a wide-bore needle is passed through the cricothyroid membrane to obtain an airway.

Excision of a **thyroglossal cyst** is through a transverse incision over it. The complete tract must be removed, and this may require excision of the central portion of the body of the hyoid bone.

Exposure of the **carotid bifurcation** and common carotid artery is by an incision along the anterior border of the sternomastoid muscle. The upper part of this incision also exposes the upper part of the deep **cervical lymph chain**.

The **parotid gland** is approached through a vertical incision along the front of the ear, extended under the lobe and along the upper anterior border of the sternomastoid muscle. The surgical approach to the **submandibular gland** is through an incision parallel with the lower jaw, but 2 cm below it, to avoid damaging the mandibular branch of the facial nerve that innervates the lower facial muscles.

Musculoskeletal System

The musculoskeletal system comprises the joints, bones, and muscles. This section considers the general and individual examination of the **muscles** and their adjacent **bones** and **joints**; neuromuscular assessment is considered in more detail with the nervous system (pages 345–92).

MUSCLES

Muscles vary in their **shape** and **texture**; for example, compare the smooth parallel fibers of the lower part of the rectus abdominis and biceps muscles, with the coarser structure of the middle fibers of the deltoid and gluteus maximus. Tendinous **intersections** may be visible, and palpable, as within the upper part of rectus abdominis, and tendons and their attachments may be easily seen and felt, e.g., the tendons over the dorsum of the wrist and hand. **Malalignment** and rupture may be obvious, and fibrous damage is palpable as stringy areas across a muscle. **Spasm** produces a smooth, slightly tender but firm swelling; this may change with heat and massage. A **hematoma** within the muscle has similar features, but is harder and more painful on examination, with increased temperature and possibly overlying redness. **Inflammation** of tendon sheaths may produce swelling and thickness of the sheath, accompanied by pain, and surrounding edema, tenderness, and local heat. **Infection** of a muscle or muscle compartment (pyomyositis), although rare, is a serious and potentially fatal event, particularly if clostridial organisms are involved.

Atrophy of muscles (page 350) may suggest disuse, injury, myopathy or neuropathy, and abnormal movements should be noted. Benign (rhabdomyomas) and malignant (rhabdomyosarcomas) muscle, and other soft tissue **tumors** are occasionally encountered (figure 1).

BONES AND JOINTS

The commonest disorders of bone and joints relate to **trauma** – fractures, dislocations, and chronic arthritic problems. However, congenital and acquired deformity (figure 2), inflammation, metabolic disorders, and tumors are encountered in an orthopedic practice. Tumors may be benign or malignant (figure 3), and bone is a common site for metastatic deposits (figure 4).

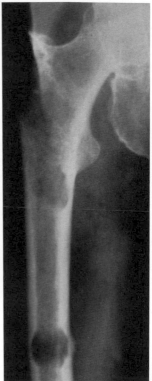

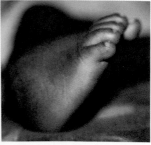

Figure 2 Club foot.

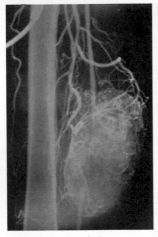

Figure 1 Vascular soft tissue tumor (rhabdomyosarcoma) of thigh.

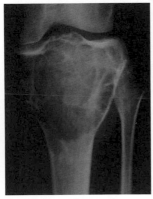

Figure 3 Giant cell tumor of upper end of tibia.

Figure 4 Multiple metastases in upper end of femur.

Routine physical examination does not include the examination of every joint. More often this is directed by a patient's history and abnormalities noted on general inspection. All students must, however, learn how to examine each joint: the principles are to **look**, **feel**, **move**, **measure**, and **x-ray**.

Inspection (Look)

A patient must be appropriately undressed; always compare right with left, and with abnormalities of other joints. Note **skin** color, rashes, creases, scars, sinuses, and **contractures**. Erythema may indicate arthritis or infection, while a rash may give important clues to underlying joint disturbances. Abnormal **shape** of a joint may reflect swelling due to effusions, synovial hypertrophy, inflammation, and bony overgrowths.

Deformity may be postural (due to abnormal posture), structural (due to tissue abnormalities), paralytic (due to muscular imbalance) or compensatory (to overcome abnormalities elsewhere). The deformity may be mobile or fixed, i.e., not changeable on passive movement; they may be symmetrical or asymmetrical. The degree of deformity may be mild (e.g., ulnar deviation of the metacarpophalangeal joint in early rheumatoid arthritis) or gross (e.g., destruction of a denervated joint in a neuropathic disorder).

Lateral deviation of the distal portion of a joint in relation to the proximal is termed a **valgus** deformity; medial deviation, a **varus** deformity. Abnormalities of bone alignment are classified as **subluxation** when the displaced parts of joint surfaces remain in contact, and **dislocation** when there is loss of contact between the two adjacent surfaces.

You should note any alteration in the shape or outline of the bone, localized swelling and evidence of tenderness. Bones may be both deformed and enlarged, as in osteitis deformans (Paget disease), or there may be alteration of their shape, as in the bowing of the tibia seen in rickets. Tendons and bursae are examined for inflammatory changes.

Palpation (Feel)

The history indicates the presence of painful sites and you must show extreme gentleness during **palpation**; watch a patient's face (also later in active and passive movement). **Tenderness** is an important sign of pathology localize its site as accurately as possible. Remember, however, that tenderness, like pain, can be referred from a damaged to a distant area. Commence with palpation of the adjacent bones, their surfaces and the joint line. There may be tenderness along this line, as with damaged menisci in the knee joint. Ligamentous tenderness may be due to tears at the joint line or the ligament attachments on either side of it.

Palpation should detect **warmth**, which may signify an active synovitis or infection, and tenderness of the joint or periarticular tissues. Stroking a limb from proximal to distal encounters a gradual cooling of temperature and abnormality can be readily appreciated; use the medial side of your hand for this maneuver.

The joint is systematically palpated for evidence of **swelling**, which may be of the skin, subcutaneous tissues, muscles, joint capsule, ligaments, synovial membrane, bursae, bone or intracapsular structures, such as an effusion or abnormal cartilages. Soft tissue swelling around the joint causes deformity, with loss of the normal contour and palpable landmarks. An **effusion** is fluctuant and, using specific tests, fluid can be made to shift within the joint. However, there may be associated inflammatory edema and surrounding inflamed tendons or a **hemarthrosis**. Synovial thickening and **synovitis** have a soft and boggy characteristic, with associated warmth and redness. Sustained pressure is usually required to produce any indentation of the inflammatory edema. These conditions untreated may lead to permanent damage to the joint surfaces.

Tenderness of bones is characteristic of **osteitis fibrosa**, **multiple myeloma**, **leukemic** infiltration of bones, **secondary** deposits and **osteomyelitis**. **Fractures** may be accompanied by swelling, deformity, crepitus, abnormal mobility, and loss of function.

Map out any areas of altered cutaneous sensation.

Movement

In examining movement of a joint, it is important to first ask the patient specifically about pain and tenderness in the joint or the limb being examined. Initially the range of **active** movements is tested *before* proceeding to a more thorough evaluation of **resisted** and **passive** movement. Asking the patient to demonstrate the full range of active movement reveals the extent of dysfunction of a joint. For example, doing up a shirt button may reveal the extent of dysfunction of a hand.

Movement of a damaged muscle or its tendons commonly produces **pain**. This pain can be demonstrated by holding a joint in the mid range of a muscle activity, while the patient forcibly contracts this muscle. As no movement takes place, any pain can be localized to a specific muscle rather than the rigid elements or other muscles acting on the joint. This **"resisted movement** technique" requires knowledge of the action of each muscle in order to stand in the appropriate position to hold and resist activity. Note is also taken of any muscle weakness. **Power** is graded on a scale of 0 to 5: 5 is normal and 0 total paralysis.

Passive movement must be undertaken with extreme gentleness and the patient's face watched during all these maneuvers. These precautions give the patient confidence to totally relax while you are testing the full range of movement in each joint. Before you start, consider how you are going to stand and hold the limb to assess the full range of joint movement, without moving your feet or grip during the process. Know the normal end points of the movements of a joint, and whether the end point is a **hard bony end point** ("close-pack"- congruence of the bony surfaces), e.g., elbow extension, and tautness of tendons and ligament of knee extension, or a **soft end point**, limited by soft tissue apposition (the "loose-pack" of non-bony congruence), e.g., knee flexion. Some springiness of the soft tissues is usually present in the mid-range of normal joint movement.

In passive movement of the hip joints, check for associated movement of the pelvis and spine, and in the shoulder, associated scapular movement. In larger joints, the distal limb is usually moved with one hand while the palm of the other rests over the joint surface. Grinding, grating or creaking sensation of the surfaces may be heard and felt, including **crepitus**, clicks, clunks, resistance, and catching or locking, suggesting irregularity of the articular cartilage or bony surfaces.

The commonest cause of limited movement is pain from the structures attached to the joint or elsewhere within the limb. It may be due to inflammatory changes. Other causes are thickening of the capsule and periarticular structures, joint effusions, muscle spasm, contractures, and bony irregularities or **ankylosis**.

Once the limit of normal movement has been assessed specific maneuvers are undertaken to identify abnormal movements and joint instability. Excessive movement may be due to lax or torn ligaments and bony deformity.

Movement involves both the neurological and musculoskeletal systems, the emphasis in the former is on tone, power, coordination and reflexes, while in the latter the emphasis is on the measurement of active and passive movement. There is, however, a considerable overlap. In this text, to avoid excessive repetition, the neurological examination considers neuromuscular abnormalities, while in this chapter movement is emphasized. In practice you need to master all techniques for assessing active, passive and resisted movement, and muscle power for use in either system.

Measurement

Loss of muscle bulk may be due to local or systemic disease; generalized wasting can be observed in the hands, by examining the interossei over the dorsum, particularly between the thumb and index finger. Limb **wasting** can be measured at fixed points along it (page 349), comparing measurements on the two sides of the body. Be sure to use the same markers on each side, and record the distance and the circumference in the patient's notes.

Measurement of the length of the whole or part of each limb establishes real or apparent shortening (page 144). The various segments are measured not only in developmental assessment, but also to demonstrate shortening due to congenital abnormalities or injuries.

Note the range of active and passive movement of a joint being examined.

Joint and Soft Tissue Injection

Acute and chronic pain in joints and soft tissues may benefit from injection of corticosteroids, local anesthetic or a combination with hyaluronidase, to enhance penetration of drugs and reabsorption of tissue fluid. This is usually a second line management, and requires precise localization of the pain, stiffness or deformity by a full history and examination.

The injection may be into a joint cavity; although there are often a number of approaches to a joint, the standard techniques illustrated avoid major neurovascular structures. Injection into ligaments and bursae is into the tender area. In persistent tenosynovitis, the injection is into the tendon sheath, rather than the tendon itself. The latter may promote tendon rupture, and injection is not usually undertaken in the tendo Achilles, as this lacks a distinct sheath.

Injection techniques are considered in this chapter, rather than a separate section, so that they can be linked to the relevant anatomy and examination.

As with all invasive techniques, an aseptic technique is used; injection is not undertaken through infected tissues and full account is taken of potential injury to neurovascular structures and adjacent organs. After the first injection of a specific drug, observe the patient for 20–30 minutes to ensure there is no hypersensitivity to the agent.

BACK

The **axial skeleton** is formed from the skull, vertebral column, ribs, and sternum. The **vertebral column** provides protection for the spinal cord, and a firm strong bilaterally symmetrical central axis for supporting muscular activity. It is formed of 33 vertebrae: 7 cervical, 12 thoracic, 5 lumbar, 5 sacral, and 4 coccygeal. The **vertebral canal** extends from the foramen magnum to the sacral hiatus. It is formed by the vertebral arches and intervening ligaments laterally and posteriorly, and anteriorly by the vertebral bodies and intervertebral discs. It houses the **spinal cord**, its **meningeal coverings** and the emerging **spinal nerves**. The number of nerves corresponds to that of the vertebrae, except in the **cervical region**, where there are eight: the first emerges above the axis, the remainder below each of the seven cervical vertebrae (but the nerve number is one greater than that of the related vertebra). The thoracic and **lumbar** spinal nerves pass beneath the pedicles of the same numbered vertebra. The **sacral** nerves pass through the sacral foramina, the dorsal roots posteriorly and the ventral anteriorly. The **coccygeal** nerves pass through the **sacral hiatus.**

The spinal cord ends opposite the first lumbar vertebra (**third in children**), and the collection of descending nerves below this level is termed the **cauda equina**. The **dural sac** descends to the level of the second sacral vertebra; this means that the lower dural sac contains the cauda equina and lower spinal nerves, but not the spinal cord. This fact is made use of clinically, as a needle can be introduced into the sac to inject substances, or sample cerebrospinal fluid, without risk of damage to the spinal cord.

The surface marking for this insertion is the supracristal plane (the uppermost level of the iliac crests – figure 5), which passes through the fourth lumbar spine. A needle is inserted above or below this spine, which is palpable (lumbar puncture). The needle passes through the skin and supraspinous ligaments and into the **extradural space** (containing

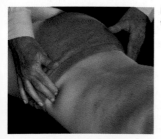

Figure 5 Supracristal plane passing through iliac crests and spine of L4.

fat and a venous plexus). Local anesthetic can be introduced at this level (**epidural anesthesia**), or the needle advanced through the meninges into the dural sac to deliver anesthetic (**spinal anesthesia**). Local anesthetic may also be introduced into the sacral hiatus (**caudal block**) to anesthetize the perineum, a technique used to suppress pain in vaginal childbirth.

In utero, the spine is curved in C fashion, with a **primary thoracic kyphosis**. After birth, a **secondary cervical lordosis** develops in relation to raising the head and the **lumbar lordosis** in relation to walking. In the upright position the vertebral column supports the weight of the head, trunk and upper limbs, and transmits it through the pelvic girdle to the lower limbs. The segmental nature of the vertebral column adds flexibility without reducing its strength. Movement between individual vertebrae is not marked but collectively there is extensive movement across the whole vertebral column. Flexion is most marked in the cervical region, rotation in the thoracic, and extension and lateral flexion in the lumbar region.

Everyone suffers from backache at some time in their life, but fortunately the vast majority of these problems are self-limiting and only challenge the difficulties of diagnosis when they are persistent, recurrent or disabling. Figure 6a–f shows some normal and abnormal radiological features.

Backache is usually musculoskeletal in origin. However, always consider the possibility of referred pain and look for other diagnostic features. Acute severe thorocolumbar and abdominal back pain can be produced by acute **aortic** lesions (both dissection and rupture), and the pain of **myocardial infarction** may pass between the scapulae; **gallbladder** disease often presents with pain below the right scapula. Pancreatic pain is typically in the upper lumbar region and other **retroperitoneal lesions**, such as neoplasms, hemorrhage and renal disease, may present in similar fashion. Pain of **gynecological** origin typically presents with low back pain; it is an important differential diagnosis.

Backache in the skeletally immature should always be considered organic and investigated, as should neurological signs, such as muscle wasting, and bladder and bowel dysfunction. Deformities may be congenital;

Figure 6 Radiology of the spine: a,b. Antero-posterior (AP) and lateral normal radiographs of cervical spine; c,d. normal and osteoarthritic spine; e. MRI of spine; f. myleogram of lower spinal cord and cauda equina, with protruding intervertebral disc compressing emerging nerves.

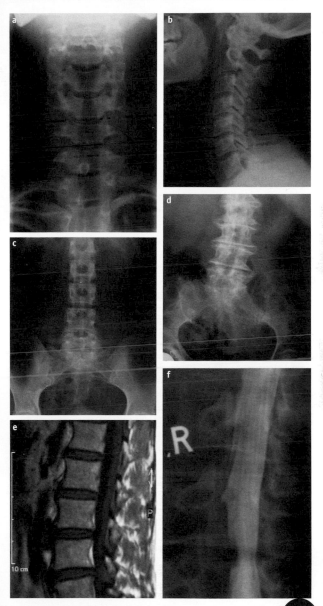

these include all forms of **spinal bifida**, ranging from spina bifida occulta, involving only a local skin abnormality, through vertebral arch defects to myeloceles and meningomyeloceles. In the latter the cord presents as a surface neurological plaque. Severe forms are commonly associated with **hydrocephalus**, in relation to the Arnold Chiari malformation (where the cerebellar hemispheres cone into the foramen magnum, and obstruct the flow of cerebrospinal fluid).

Vertebral deformities include hemivertebrae, spondylolisthesis, and sacral agenesis. Increased thoracic kyphosis is a phenomenon of aging and is accentuated in osteoporosis, Scheuermann disease, ankylosing spondylitis, and Parkinson and Paget diseases. Acute angulation of the spine with prominent abnormal spinous processes (gibbus) may be due to congenitally abnormal vertebrae, trauma, and destructive infections, such as tuberculosis. The lumbar lordosis may be accentuated in protrusion of an intervertebral disc, osteomyelitis, and spondylolisthesis.

Scoliosis (lateral curvature of the spine) may be postural (this is common in adolescent girls and corrected in flexion) or compensatory (secondary to previous thoracic surgery, hip pathology or leg length discrepancy), in the latter the curve corrects on sitting down, or sciatic (list – due to muscle spasm – the convexity is usually directed to the side of the offending intervertebral disc protrusion). Structural indicates a fixed bony abnormality; it is usually accompanied by rotation and a prominent rib hump deformity. It may be related to the aging process, including osteoporosis associated with a crush vertebral fracture.

Spinal stenosis may be related to osteoarthritic changes, particularly involving the lumbar region, and compressing the spinal cord and emerging spinal nerves. Vertebral osteomyelitis usually commences in the disc, and progresses to end plate destruction and paravertebral abscess formation. There may be collapse of the infected vertebra with severe angular kyphosis. A **psoas abscess** tract, secondary to vertebral infection, passes along the psoas sheath, to present as a lump below the inguinal ligament; it is a feature of tuberculous disease.

Spinal tumors may originate in the spinal cord, particularly meningiomas and peripheral nerve neuromas, or they may be benign or malignant bone tumors. Benign tumors include osteoid osteomas, giant cell tumors and osteochondromas. Malignant tumors are predominantly metastases: common primary sites are the lung, breast, prostate, kidney, thyroid and, less commonly, lymphomas and from the gastrointestinal tract. Biopsy is frequently necessary to reach a diagnosis.

Spinal fractures may be divided into **compression**, **burst**, **flexion-distraction injuries**, and **fracture dislocations**. In the latter the spinal cord is subject to injury, with initial flaccidity and areflexia below the level of the injury.

When taking **a history of back** or **spinal pain**, try to differentiate between pain limited to the lower back and leg pain. In deformity, note the age of onset and the rate of progression, together with precipitating factors and the general state of the patient's health. Note whether the pain is related to coughing and movement, and its relieving factors. Determine whether any medicolegal claims are outstanding from injury, and the mental and psychological state of the patient.

Observe the patient throughout the consultation, including the history taking and when undressing: note body proportions, congenital syndromes, deformities, evidence of endocrine or metabolic disease, and **gait**. An **antalgic gait** is when the patient spends more time on one leg than the other, indicating pain related to the other; it is particularly suggestive of hip and knee pathology. A **flexed gait** is suggestive of spinal stenosis (there may also be a **simian stance** with flexion of the spine, hips, and knees). A **shuffling gait** often indicates a neurological abnormality, while **spasticity** may produce a **hemiplegic** (unilateral) or **scissors** (bilateral) gait. A **short gait** (shoulder dipping on the short side) becomes a **Trendelenburg gait** (sideway dipping of the shoulder) when there is weak adduction; the latter becomes a **waddling gait** when the abnormality is bilateral.

Inspection

The spine is initially examined in the standing position with the hands relaxed at each side. The entire posterior aspect of the trunk should be exposed, the subject wearing small briefs and being barefooted. Observe the posture from behind and from each side (figure 7). The details of the posterior spinal muscles are shown in figure 8 and table 1. Note the natural cervical, thoracic, and lumbar curvatures. The thoracic curvature may be more pronounced with increased age; abnormal prominence is termed **kyphosis**. The lumbar curve is more marked in females and excessive curvature is termed **lordosis**. Note any scoliosis.

Bony landmarks are the spinous processes, the angles of the scapulae, the ribs, and the crests and posterior superior iliac spines of the pelvis. A shallow pit (dimple of Venus) may be present over the posterior superior iliac spine, particularly in the female. The spines should be in the midline and the two sides of the body symmetrical. The **vertebra**

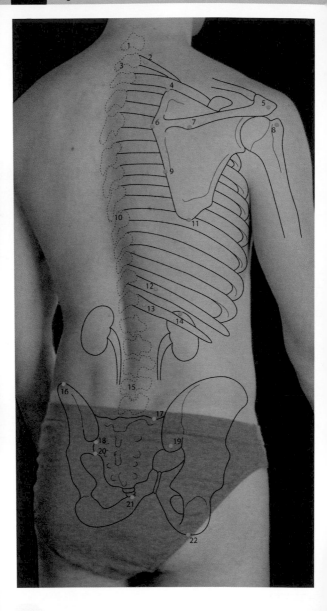

Figure 7
Vertebral column.

1. Vertebra prominens of C7
2. First rib
3. Spine of T1
4. Superior, 6. medial, and 11. inferior, angles of scapula
5. Acromion
7. Spine of scapula, with medial expansion (tubercle)
8. Greater tuberosity of humerus
9. Medial border of scapula
10. Spine of T7, extending downward by more than a vertebra in depth
12. Eleventh and 13. twelfth ribs
14. Upper pole of right kidney
15. Spine of fourth lumbar vertebra (supracristal plane)
16. Iliac crest
17. Lateral part (ala) of sacrum
18. Sacroiliac joint
19. Posterior superior iliac spine (marked by dimple of Venus)
20. Posterior inferior iliac spine
21. Tip of coccyx
22. Ischial tuberosity

prominens is the spine of C7. Note any steps in the spinous processes, indicating abnormalities of the underlying vertebra.

Palpation

Before commencing to palpate, ask the patient to point out any site of discomfort. It may be appropriate to mark this site to direct attention in the examination and ensure consistency of the witness.

Altered sensation on either side of the midline can be demonstrated by simultaneous digital dragging or pinching of the skin on each side. Palpation of the muscles on either side, particularly in the lumbar region, assesses the presence of spasm: lumbar spasm may also be accompanied by loss of the normal lumbar lordosis.

The vertebral spines can be felt in a thin subject from C6 down to the sacrum, and the tips of the index finger can be inserted between and over them to locate any tender spots. Palpate the cervical, thoracic, and lumbar spines (figure 9a–c) and the sacroiliac joints (figure 9d). Palpate on either side, over the transverse processes, the intervertebral joints and paravertebral muscle, to assess tone, spasm, and tenderness. Assess paravertebral tone in the cervical, thoracic, and lumbar regions, and the buttock (figure 10a–d).

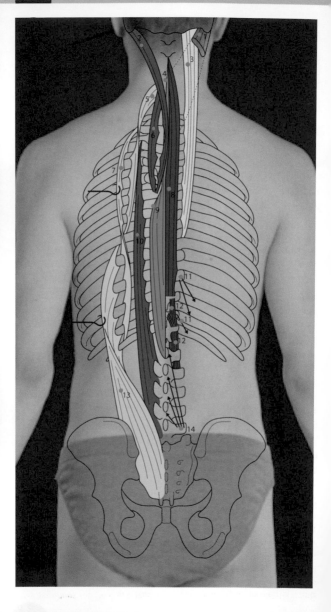

Figure 8
Posterior spinal muscles.

Iliocostalis (green): 5. cervicis, 7. thoracis, 13. lumborum
Longissimus (red): 2. capitis, 6. cervicis, 10. thoracis
Spinalis (blue): 4. cervicis, 9. thoracis
Semispinalis 8. (purple): length of thoracic and cervical spine, 3. (yellow) capitis
  1. Spenius capitis
11. Levatores costarum: to adjacent or lower rib
12. Intertransverse, interspinous, rotators: close to midline, length of spine
14. Multifidus: across one or more vertebra, length of spine

First apply digital pressure over a symptomatic, or suspected abnormal area. If no tenderness is elicited, increase the pressure by using both thumbs. Progress to percussion, at first with a single fist thump, and then a more pronounced double hand thumb over the spines, and on each side (figure 11a–d).

Posteriorly, pressure is applied over the iliac crests, sacroiliac joints, the sacrum and the ischial tuberosities, to identify pelvic pain (figure12a–c).

Anteriorly, palpate the iliac crests, the anterior superior iliac spines, and pubic tubercles of the pelvis (figure 13a,b). The integrity of the pelvis is examined by side to side compression of the iliac bones, pressure on the pubis in the sagittal plane and simultaneous backwards pressure on the two iliac crests (figure 14a,b).

Limitation of straight leg raising is determined by lifting the patient's heel from the lying position; it indicates tension in the radicals of the sciatic nerve and may be indicative of a lumbar disc abnormality. The sign may be accentuated by simultaneous raising of the head and dorsiflexion of the ankle (figure 15a–c).

Tension can be applied to the femoral nerve by passively flexing each knee in turn in the prone position (femoral nerve stretch test – figure 16).

Movement

The **center of gravity** lies in front of the second piece of the sacrum; gravity therefore promotes flexion. Cervical flexion is also produced by the infrahyoid and sternomastoid muscles and, in the thoracic and lumbar regions, by the rectus abdominis and oblique muscles of the abdominal wall. Extension is by the powerful erector spinae muscle group (table 1). Lateral flexion is by the abdominal wall muscles, supported by quadratus lumborum; rotation is by the abdominal wall muscles and obliquely placed muscles within the erector spinae muscle mass.

Head movements are by the suboccipital muscles, and the superficial neck muscles (sternomastoid, trapezius, splenius) produce rotation and lateral flexion.

Table 1 DEEP MUSCLES OF THE BACK

The bulk of the deep extensor muscle mass of the back is formed from the **erector spinae** muscle group.

This produces the longitudinal bulge on each side of the midline that extends from the sacrum to the occiput and, in the thoracic region, reaches the angles of the ribs. A deeper **transversospinalis** group of muscles fills the groove between the spines and the transverse processes, and superiorly, the erector spinae are overlain by the two **splenius** muscles on each side, as well as by the superficial muscles (trapezius, latissimus dorsi, the rhomboids, and serratus posterior muscles).

The following table provides a summary of the attachments of these three deep muscle groups, but there is often variation, with absence, overlap, and fusion of the various parts.

The muscle mass as a whole extends the back and, on each side, rotates the trunk to the same side: similar head movements are produced by muscles from these groups that are attached to the skull. Head movements are supplemented by another group of short **suboccipital** muscles, passing between the skull, the atlas, and the axis. Collectively, the muscle mass also plays an important role in posture and stabilizing the vertebral column and rib cage. Its nerve supply is segmental, from the **dorsal rami of the spinal nerves**.

MUSCLE	INFERIOR ATTACHMENT	SUPERIOR ATTACHMENT
Splenius capitis	The spines T4-C7 and the lower half of the ligamentum nuchae	Mastoid process and below the lateral third of the superior nuchal line of the temporal bone
Splenius cervicis	Spines T6-3	Posterior tubercles of the TP C1-3
Erector spinae (sacrospinalis) Comprises three longitudinal muscle groups, each with three named components: Iliocostalis (most		

Table 1 continued

MUSCLE	INFERIOR ATTACHMENT	SUPERIOR ATTACHMENT
lateral of the three groups):		
Iliocostalis lumborum	Median crest and posterior sacrum, and adjacent iliac crest	Inferior border of the angles of ribs 6-12
Iliocostalis thoracis	Upper border of the angles of ribs 12-6, medial to the lumborum attachment	Angles of ribs 1-6 and the TPC7
Iliocostalis cervicis	Angles of ribs 6-3, medial to the thoracis attachment	Posterior tubercles of the TP C4-6
Longissimus (intermediate group):		
Longissimus thoracis	TP and accessory processes L5-1, thoracolumbar fascia	TP T1-12, between tubercles and angles of ribs 3-12
Longissimus cervicis	TP T5-1	Posterior tubercles TP C2-6
Longissimus capitis	TP T5-1 and articular processes C7-4	Posterior margin of the mastoid process of the temporal bone
Spinalis (medial group):		
Spinalis thoracis	Spines L2-T11 (indistinct)	Spines T 2-8
Spinalis cervicis	Spines T2-C7 (indistinct)	Spine C2
Spinalis capitis	Blends with semispinalis capitis	
Transversospinalis Comprises three muscle groups passing obliquely upwards from the transverse processes to the spines above: others pass between adjacent vertebrae, and the vertebrae and the ribs. Semispinalis extends from the lower thorax to the skull, crossing 4-6 vertebrae:		
Semispinalis thoracic	TP T10-6	Spines C6-T4
Semispinalis cervicis	TP T6-1	Spines C2-5
Semispinalis capitis	TP T7-C7 and articular processes C6-4	Medial part of the occipital bone, between the inferior and superior nuchal lines

Table 1 continued

MUSCLE	INFERIOR ATTACHMENT	SUPERIOR ATTACHMENT
Multifidus	Along the length of the spine, from the back of the sacrum, the lumbar mamillary processes, TP T12-1 and the articular processes C7-4	Spines of one to four vertebrae above, reaching C2
Rotatores thoracis	TP T12-2	Lamina of usually the vertebra above
Rotatores lumborum and cervicis	Similar attachments to thoracis	Both inconstant
Levator costarum	Upper edge of all ribs, between the tubercle and the angle	TP C7-T11, slips from one and two ribs below
Intertransversarii	Pass between adjacent vertebrae, best developed in the cervical region	(Also an anterior group, supplied by the ventral rami of the spinal nerves)
Interspinalis	On either side of the midline, best developed in the cervical region, where they may also span more than one vertebra	
Suboccipital muscles form the suboccipital triangle, the floor of which is crossed by the posterior arch of the atlas, the dorsal ramus of C1 and the vertebral artery:		
Rectus capitis posterior major	Spine of the axis	Inferior nuchal line, and the occipital bone below it, the major lying lateral to the minor
Rectus capitis posterior minor	Posterior tubercle of the atlas	
Oblique capitis inferior	Spine of the axis	TP atlas
Oblique capitis superior	TP atlas	Lateral part of the occipital bone, between the inferior and superior nuchal lines

TP transverse process; C cervical; T thoracic; L lumbar

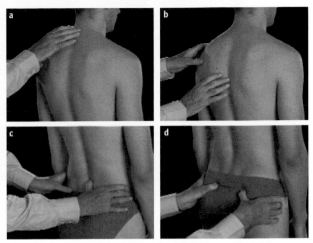

Figure 9 a,b,c,d. Palpation of spines of vertebra and sacroiliac joints.

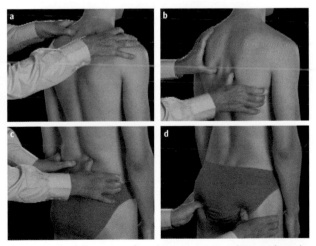

Figure 10 a,b,c,d. Assessment of muscle tone in erector spinae muscles and buttocks.

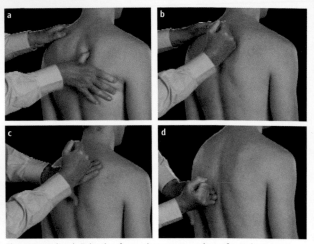

Figure 11 a,b,c,d. Palpating for tenderness over spines of vertebrae and paravertebral muscles.

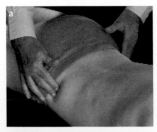

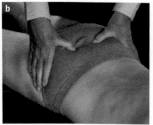

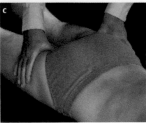

Figure 12 a. Posterior examination of pelvis: iliac crests; b. sacroiliac joints; c. ischial tuberosities, pressure is applied to these areas to assess deep tenderness.

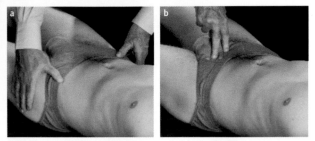

Figure 13 a. Anterior superior iliac spines, and b. pubic tubercles.

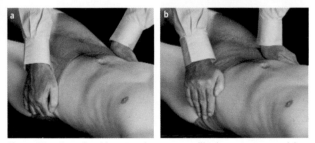

Figure 14 a. Inward and b. outward pressure on iliac bones to assess pelvic integrity.

Scoliosis may be mild and postural in nature, and can be overcome by asking the subject to place each hand on the opposite shoulder and to lean forward (figure 17). The latter movement also accentuates a pathological scoliosis. Scoliosis is produced by rotation of the bodies of the vertebrae, so that the spine points to the concavity of the curve: **kyphosis and scoliosis are thus often combined.**

Active and passive movements of the cervical spine are often assessed independently to the rest of the back. To test **flexion**, ask the patient to put their chin on their chest (normal 45 degrees) and then **extension** by looking upward and backward (45 degrees). **Lateral flexion** is by approximating the ear to the adjacent shoulder on each side; it is approximately 45 degrees. **Rotation** is assessed by looking over each shoulder and is normally 75 degrees in each direction (figure 18a–k). Combined movements of the sternomastoid muscles of the two sides

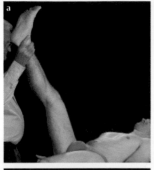

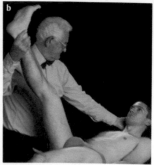

Figure 15 a. Straight leg raising; signs accentuated by b. neck flexion and c. dorsiflexion of foot.

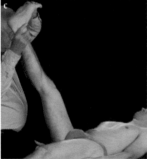

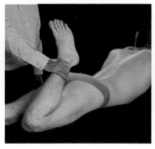

Figure 16 Femoral nerve stretch test.

Figure 17 Trunk flexion with hands on opposite shoulders; note any asymmetry of scoliosis.

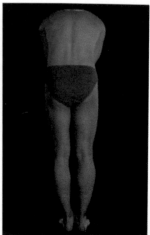

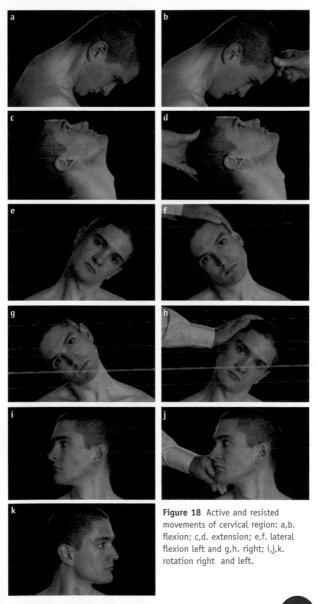

Figure 18 Active and resisted movements of cervical region: a,b. flexion; c,d. extension; e,f. lateral flexion left and g,h. right; i,j,k. rotation right and left.

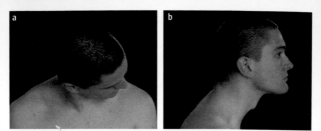

Figure 19 a,b. Combined neck movements: looking under table; and chin protrusion.

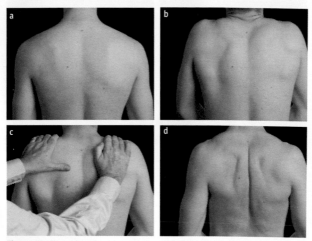

Figure 20 Shrugging shoulders: a. at rest; b. raised; c. resisted; d. bracing shoulders.

produce other head and neck movements such as looking under tables, raising the head from the horizontal, and protruding the jaw (figure 19a,b).

Shrugging and **bracing** the shoulders is primarily brought about by the muscles of the pectoral girdle (figure 20a–d).

Much of the apparent flexion on leaning forward to touch one's toes with straight legs (figure 21) takes place at the atlanto-occipital and hip joints. In the cervical region flexion straightens the cervical curve. There is little flexion in the thoracic spine but flexion is maximal in the lumbar

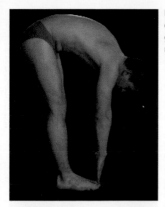

Figure 21 Touching toes – the distance of finger tips from the ground is a useful measure in monitoring progress.

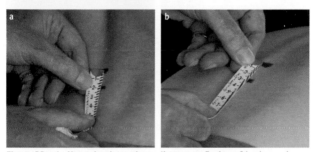

Figure 22 a,b. Measuring interspinous distance on flexion of lumbar region.

region. The distance of the fingertips from the ground on bending forward varies with age and between individuals. This distance can be used to determine the point of onset of pain, and to monitor progress of any limitation of movement.

The spines can be marked and the distance in between any chosen levels measured with a tape measure before and after flexion (figure 22a,b).

Trunk flexion can be observed and resisted, as in sitting up from the horizontal (figure 23a,b). Assess extension by leaning backwards (figure 23c). Assess lateral flexion by asking the subject to slide a hand down each thigh in turn (figure 23d,e). Rotation can be masked by pelvic movement, and you have to hold the pelvis whilst the subject turns their head and shoulders maximally to each side; more conveniently, test the movement with the subject sitting down (figure 23f,g).

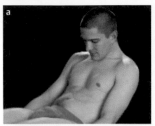

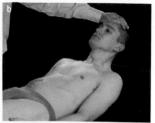

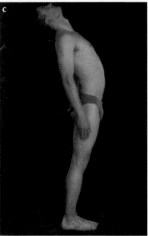

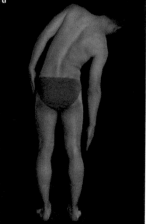

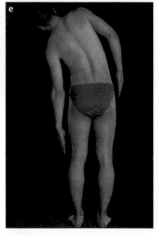

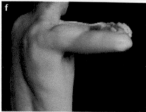

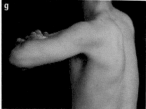

Other essential components of the examination of back pain are a neurological assessment, and a rectal and/or vaginal examination to ensure that pathology within the pelvis is not causing the symptom. Lumbar puncture is considered on page 368.

The surgical approach to the spinal cord is through dorsal midline incisions, removing one or more laminae (laminectomy) to reach the extradural space, and the dura and its contents. With improved imaging and telescopic devices, minor disc protrusions are increasingly being managed by minimally invasive surgery, to remove the protruded annulus fibrosus and relieve nerve pressure.

UPPER LIMB

Injuries of the upper limb are commonly due to falls on the outstretched arm; the resultant fractures vary with age. The clavicle may be fractured at any age, the common site is at the junction of the middle and lateral thirds. Young adults, undertaking rigorous sporting and other activities, fracture the neck of the humerus, endangering the axillary nerve; severe trauma may also produce a spiral fracture of the humerus, with damage to the radial nerve.

In childhood, falls may produce a **supracondylar** fracture, through the thin transverse layer of bone above the condyles of the humerus. A serious complication of this injury is entrapment of the brachial artery during reduction. Great care must be taken to monitor the radial pulse, the perfusion of the hand, and the sensation of the median nerve in these children. Forearm fractures in the child (figure 24) may be of the **greenstick** variety, where only one side of a bone breaks, the other side bending, with angulation of the forearm; this may occur in one or both forearm bones.

Upper limb falls may also produce wrist fractures. In children, they produce fracture of the **radial epiphysis**. In young adults, fracture of the **scaphoid** (figure 25) is more common, and must be identified, as the bone is prone to non-union giving long-standing wrist weakness. Persistent tenderness over the proximal scaphoid, in the anatomical snuffbox, is a useful diagnostic sign. In the elderly, falling on the wrist characteristically produces a **Colles'** fracture (figure 26). This is through

Figure 23 Trunk movement: a,b. active and resisted flexion; c. extension; d,e. lateral flexion to right and left; f,g. trunk rotation to right and left (subject seated to exclude pelvic rotation in the assessment).

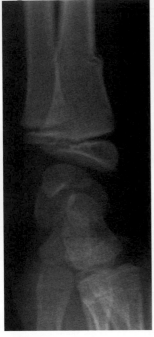

Figure 24 Fracture of lower radius in a child.

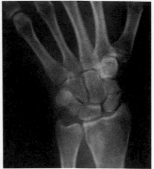

Figure 25 Non-union of scaphoid fracture; note bone in two segments.

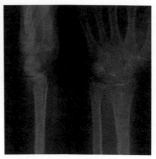

Figure 26 Colles' fracture.

the distal radius, with posterolateral angulation, posterolateral displacement, and impaction of the distal fragment.

Dislocations in the upper limb include the **shoulder joint**, which occurs with the arm abducted; the displacement is through the unsupported inferior capsule and the axillary nerve is at risk. Dislocation of the **radial head** occurs in children, before the conical shape of the radial head has expanded to fit the annular ligament. In the hand, the lunate may be dislocated, and dislocations of the phalanges are common sporting injuries.

The initial application of a few simple tests may serve to localize upper limb abnormalities. These may for example include picking up objects, writing, asking the patient to put their hands together, as in praying, or to comb their hair. Functional limitation and problems then usually become apparent, and direct the subsequent examination. A full regional examination includes inspection, palpation, and movement of all joints, and examination of periarticular structures. Assessment of muscle power and neurological function should also be carried out.

Shoulder Girdle

Shoulder movements are composite, involving the ball and socket articulation at the shoulder (glenohumeral) joint, together with movements between the scapula and clavicle, and the thorax. The shoulder girdle muscles are detailed in tables 2 & 3, and figure 27 shows the muscles of the superior aspect of the shoulder.

Table 2 **MUSCLES OF THE ANTERIOR ASPECT OF THE SHOULDER GIRDLE (CLAVICLE, SCAPULA, AND HUMERUS TO TRUNK)**

MUSCLE	PROXIMAL ATTACHMENT	DISTAL ATTACHMENT	FUNCTION	NERVE SUPPLY
Subclavius	Costochondral junction of the first rib	Under surface of the middle of the clavicle	Stabilization of the clavicle	C5,6
Pectoralis minor	Anterior surface of the third to fifth ribs	Coracoid process of the scapula	Stabilization of the scapula	Medial and lateral pectoral (C6,7,8)
Pectoralis major	Two heads. Clavicular: medial anterior half of the clavicle. Sternocostal: anterior sternum, upper six costal cartilages and the external oblique aponeurosis	Intertubercular groove of the humerus (forming anterior fold of the axilla): clavicular head anterior; sternal fibers spiral beneath costal fibers, forming second and third layers	Adduction and medial rotation of the humerus, flexion from the extended and extension from the flexed position (as in climbing)	Medial and lateral pectoral (C5,6,7,8,T1)

Table 3 **MUSCLES OF THE SUPERIOR AND POSTERIOR ASPECT OF THE SHOULDER GIRDLE (TRUNK TO SCAPULA)**

MUSCLE	PROXIMAL ATTACHMENT	DISTAL ATTACHMENT	FUNCTION	NERVE SUPPLY
Trapezius	Superior nuchal line of the occipital bone, ligamentum nuchae, C7 and all thoracic spines and supraspinous ligaments	Lateral posterior third of the clavicle, acromion and spine of scapula	Upper fibers elevate, middle fibers retract, lower fibers depress and combined fibers rotate the scapula, the head is extended when the scapula is fixed	Spinal accessory, cervical plexus (C3,C4)
Latissimus dorsi	Spines of the lower six thoracic vertebrae, thoracolumbar fascia, posterior iliac crest, lower four ribs and inferior angle of the scapula	Intertubercular groove of the humerus (tendon spirals around teres major, producing the posterior axillary fold)	Adduction and medial rotation of the humerus, extension from the flexed position, as in climbing	Thoracodorsal (C6,7,8)
Levator scapulae	Transverse processes of the upper four cervical vertebrae	Medial border of the scapula above the spine	Elevation of the scapula	Dorsal scapula (C3,4,5)
Rhomboids (major and minor)	Spines of C7 and upper five thoracic vertebrae, and supraspinous ligaments	Medial border of the scapula opposite and below the spine	Retraction of the scapula	Dorsal scapula (C4,5)
Serratus anterior	External surface of the lateral aspect of the upper eight ribs (interdigitating with the external oblique in its lower half)	Anterior surface of the medial border of the scapula	Protraction (pushing forwards) and rotation of the scapula, retains scapula against the chest wall	Long thoracic (C5,6,7)

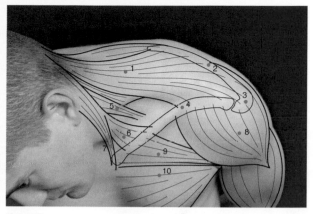

Figure 27
Superior aspect of shoulder girdle.

1. Trapezius
2. Spine of scapula
3. Acromion
4. Clavicle
5. Scalenus anterior

6. Clavicular and 7. sternal heads of sternomastoid
8. Deltoid
9. Clavicular and 10. sternal heads of pectoralis major

Scapula

The scapula is raised, as in a **shrug** of the shoulders, by the trapezius and levator scapulae muscles (figure 28a,b).

Drawing the scapula medially (**bracing** the shoulders) is by the central fibers of the trapezius and the rhomboid muscles (figure 28c). Downward movement of the scapula is primarily the effects of gravity on the weight of the arm and contributed to by the lower fibers of trapezius and latissimus dorsi. The scapula is drawn forward around the chest and retained on the chest wall by the serratus anterior (figure 28d). Absence, weakness or paralysis of this muscle produces winging of the scapula.

The scapula is closely linked to movements of the shoulder joint (see below). In abduction, the various fibers of the trapezius **rotate** the bone and, in adduction, the pectoral and lattisimus dorsi muscles pass directly from the trunk to the humerus, as well as to their scapular attachments; the short scapular muscles all contribute to its stability.

The **sternoclavicular joint**, the **clavicle**, the **acromioclavicular joint**, the **subacromial bursa**, the **bicipital groove** and the **head of the humerus**

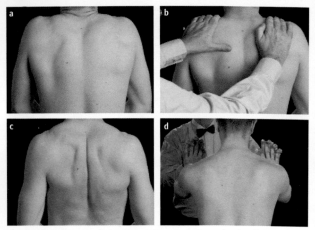

Figure 28 Movements of shoulder girdle: a,b. active and resisted shrugging of shoulders; c. bracing of shoulders; d. forward movement by serratus anterior.

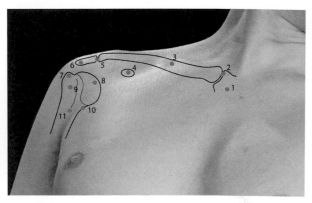

Figure 29
Anatomy of the anterior shoulder girdle.

1. Manubrium
2. Sternoclavicular joint
3. Clavicle
4. Corocoid process
5. Acromioclavicular joint
6. Acromion
7. Greater tuberosity
8. Head of humerus
9. Lesser tuberosity
10. Surgical neck of humerus
11. Bicipital groove

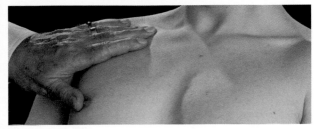

Figure 30 Palpation of subcutaneous anterosuperior surface of clavicle.

are palpable (figure 29); the clavicle is palpable along its length anteriorly (figure 30).

In figure 31a, the thumbnail lies in the sternoclavicular joint, the sternal head of the sternomastoid muscle lies medially. The joint is injected through an anterior approach (figure 31b).

In figure 32a, the thumbnail lies in the acromioclavicular joint. The joint is injected through an anterior or superior approach (figure 32b).

The **coracoid process** of the scapula projects forward just below the clavicle and is palpable through the anterior fibers of the deltoid muscle (figure 33a). Injection of the attached tendons is through an anterior

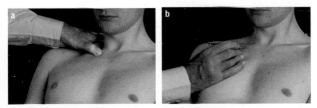

Figure 31 a,b. Palpation and injection of sternoclavicular joint.

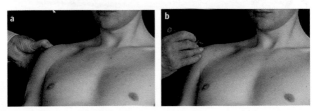

Figure 32 a,b. Palpation and injection of acromioclavicular joint.

103

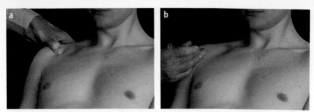

Figure 33 a,b. Palpation and injection of corocoid process.

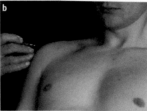

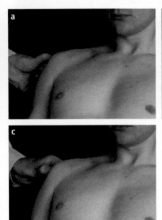

Figure 34 a,b. Palpation and injection of subacromial bursa; c. palpation of greater tuberosity.

approach onto the bone, thus avoiding the axillary vessels and the cords of the brachial plexus that lie below it (figure 33b).

In figure 34a, the thumbnail is inserted beneath the acromion, over the **subacromial bursa**, and above the **supraspinatus tendon** and greater tuberosity. The bursa is injected through a lateral approach (figure 34b). The greater tuberosity lies just below this level, where it can be palpated (figure 34c), and the attached tendons injected.

The **greater and lesser tuberosities** of the humerus are separated by the **bicipital groove**, containing the long tendon of the biceps muscle, its sheath and its bursa (figure 35a). Injections into the sheath are made at this level (figure 35b). Injection into the shoulder joint cavity is through a posterior approach, the needle passing through the fibers of deltoid and teres minor (figure 36).

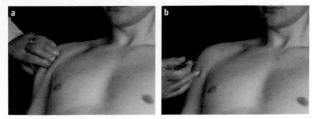

Figure 35 a,b. Palpation and injection of long head of biceps in bicipital groove.

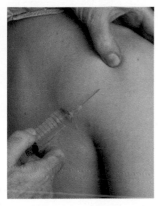

Figure 36 Injection of shoulder joint; needle passed through fibers of deltoid and teres minor.

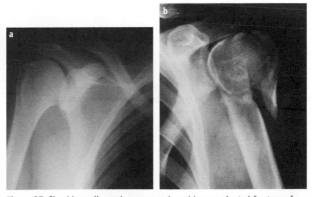

Figure 37 Shoulder radiographs: a. normal, and b. comminuted fracture of surgical neck of humerus.

Table 4 MUSCLES OF THE SHOULDER JOINT AND UPPER ARM

MUSCLE	PROXIMAL ATTACHMENT	DISTAL ATTACHMENT	FUNCTION	NERVE SUPPLY
Deltoid	Lateral third of the clavicle, acromion and spine of the scapula	Deltoid tuberosity of humerus (the central, acromial fibers are multipenate and palpable)	Anterior fibers flex and medially rotate, middle fibers abduct and posterior fibers extend and laterally rotate the humerus	Axillary (C5,6)
Sub-scapularis	Subscapular fossa on the anterior surface of the scapula (subscapular bursa between)	Lesser tuberosity of the humerus	Medial rotation	Upper and lower subscapular (C5,6,7)
Supra-spinatus	Supraspinous fossa on the posterior surface of the scapula	Greater tuberosity of the humerus	Abduction	Supra-scapular (C4,5,6)
Infra-spinatus	Infraspinous fossa on the posterior surface of the scapula	Greater tuberosity of the humerus	Lateral rotation	Supra-scapular (C5,6)
Teres minor	Lateral border of scapula	Greater tuberosity of the humerus	Lateral rotation	Axillary (C5,6)
Teres major	Inferior angle of scapula	Intertubercular groove of the humerus (forming the posterior axillary fold)	Adduction and medial rotation of the humerus	Lower subscapular (C6,7)
Coraco-brachialis	Tip of the coracoid process	Medial border, mid-shaft of the humerus	Abduction and flexion of the humerus	Musculo-cutaneous (C5,6)

Table 4 continued

MUSCLE	PROXIMAL ATTACHMENT	DISTAL ATTACHMENT	FUNCTION	NERVE SUPPLY
Biceps	Two heads. Long: supraglenoid tubercle of the scapula (passing within a synovial sheath through the shoulder joint and intertubercular groove of the humerus) Short: tip of the coracoid process	Radial tuberosity of the radius (with bursa between)	Supination and elbow flexion	Musculo-cutaneous (C5,6)
Brachialis	Lower half of the anterior surface of the humerus	Coronoid process of the ulna	Elbow flexion	Musculo-cutaneous (C5,6)
Triceps	Three heads. Long: infra-glenoid tubercle of the scapula Lateral: posterior humerus above radial groove Medial: posterior humerus below radial groove	Olecranon process of the ulna	Elbow extension	Radial nerve (C6,7,8)

Shoulder

Swelling of the shoulder joint may be visible due to a joint effusion, or synovial thickening. Deformity of the joint and fractures and dislocations are usually obvious (figure 37a,b). Table 4 provides details of the muscles of the shoulder and figure 38a–d illustrations of the anterior and posterior bones and muscles of the upper limb.

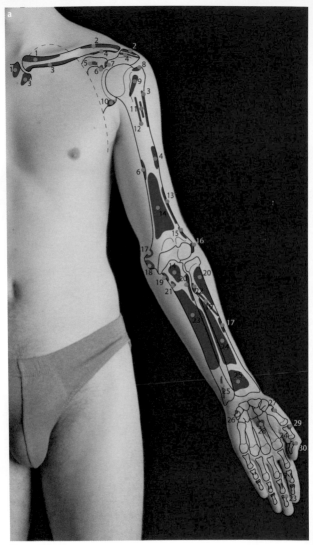

Figure 38a
Upper limb anatomy: anterior bones and muscle attachments.

1. Sternal and clavicular heads of sternomastoid
2. Clavicular and acromial attachments of trapezius
3. Sternal and clavicular heads of pectoralis major, and laterally to outer lip of bicipital groove
4. Clavicular and acromial attachments of deltoid: distally to midshaft humerus
5. Pectoralis minor
6. Coracobrachialis: distally to medial humeral midshaft
7. Short head of biceps
8. Supraspinatus
9. Subscapularis
10. Long head of triceps
11. Latissimus dorsi: rotates around teres major to floor of bicipital groove
12. Teres major
13. Brachioradialis
14. Brachialis
15. Extensor carpi radialis longus
16. Common extensor origin
17. Pronator teres: distally to lateral radial midshaft
18. Common flexor origin
19. Flexor digitorum superficialis: distal split onto middle phalanx
20. Supinator: from lateral ulna around posterior aspect of upper radius
21. Ulnar head of pronator teres
22. Radial attachment of biceps
23. Flexor digitorum profundus: to distal phalanx
24. Flexor pollicis longus: to base of distal phalanx
25. Pronator quadratus: between adjacent radius and ulna
26. Flexor carpi ulnaris
27. Abductor pollicis longus
28. Tendons of extensor carpi radialis longus and brevis
29. Extensor pollicis brevis
30. Extensor pollicis longus

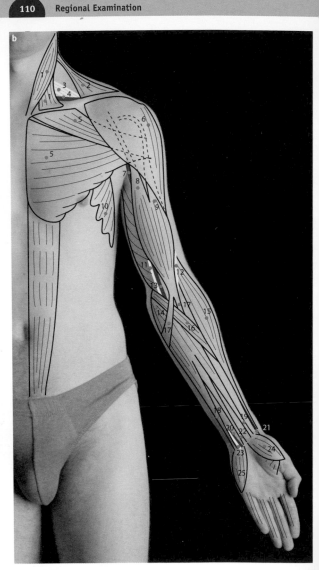

Figure 38b
Upper limb anatomy: anterior muscles.

1. Sternal and clavicular heads of sternomastoid
2. Trapezius
3. Brachial plexus
4. Subclavian artery
5. Sternal and clavicular heads of pectoralis major
6. Deltoid
7. Axillary artery
8. Biceps, short head
9. Biceps, long head
10. Serratus anterior
11. Median nerve
12. Radial nerve
13. Brachial artery
14. Common flexor origin
15. Brachioradialis
16. Pronator teres
17. Biceps tendon and aponeurosis
18. Flexor carpi ulnaris
19. Flexor carpi radialis
20. Ulnar artery
21. Radial artery
22. Palmaris longus, overlying median nerve at wrist
23. Ulnar nerve
24. Thenar muscles
25. Hypothenar muscles

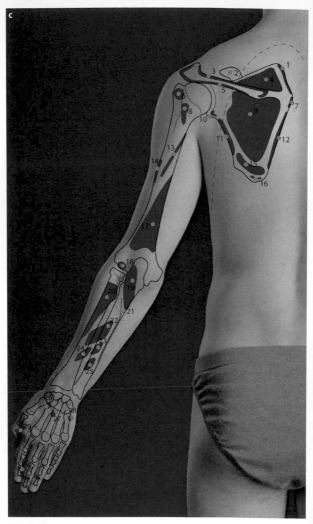

Figure 38c
Upper limb anatomy: posterior bones and muscle attachments.

1. Levator scapulae
2. Coracoid process
3. Trapezius
4. Supraspinatus
5. Deltoid: spine and acromion, to 14. deltoid tuberosity of humerus
7.12. Rhomboideus minor and major
8, 11. Teres minor
9,6. Infraspinatus
10. Long head of triceps
13. Lateral and 17. medial heads of triceps
15. Teres major
16. Latissimus dorsi
18.19. Anconeus
20. Supinator
21. Linear attachment on subcutaneous border of ulna of extensor carpi ulnaris, flexor carpi ulnaris, and flexor digitorum profundus
22. Abductor pollicis longus
23. Extensor pollicis longus
24. Extensor pollicis brevis
25. Extensor indicis
26. Extensor carpi radialis longus
27. Extensor carpi radialis brevis
28. Extensor carpi ulnaris (through pisometacarpal ligament)
29. Extensor pollicis longus
30. Extensor digitorum longus

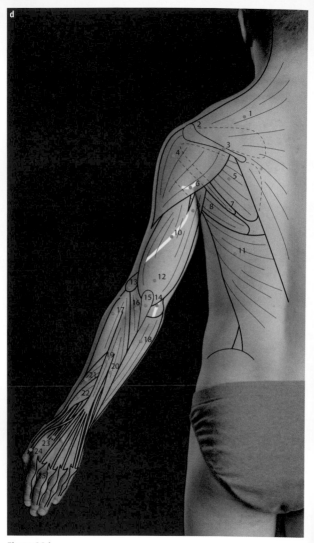

Figure 38d
Upper limb anatomy: posterior muscles.

1. Trapezius
2. Acromion
3. Spine of scapula
4. Deltoid
5. Infraspinatus
6. Axillary nerve: impalpable but important relation to surgical neck of humerus
7. Teres minor
8. Teres major
9. Long head of triceps, 12. tendon to upper border of olecranon
10. Radial nerve: palpable through the fibers of triceps
11. Latissimus dorsi
12. Lateral epicondyle
13. Lateral epicondyle
14. Ulnar nerve: lying on back of medial epicondyle
15. Olecranon process
16. Anconeus
17. Brachioradialis and common extensor muscles
18. Common flexor muscles
19. Extensor digitorum longus
20. Extensor carpi ulnaris
21. Abductor pollicis longus
22. Extensor pollicis brevis
23. Tendons of extensor carpi radialis longus and brevis
24. Extensor pollicis longus
25. Dorsal digital expansion over metacarpophalangeal joints

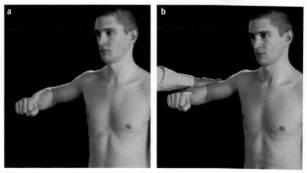

Figure 39 Active and resisted: a,b. flexion and c,d. extension of the shoulder.

Figure 40 a,b. Active and resisted shoulder abduction.

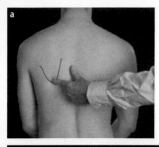

Figure 41 a,b,c. Relative scapular and shoulder joint movement in abduction; inferior angle of scapula, in anatomical position, overlies seventh intercostal space.

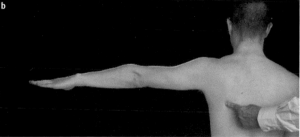

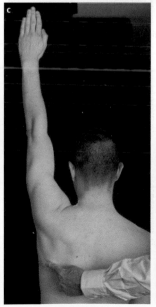

Figure 42
Active movement of pectoralis major and latissimus dorsi in palmar compression.

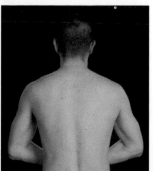

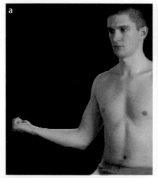

Figure 43 a,b. Active and resisted adduction of shoulder.

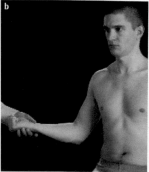

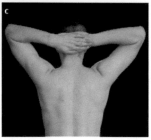

Figure 44 a,b,c. Active and resisted external rotation of shoulder.

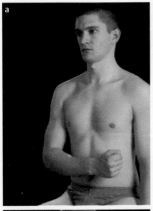

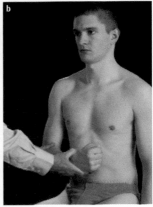

Figure 45 a,b,c. Active and resisted internal rotation of shoulder.

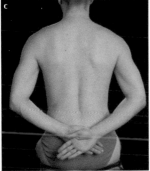

The shoulder joint allows flexion, extension, abduction, adduction, external and internal rotation, and circumduction. **Flexion** (figure 39a,b) is possible to 180 degrees when the arm is swung forward as in marching. This involves some scapular movement, the glenohumeral joint contributing about 90 degrees. **Extension** (figure 39c,d) of the shoulder is possible to 65 degrees, when the arm is swung backward.

Arm **abduction** takes place at both the glenohumeral joint and through scapular rotation. On its own, assessed by fixing the scapula, the former is to 90 degrees (figure 40a,b). When the movement of the scapula is included 180 degrees is possible; however, there is also external rotation of the shoulder joint for the greater tuberosity to clear the acromion. The scapular movement in abduction can be observed from behind,

Table 5 **SUPERFICIAL MUSCLES OF THE ANTERIOR (FLEXOR) COMPARTMENT OF THE FOREARM**

MUSCLE	PROXIMAL ATTACHMENT	DISTAL ATTACHMENT	FUNCTION	NERVE SUPPLY
Pronator teres	Flexor origin of the humerus: additional head forms from the coronoid process of the ulna	Distal lateral surface of the radius (forms the medial margin of the cubital fossa)	Pronation	Median (C6,7)
Flexor carpi radialis	Flexor origin of the humerus	Bases of the second and third metacarpals	Flexion and abduction of the wrist	Median (C6,7)
Palmaris longus	Flexor origin of the humerus	Palmar aponeurosis and the flexor retinaculum	Flexion of the wrist	Median (C6,7,8)
Flexor carpi ulnaris	Flexor origin of the humerus, medial olecranon and posterior border of the ulna	Pisiform, hamate, and base of the fifth metacarpal	Flexion and adduction of the wrist	Ulnar (C7,8)
Flexor digitorum super-ficialis (inter-mediate group)	Flexor origin of humerus, adjacent anterior surfaces of radius and ulna, and intermuscular septum	Sides of the shaft of the middle phalanges of the four fingers	Flexion of the wrist, meta-carpophalangeal and proximal interphalangeal joints	Median (C7,8,T1)

noting the position of the inferior angle, at rest, at 90 degrees, and at 180 degrees abduction (figure 41a–c).

The pectoralis major and latissimus dorsi muscles are powerful adductors from the abducted position, as in raising the body from an overhead bar, pulling objects toward you and in the follow through of a tennis serve. They can be tested and palpated by asking the subject to press their hands together (figure 42) or downward on their hips.

Table 6 **DEEP MUSCLES OF THE ANTERIOR (FLEXOR) COMPARTMENT OF THE FOREARM**

MUSCLE	PROXIMAL ATTACHMENT	DISTAL ATTACHMENT	FUNCTION	NERVE SUPPLY
Flexor pollicis longus	Anterior shaft of the radius and the adjacent interosseous membrane	Anterior aspect of the base of the distal phalanx of the thumb	Flexion of the joints of the thumb	Median (C8,T1)
Flexor digitorum profundus	Coronoid process, posterior border, and medial and anterior surfaces of the ulna, and interosseous membrane	Anterior aspect of the bases of the distal phalanges of the fingers	Flexion of the distal interphalangeal joints and, to a lesser extent, the wrist and other digital joints	Anterior interosseous branch of the median, and the ulnar (C8,T1)
Pronator quadratus	Lateral surface of the distal radius	Medial surface of the distal ulna	Pronation	Median (C8,T1)

Adduction (figure 43a,b) is possible to 50 degrees in a normal joint, when the elbow is carried forward across the front of the chest.

External rotation (figure 44a–c) is to 60 degrees. This is assessed with a flexed elbow, placing the hand behind the head. The movement, however, combines abduction with external rotation.

Internal rotation of the shoulder joint is stopped when the flexed forearm meets the trunk. However, resisted movement can be tested in this position (figure 45a,b); ask the subject to scratch the middle of their back, with the thumb as high as possible, to check the full rotation of 90 degrees (figure 45c).

Elbow

The details of forearm muscles are given in tables 5-8. The relation of the epicondyles to the olecranon is best seen posteriorly (figure 46a,b); the shape of the triangle joining these structures changes in height in extension and flexion.

Table 7 SUPERFICIAL MUSCLES OF THE LATERAL AND POSTERIOR (EXTENSOR) COMPARTMENT OF THE FOREARM

MUSCLE	PROXIMAL ATTACHMENT	DISTAL ATTACHMENT	FUNCTION	NERVE SUPPLY
Brachio-radialis	Upper two-thirds of the lateral supra-condylar ridge and lateral intermuscular septum of the humerus	Base of the styloid process of the radius (forms the lateral margin of the cubital fossa)	Flexion of the elbow (optimal action in the midprone position)	Radial (C5,6,7)
Extensor carpi radialis longus	Lower third of the supra-condylar ridge of the humerus	Base of the second metacarpal	Extension and abduction of the wrist	Radial (C6,7)
Extensor carpi radialis brevis	Common extensor origin on the lateral epicondyle of the humerus	Base of the third metacarpal	Extension and abduction of the wrist	Radial (C7,8)
Extensor digitorum	Common extensor origin on the lateral epicondyle of the humerus	Via the dorsal digital expan-sion to the posterior sur-faces of phalanges of the fingers	Extension of finger and wrist joints	Radial (C7,8)
Extensor digiti minimi	Common extensor origin on the lateral epicondyle of the humerus	Dorsal digital expansion of the little finger	Extension of the little finger	Radial (C7,8)
Extensor carpi ulnaris	Common extensor origin on the lateral epicondyle of the humerus	Base of the fifth metacarpal	Extension and adduction of the wrist	Radial (C7,8)
Anconeus	Posterior aspect of the lateral epicondyle of the humerus	Lateral side of the olecranon process of the ulna (develop-mentally part of the triceps)	Elbow extension	Radial (C7,8)

Table 8 **DEEP MUSCLES OF THE LATERAL AND POSTERIOR (EXTENSOR) COMPARTMENT OF THE FOREARM**

MUSCLE	PROXIMAL ATTACHMENT	DISTAL ATTACHMENT	FUNCTION	NERVE SUPPLY
Supinator	Deep and superficial heads, from the extensor origin on the lateral epicondyle of the humerus and the proximal posterior ulna	Anterolateral surface of the proximal third of the radius (the posterior interosseous nerve lies between the heads)	Supination	Radial (C5,6)
Abductor pollicis	Posterior proximal surfaces of the radius and ulna, and the interosseous membrane	Lateral aspect of the base of the first metacarpal	Abduction of the thumb and wrist	Radial (C7,8)
Extensor pollicis longus	Posterior shaft of the ulna and interosseous membrane	Base of the distal phalanx of the thumb	Extension of the thumb and abduction of the wrist	Radial (C7,8)
Extensor pollicis brevis	Distal shaft of the radius and interosseous membrane	Base of the proximal phalanx of the thumb	Extension of the thumb and abduction of the wrist	Radial (C7,8)
Extensor indicis	Posterior surface of the ulna and interosseous membrane	Dorsal digital expansion of the index finger	Extension of the index finger and wrist	Radial (C7,8)

A number of bony points in the elbow and superior radioulnar joints are palpable. These include the lateral and medial epicondyles, the supracondylar ridges, the olecranon and the head of the radius. The

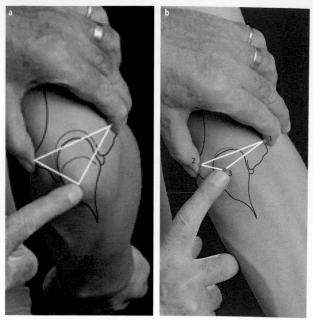

Figure 46 Relative position of olecranon to epicondyles in: a. elbow flexion and b. extension.
1. Lateral epicondyle
2. Medial epicondyle
3. Olecranon process

coronoid process can be palpated with deep pressure in the cubital fossa. The ulnar nerve can be palpated behind the medial epicondyle; the ulna has a palpable posterior subcutaneous border (figure 47a–e).

Figure 48a–c shows the normal lateral radiograph of the elbow, and the disruption that occurs in a dislocation or a comminuted fracture.

The common extensor origin, from the lateral epicondyle, is injected for the condition of tennis elbow (figure 49a) and the olecranon bursa over the proximal ulna (figure 49b). The elbow joint can be injected

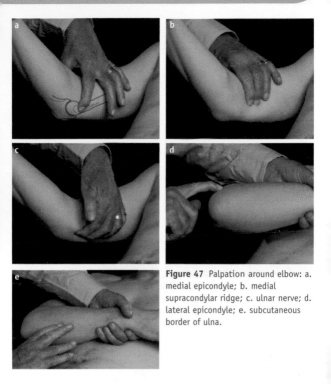

Figure 47 Palpation around elbow: a. medial epicondyle; b. medial supracondylar ridge; c. ulnar nerve; d. lateral epicondyle; e. subcutaneous border of ulna.

through a posterolateral approach, lateral to the tendon of triceps (figure 50).

The elbow is a hinge joint and the zero position is when the arm is fully extended (figure 51a,b); normal **flexion** is to approximately 150 degrees (figure 51c,d). Early synovitis may limit these movements.

Pronation (figure 52a,b) and **supination** (figure 52c,d) may be tested with the elbow flexed to 90 degrees; about 80 degrees of supination and 80 degrees of pronation are possible. Pronation and supination take place at both the superior and inferior radioulnar joints.

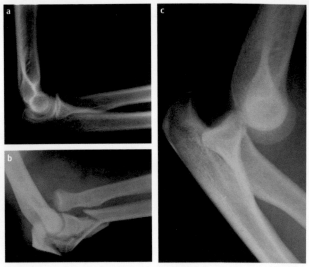

Figure 48 Lateral radiographs of elbow: a. normal; b. comminuted fracture; and c. dislocation.

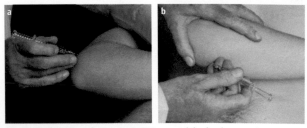

Figure 49 Injection of: a. common extensor origin; b. olecranon bursa.

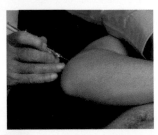

Figure 50 Injection of elbow joint, lateral to triceps tendon.

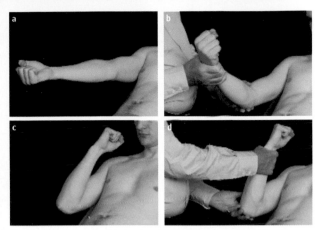

Figure 51 Active and resisted: a,b. extension and c,d. flexion of the elbow.

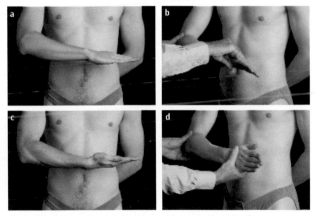

Figure 52 Active and resisted: a,b. pronation and c,d. supination.

Wrist and Hand

Wrist movements occur both at the wrist (radiocarpal) joint and the midcarpal joint. Flexion is predominantly at the midcarpal joint, and produced by the long digital flexor tendons, flexor carpi radialis, and flexor carpi ulnaris. Extension is predominantly at the radiocarpal joint;

Table 9 MUSCLES OF THE HAND

MUSCLE	PROXIMAL ATTACHMENT	DISTAL ATTACHMENT	FUNCTION	NERVE SUPPLY
Thenar: Abductor pollicis brevis	Tubercle of the scaphoid and the adjacent flexor retinaculum	Lateral aspect of the base of the proximal phalanx of the thumb	Abduction of the thumb	Median (C8,T1)
Flexor pollicis brevis	Ridge of the trapezium and the adjacent flexor retinaculum	Lateral aspect of the base of the proximal phalanx of the thumb	Flexion of the thumb	Median (C8,T1)
Opponens pollicis	Ridge of the trapezium and the adjacent flexor retinaculum	Whole length of the lateral surface of the first metacarpal	Opposition of the thumb to the fingers	Median (C8,T1)
Adductor pollicis	Oblique head: palmar surface of the capitate and the second and third metacarpals Transverse head: palmar surface of the third metacarpal	Medial aspect of the base of the proximal phalanx of the thumb	Adduction of the thumb	Ulnar (C8,T1)
Hypothenar: Abductor digiti minimi	Pisiform bone	Medial aspect of the base of the proximal phalanx of the little finger	Abduction of the little finger	Ulnar (C8,T1)
Flexor digiti minimi	Hook of the hamate and the adjacent flexor retinaculum	Medial aspect of the base of the proximal phalanx of the little finger	Flexion of the little finger	Ulnar (C8,T1)

Table 9 continued

MUSCLE	PROXIMAL ATTACHMENT	DISTAL ATTACHMENT	FUNCTION	NERVE SUPPLY
Opponens digiti minimi	Hook of the hamate and adjacent flexor retinaculum	Whole length of the medial surface of the fifth metacarpal	Opposition of the little finger, deepening the hollow of the palm	Ulnar (C8,T1)
Palmar and dorsal interossei: the four muscles of each group are numbered from the lateral side	Shafts of the metacarpals: palmar by single heads from the palmar surface of the first, second, fourth, and fifth; the larger dorsal by two heads from the adjacent sides of the meta-carpals	Sides of the base of the proximal phalanges and the dorsal digital expansions – the arrangement is linked to their function	Movements are around the axial line of the middle finger. Palmar adduct (PAD) and dorsal abduct (DAB) the fingers	Ulna (C8,T1)
Lumbricals: four slender muscles of the palm	Lateral side of the four tendons of the flexor digitorum profundus	Lateral aspect of the dorsal digital expansion of the same fingers	Acting with the interossei, flexion of the proximal, and extension of the middle and distal interphalangeal joints	Lateral two-median (C8,T1) Medial two-ulnar (C8,T1)

it is produced by the long digital extensors, combined with the radial and ulnar carpal extensors. Abduction occurs mainly at the midcarpal and adduction mainly at the radiocarpal joint; they are produced mainly by the flexor and extensor carpi ulnaris (adduction), and extensor carpi radialis longus and brevis, and flexor carpi radialis (abduction).

Normal **hand function** is dependent on the integrated activity of many muscles and joints, as well as intact sensory and motor function (page 348). The details of the small muscles of the hand are considered in table 9.

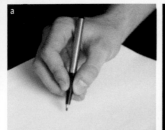
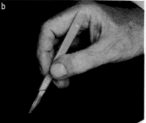
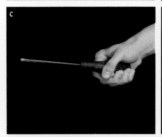
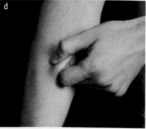
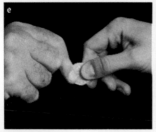
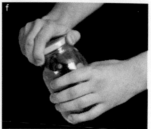
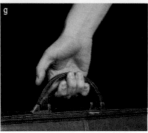

Figure 53 Hand movements: a. holding pen; b. holding scalpel; c. holding screwdriver; d.e. pinch-grips of flesh and coins; f. opening jamjars; g. carrying briefcase.

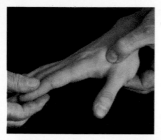

Figure 54 Assessing wasting of first dorsal interossei.

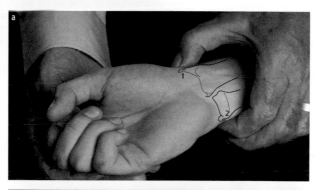

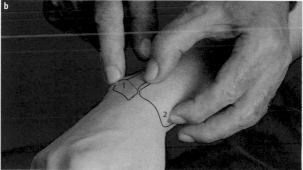

Figure 55 Relative position of radial styloid (lateral) and ulnar styloid (medial) in: a. supination: radial styloid approximately 1 cm distal to that of ulna; b. pronation: radial styloid medial and head of ulna lateral.

a
1. Radial styloid
2. Ulnar styloid

b
1. Head of ulna
2. Radial styloid

131

This activity is assessed throughout the examination in the patient's ability to unbutton and undress, and noting any difficulty or associated pain. Other practical measures to assess ability are: holding a pen, scalpel or screwdriver, the pinch-grip of flesh or coins, opening a jam jar or carrying a brief case (figure 53a–g).

Note any wasting, particularly of the first dorsal interosseus (figure 54), and the interossei deep to the extensor tendons.

In the anatomical position (with the palm facing forward in full supination – figure 55a), the radial and ulnar **styloid processes** can be palpated. The radial styloid is approximately 1 cm distal to that of the ulna. This is an important relationship, since fractures of the lower end of the radius are common, and **impaction** displaces the radial styloid proximally, so that the two styloid processes often end up at the same level.

In pronation (figure 55b), the radial styloid process is still palpable, but on the medial side of the wrist – it is the **head**, and not the styloid process, of the ulna that is now palpable on the lateral side. Injection into the wrist joint is from the dorsal surface, just medial to the dorsal tubercle, where the extensor pollicis longus turns laterally around it (figure 56).

Inspect the wrist for erythema, swelling, deformity, and muscle wasting. A boggy swelling may signify the presence of synovitis or an effusion. When abnormalities exist, **palpate** for tenderness and observe active movement, and examine resisted and then passive movement, of each joint. Palpate the dorsal surface of the wrist with both thumbs, supporting the joint underneath with your index fingers.

The anatomical **snuffbox** (figure 57) overlies the lateral aspect of the wrist joint, the scaphoid, trapezium and the base of the first metacarpal.

Figure 56 Injection of wrist joint.

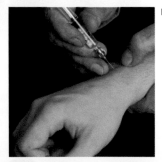

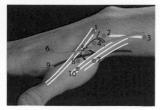

Figure 57 Anatomical snuffbox.
1. Extensor pollicis longus
2. Distal end of radius
3. Radial nerve
4. Scaphoid
5. Trapezium
6. Cephalic vein
7. Abductor pollicis longus
8. Base of first metacarpal
9. Radial artery
10. Extensor pollicis brevis

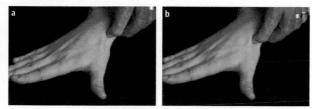

Figure 58 Pressure applied to: a. wrist joint and b. scaphoid.

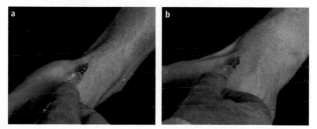

Figure 59 a. Injection of abductor pollicis longus and extensor pollicis brevis, and b. extensor pollicis longus, over anterior and posterior snuffbox.

Fractures of the scaphoid can be easily missed and an important physical sign is persistent tenderness over the bone at this site.

Examine the lateral aspect of the wrist joint (figure 58a), palpate and apply **pressure** to the scaphoid (figure 58b) to search for tenderness. This is a common site for synovitis of the tendons on either side of the snuffbox, after unusual activity (De Quervain's synovitis). The tendons may require injection: abductor pollicis longus and extensor pollicis brevis (figure 59a) and extensor pollicis longus (figure 59b).

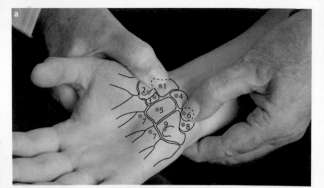

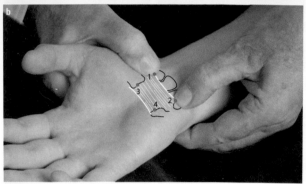

Figure 60 a,b. Bony attachments of flexor retinaculum.

a
1. Right thumb on tubercle of scaphoid
2. Ridge of trapezium
3. Trapezoid
4. Lunate
5. Capitate
6. Left thumb on pisiform
7. Bases of metacarpals
8. Triquetral
9. Hook of the hamate

b
1. Right thumb on tubercle of scaphoid
2. Left thumb on pisiform
3. Ridge of trapezium
4. Hook of the hamate

The **flexor retinaculum** is attached to four palpable bony structures at the wrist (figure 60a,b). It is only the size of a postage stamp, but has important clinical implications, as the median nerve passes beneath it and can be compressed, particularly after injury or with arthritic changes of the wrist or carpal bones. The proximal bony attachments are the tubercle of the scaphoid and the pisiform bone, and the distal ridge of the trapezium and the hook of the hamate. Palpation at these sites also identifies other abnormalities of the carpal bones: dorsal pressure may locate tenderness, in particular note tenderness or deformity of the lunate bone; it is subject to dislocation.

Apply pressure over the palm of the hand where the median nerve passes from under the flexor retinaculum (figure 61a). Injection of the nerve and the carpal tunnel may be proximal or distal to the retinaculum (figure 61b,c). Further distally in the palm, there may be thickening of a **Dupuyteren's contracture** (page 11) or the palpable nodule and clicking of a **trigger finger**. The latter may respond to injection (figure 61d), but often requires surgical incision of the tendon sheath.

Side to side pressure across the metacarpal heads or anteroposterior over individual joints (figure 62a,b) may elicit tenderness and can be early signs of inflammatory disease.

The interphalangeal joints are very superficial and pressure can be applied across them to detect tenderness (figure 62c,d).

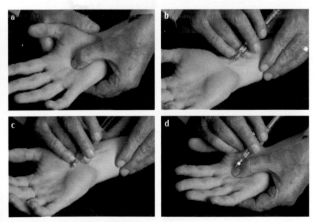

Figure 61 a. Pressure over flexor retinaculum; b. injection proximal and c. distal to flexor retinaculum, and d. into trigger finger.

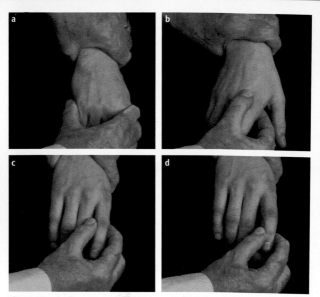

Figure 62 a,b. Pressure applied to metacarpal heads and c,d. interphalangeal joints.

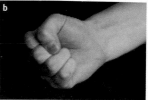

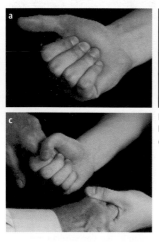

Figure 63 Position of fingers in: a. loose and b. tight grip, and assessing c. power grip.

Gently passively flex and extend the patient's fingers while palpating the flexor tendons to detect crepitus or restriction of movement from tenosynovitis.

When assessing the **grip**, note that the flattened fingers angle toward the line of the middle finger (figure 63a). When making a fist, the hand is more compact, functional and angular (figure 63b).

When assessing the power of the grip, compare the two sides; give the patient two fingers to grip in each hand (figure 63c – three fingers could end up with a personal crush injury!).

Examine **wrist flexion** by asking the patient to approximate the dorsum of their hands together and to flex the wrists, it is approximately 90 degrees (figure 64a–c).

Extension of the wrist joint is from 85–90 degrees; ask the patient to put their palms together in the praying position, and then extend the wrists (figure 64d–f).

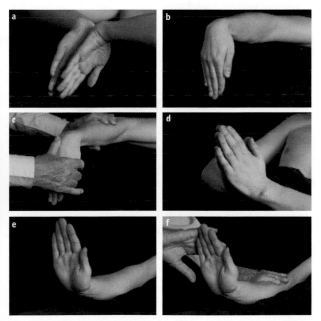

Figure 64 Active and resisted wrist: a,b,c. flexion, and d,e,f. extension.

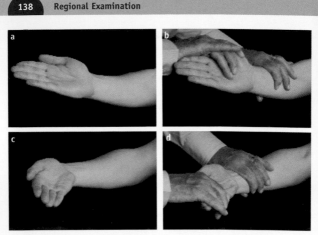

Figure 65 Active and resisted: a,b. radial and c,d. ulnar deviation.

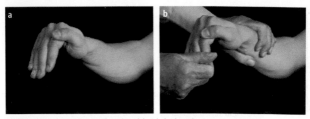

Figure 66 a,b. Active and resisted lumbrical action.

Radial and ulnar **deviation** at the wrist are about 20–50 degrees and 90 degrees respectively (figure 65a,b). Similar ranges should be achieved in active and passive movements.

The combined action of the long flexors and extensors, linked by the **lumbricals**, produces flexion at the metacarpophalangeal joints and extension at the interphalangeal joints. Assessing the power of this movement reflects lumbrical activity; they are supplied by both median and ulnar nerves, on the respective sides of the hand (figure 66a,b).

Flexion of the **metacarpophalangeal** joints, with the fingers straight, is to 90 degrees; flexion at the proximal **interphalangeal** joint is approximately 90 degrees but increases to 120 degrees when the distal interphalangeal joint is fully extended. Flexion of the distal

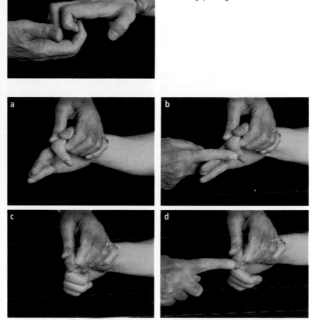

Figure 67 Assessment of finger flexion by pulling claw.

Figure 68 Active and resisted extension of: a,b. proximal and c,d. distal interphalangeal joints.

interphalangeal joint is approximately 80 degrees. Active flexion is assessed by asking the subject to make a fist; resisted flexion is by pulling on clawed fingers, either of the subject's two hands or against your own claw (figure 67).

Extension of the proximal and distal interphalangeal joints is to zero (figure 68a–d). There should be no hyperextension at the proximal interphalangeal joint, but often some laxity at the distal. The capacity to hyperextend should be noted, as hypermobility of the joints may indicate Marfan or Ehlers-Danlos syndromes.

Abduction of the **little finger** and **thumb** can be compared on the two sides by pressing the equivalent digits together, with a rigid outstretched hand (figure 69a,b).

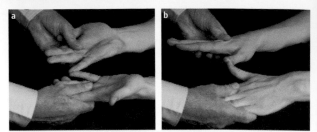

Figure 69 Assessment of abduction of a. little fingers and b. thumbs.

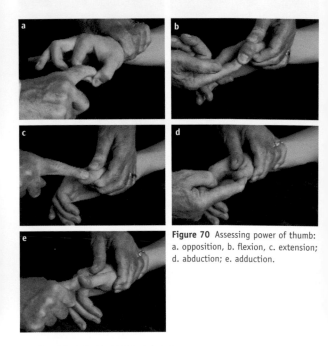

Figure 70 Assessing power of thumb: a. opposition, b. flexion, c. extension; d. abduction; e. adduction.

Assess the power of **opposition** of the thumb to the pulp of the fingers by trying to separate this contact (figure 70a). Figure 70b–e shows the examination of other thumb movements.

Gripping between the thumb and the side of the index finger is supported by the adductor pollicis muscle (the only thenar muscle to be supplied by the ulnar nerve). In ulnar nerve injury, weakness of this

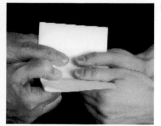

Figure 71 Froment's sign.

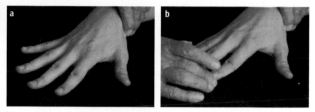

Figure 72 a,b. Active and resisted abduction of dorsal interossei.

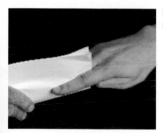

Figure 73 Resisted adduction of palmar interossei.

muscle is compensated for by flexion at the interphalangeal joint, as seen in the right thumb of the subject on the left in figure 71; this is known as **Froment's** sign.

The dorsal **interossei** abduct the fingers (DAB); assess their power by asking the patient to keep the fingers spread apart against resistance (figure 72a,b). The palmar interossei adduct (PAD); this is tested by gripping paper between adjacent fingers (figure 73).

LOWER LIMB

Hip Joint

Initial assessment of the hip joint is with the patient lying flat and straight on a couch, in the supine position, with a single head pillow and wearing briefs. The neutral position of the hip is in extension with the patella pointing forward. Although the muscles and bones around the joint limit the value of **inspection** and **palpation**, an abnormal posture of the limb may indicate pain, deformity, and altered mobility. Observe the symmetry of skin creases, and the contour of the thighs and buttocks in each part of the examination. The anterior surface marking of the joint is just inferior and posterior to the midinguinal point and pressure at this site may reveal joint tenderness.

The **greater trochanter** is palpable and is on, or just below, a line joining the anterior superior iliac spine with the **ischial tuberosity** (**Nelaton's line** on a lateral hip radiograph).

The relative position of the two hip joints can be roughly compared, by placing your thumbs on the anterior superior iliac spines and your middle fingers on the greater trochanters (figure 74 – other pelvic landmarks are considered with the spine – page 91). Figure 75a shows a normal anteroposterior radiograph of the pelvis and hip joints; note the shortening of the femoral neck associated with fracture of the neck of the femur in figure 75b.

With the subject lying on a couch, the intersection point of the line passing vertically backward through the anterior superior line and the horizontal line through the greater trochanter is approximately 4 cm from the trochanter in the adult. Reduction of this distance may indicate abnormalities of the neck of the femur. The triangle of this intersection point and the two bony markings make up **Bryant's triangle** (figure 76).

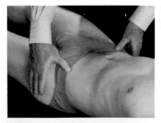

Figure 74 Relative positions of greater trochanters.

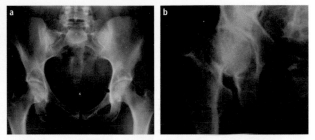

Figure 75 a. Anteroposterior radiograph of normal pelvis and hip joints; b. fractured neck of right femur, compare radiographs, note the shortened neck in fractured bone.

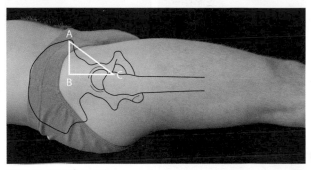

Figure 76 Bryant's triangle.
Bryant's triangle: with patient supine, perpendicular line AB from anterior superior iliac spine joins horizontal from greater trochanter – compare BC on two sides for shortening of femoral neck.

Abnormalities of the hip joint may alter leg length and there may be true and/or apparent **shortening**; the latter is due to abnormal tilting of the pelvis. First ask the patient to lie straight on the bed. True shortening is measured between the anterior superior iliac spine and the medial malleolus on each side (figure 77a,b), or an equivalent position on each leg, such as the medial femoral condyle or the patella. Apparent shortening is between the umbilicus or sternal angle and each medial malleolus (figure 77c,d).

When both knees are bent and the feet placed together on the couch, differences of leg length can also be demonstrated by differences in the position of the two knee joints, and whether the difference is above or below the knee (figure 78).

143

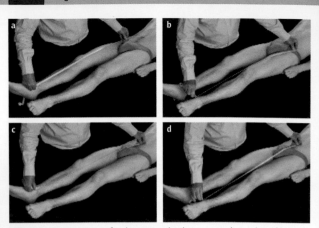

Figure 77 Measurement of: a,b. true, and c,d. apparent shortening of lower limb.

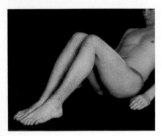

Figure 78 Assessment of relative lengths of above- and below-knee limb segments.

Examine for abnormal mobility of the hip joint by gripping the flexed thigh with both hands, and feeling the presence of any **telescopic** movement, when pulling and pushing along the length of the limb.

Movement
Tables 10-13 provide details of the muscles of the thigh and buttock, and figure 79a–d shows the bones and muscles of the region. Hip joint abnormalities can have a marked effect on **gait**. This can also be produced by musculoskeletal abnormalities elsewhere in the spine, pelvis and lower limbs, and painful soft tissue conditions. Interpretation is therefore dependent on a detailed general examination, directed by the patient's history.

Table 10 **MUSCLES OF THE GLUTEAL REGION (BUTTOCK)**

MUSCLE	PROXIMAL ATTACHMENT	DISTAL ATTACHMENT	FUNCTION	NERVE SUPPLY
Tensor fasciae latae	Anterolateral part of the iliac crest	Iliotibial tract (a broad thickening of the fascia lata, passing between the iliac crest and the upper end of the tibia)	Flexes and abducts the hip joint, and extends and stabilizes the knee joint through the iliotibial tract	Superior gluteal (L4,5)
Gluteus maximus	Postero-external surface of the ilium, sacrotuberous ligament and the sacrum	The majority of the fibers are attached to the iliotibial tract and some to the posterior upper femur	Extends and assists in lateral rotation of the hip, and raising the trunk from the stooping position	Inferior gluteal (L5,S1,2)
Gluteus medius	Gluteal surface of the ilium, deep to the gluteus maximus	Greater trochanter of the femur	Strong abductor and weak medial rotator of the hip joint	Superior gluteal (L5,S1)
Gluteus minimus	Gluteal surface of the ilium deep to the gluteus medius	Greater trochanter of the femur	Strong abductor and weak medial rotator of the hip joint	Superior gluteal (L5,S1)
Piriformis	Anterior surface of the sacrum	Greater trochanter of the femur	Lateral rotator of the hip joint	Sacral plexus (L5,S1,2)
Obturator internus	Inner surface of the obturator membrane and adjacent bone	Medial surface of the greater trochanter of the femur	Lateral rotation and abduction of the hip joint	Sacral plexus (L5,S1)

continued

Table 10 continued

MUSCLE	PROXIMAL ATTACHMENT	DISTAL ATTACHMENT	FUNCTION	NERVE SUPPLY
Quadratus femoris	Tuberosity of the ischium	Intertrochanteric crest and posterior femur	Stabilization of the hip joint, weak lateral rotator	Sacral plexus (L5,S1)
Obturator externus	Outer surface of the obturator membrane and adjacent bone	Greater trochanter of the femur	Stabilization of the hip joint, weak lateral rotator	Obturator (L3,4)

Table 11 **MUSCLES OF THE POSTERIOR (FLEXOR) COMPARTMENT OF THE THIGH**

MUSCLE	PROXIMAL ATTACHMENT	DISTAL ATTACHMENT	FUNCTION	NERVE SUPPLY
Biceps femoris	Two heads. Long: ischial tuberoisty Short: linea aspera and lateral supracondylar line of the femur	The two heads join to form a tendon that is attached to the head of the fibula	Extension of the hip, strong flexor of the knee and lateral rotation in the unlocked position	Sciatic (L5,S1,2)
Semitendinosus	Ischial tuberosity	Upper medial surface of the tibia	Extension of the hip, strong flexor of the knee and medial rotation in the unlocked position	Sciatic (L5,S1,2)
Semimembranosus	Ischial tuberosity	Posterior aspect of the medial tibial condyle	Extension of the hip, strong flexor of the knee and medial rotation in the unlocked position	Sciatic (L5,S1,2)

Table 12 **MUSCLES OF THE MEDIAL (ADDUCTOR) COMPARTMENT OF THE THIGH**

MUSCLE	PROXIMAL ATTACHMENT	DISTAL ATTACHMENT	FUNCTION	NERVE SUPPLY
Pectineus	Anterosuperior aspect of the pubis	Posteromedial femur below the lesser trochanter	Weak adduction and flexion of the hip	Femoral and obturator (L2,3)
Adductor longus	Anterior aspect of the body of the pubis	Linea aspera of the middle third of the femur	Adduction and weak medial rotation of the femur	Obturator (L2,3,4)
Adductor brevis	Body and inferior ramus of the pubis	Upper half of the linea aspera of the femur	Adduction and weak medial rotation of the femur	Obturator (L2,3,4
Adductor magnus	Ischiopubic ramus and the ischial tuberosity	Gluteal tuberosity, linea aspera, medial supracondylar line and the adductor tubercle of the femur	Powerful adduction, lateral rotation and extension of the femur; the adductors are active in posture and synergistic in gait	Obturator (L2,3,4)
Gracilis	Lower border of the ischiopubic ramus	Upper medial surface of the tibia	Weak adduction of the hip	Obturator (L2,3)

Note during your initial acquaintance with the patient the rhythm and timing of each step, and the pressure applied on each foot. Inadequate gluteal muscles and congenital dislocation of the hip joint produce waddling gaits. Other common neurological abnormalities are the shuffling gait of Parkinson's, spastic hemiplegia, the paralysis of lower motor neuron lesions, and the incoordination of cerebellar disease.

Compensatory movement of the pelvis can mask abnormalities of hip movement; various maneuvers are thus required to distinguish between the two components. Active and passive movements in each direction

Table 13 MUSCLES OF THE ANTERIOR (EXTENSOR) COMPARTMENT OF THE THIGH

MUSCLE	PROXIMAL ATTACHMENT	DISTAL ATTACHMENT	FUNCTION	NERVE SUPPLY
Sartorius	Anterior superior iliac spine	Upper medial surface of the tibia (the longest muscle in the body; *Say Grace before Tea)	Weak flexion and lateral rotation of the hip, and knee flexion (cross-legged position)	Femoral (L2,3)
Quadriceps: four heads: a. Rectus femoris	Two heads: Anterior inferior iliac spine Ilium, just above the acetabulum	As a single tendon to the upper border of the patella	Powerful extensor of the knee and flexor of the hip	Femoral (L2,3,4)
b. Vastus lateralis	Greater trochanter and the linea aspera of the femur	Base and lateral border of the patella	Powerful extensor of the knee	Femoral (L1,2,3)
c. Vastus intermedius	Anterior and lateral two-thirds of the shaft of the femur	Upper and lateral border of the patella	Powerful extensor of the knee	Femoral (L1,2,3)
d. Vastus medialis	Wide aponeurosis to the lesser trochanter, linea aspera and medial supracondylar line of the femur	Medial border of the patella: the patella is a sesamoid bone within the quadriceps tendon, this is extended as the patellar ligament to the tibial tubercle	Powerful extensor of the knee; its lower horizontal fibers prevent lateral dislocation of the patella	Femoral (L1,2,3)

*Sartorius attachment anterior to Gracilis that is anterior to semiTendinosus on upper tibia

are examined concurrently to avoid frequent repositioning the patient. The ipsilateral hand is used to hold the leg during passive movement while the other is used to feel for pelvic movement.

Hip **flexion** is limited by thigh contact with the trunk and is normally 90–100 degrees (figure 80a–d); it is increased when combined with knee flexion, due to relaxation of the hamstring muscles. Passive flexion also increases the range.

Some apparent hip flexion is due to flexion of the lumbar spine and pelvic tilting. This can be confirmed by placing your hand, palm downward, behind the lumbar curve during active and passive hip flexion.

Fixed flexion of the hip joint may limit flexion. The amount of this fixed flexion can be assessed by **Thomas' test** (figure 81). In this the normal hip is flexed until the lumbar curve is just flattened. This is determined by your left hand placed behind the lumbar spine. At this point, the number of degrees of elevation of the contralateral hip from the horizontal denotes the degree of fixed flexion.

Abduction and **adduction** (figure 82a–d) are tested after raising the heel clear of the contralateral leg. Monitor pelvic movement by placing your left hand on one, or across both, anterior superior iliac spines. The movements are 45 degrees abduction and 30 degrees adduction, from a plane at right angles to a line through the two anterior superior iliac spines.

Rotation can be assessed in both flexion and extension. In the former, the hip and knee are both flexed to 90 degrees and the foot moved medially (external rotation – figure 83a,b) and laterally (internal rotation – figure 83c,d), they are respectively 45 and 20 degrees. In extension, the subject lies prone and rotation is assessed with the knee flexed to 90 degrees.

Extension of the hip joint is 10–20 degrees and can be tested with the patient lying on the contralateral side, or lying prone and lifting the leg off the couch (figure 84a–d).

Examination of the hip is completed by observing the patient **standing**, **walking**, and **running** (figure 85a–c). The act of standing and the stance should be observed for discomfort and disability.

Overleaf
Figure 79 Lower limb anatomy: a. anterior, b. posterior and c,d. lateral thigh bones and muscles.

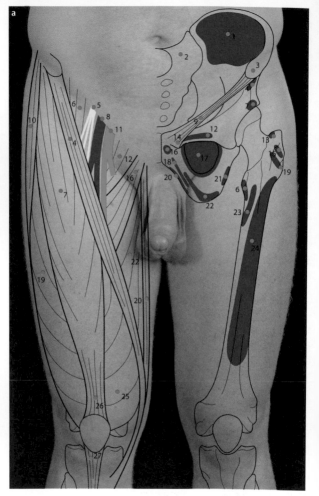

a

1. Iliacus
2. Lateral part (ala) of sacrum
3. Anterior superior iliac spine
4. Sartorius
5. Femoral nerve
6. Iliopsoas
7. Straight head of rectus femoris
8. Femoral artery
9. Inguinal ligament
10. Tensor fasciae latae
11. Femoral vein
12. Pectineus
13. Piriformis
14. Pubic tubercle
15. Gluteus minimus
16. Adductor longus
17. Obturator externus
18. Adductor brevis
19. Vastus lateralis
20. Gracilis
21. Quadratus femoris
22. Adductor magnus
24. Vastus intermedius
25. Vastus medialis
26. Quadriceps tendon
27. Patellar tendon

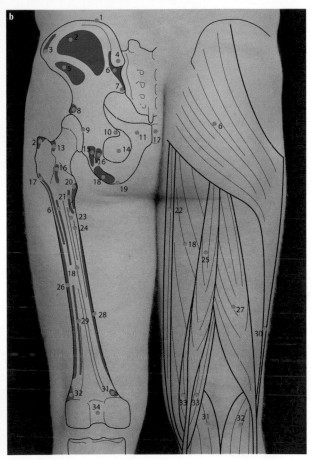

1. Iliac crest
2. Gluteus medius
3. Tensor fasciae latae
4. Posterior superior iliac spine
5. Gluteus minimus
6. Gluteus maximus; sacrum and ilium to gluteal tuberosity on femur
7. Posterior inferior iliac spine
8. Rectus femoris, oblique head
9. Acetabular rim
10. Spine of ischium
11. Body of pubis – posterior aspect
12. Symphysis pubis
13. Obturator externus
14. Obturator foramen
15,16. Hamstrings
17. Vastus lateralis
18. Adductor magnus
19. Ischial tuberosity
20. Iliopsoas
21. Pectineus
22. Gracilis
23. Adductor brevis
24. Adductor longus
25. Semitendinosus
26. Vastus intermedialis
27. Biceps
28. Vastus medialis
29. Short head of biceps
30. Iliotibial tract
31. Gastrocnemius, medial head
32. Gastrocnemius, lateral head
33. Semimembranosus
34. Intercondylar notch

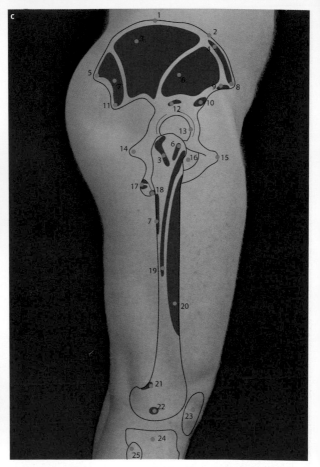

1. Iliac crest
2. Tubercle - palpable projection: intertubercular line, an abdominal marker
3. Gluteus medius: outer ilium to greater trochanter
4. Tensor fasciae latae
5. Posterior superior iliac spine
6. Gluteus minimus
7. Gluteus maximus: from posterior ilium and

    sacrum, to tuberosity on femur
8. Anterior superior iliac spine
9. Sartorius
10. Straight and 12. oblique heads of rectus femoris
11. Posterior inferior iliac spine
13. Head of femur
14. Spine of ischium
15. Symphysis pubis
16. Obturator foramen

17. Hamstring muscles from ischial tuberosity
18. Adductor magnus from ischial tuberosity
19. Vastus lateralis
20. Vastus intermedius
21. Lateral head of gastrocnemius
22. Popliteus: to lateral aspect lateral femoral condyle
23. Patella
24. Lateral tibial condyle
25. Head of fibula

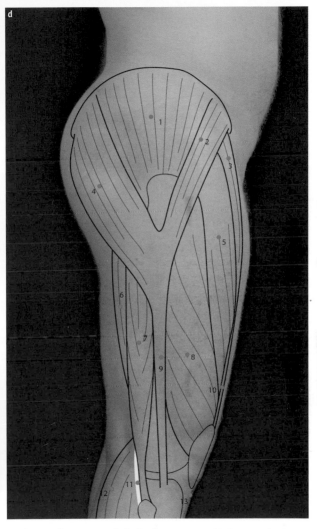

1. Gluteus medius
2. Tensor fasciae latae
3. Sartorius
4. Gluteus maximus
5. Rectus femoris

6. Semitendinosus
7. Biceps femoris
8. Vastus lateralis
9. Iliotibial tract
10. Quadriceps tendon

11. Common peroneal nerve
12. Lateral head of
    gastrocnemius
13. Patellar tendon

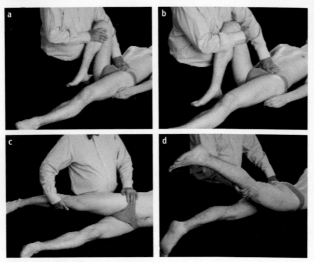

Figure 80 a.b.c.d. Active and resisted hip flexion.

Figure 81 Thomas' test

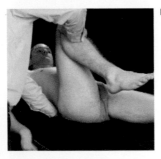

When standing on one leg (figure 86) the opposite side of the pelvis is raised by abduction of the hip joint on the weight-bearing leg. This can be confirmed when standing behind the patient, comparing the buttock creases and palpating the two anterior superior iliac spines. In some hip joint abnormalities, abduction is lost and, on standing on one leg, the opposite side of the pelvis drops. This is known as a positive **Trendelenburg sign**.

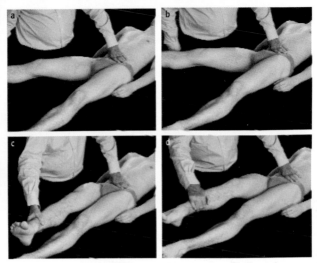

Figure 82 Active and resisted hip: a,b. abduction and c,d. adduction.

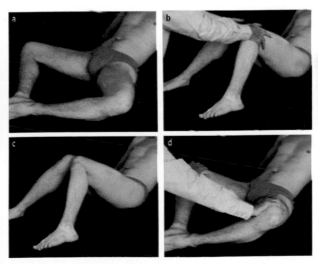

Figure 83 Active and resisted: a,b. external rotation, and c,d. internal rotation of hip.

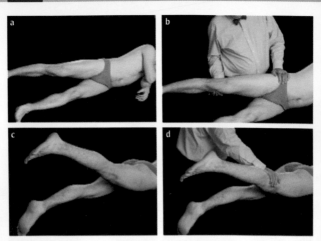

Figure 84 a,b,c,d. Active and resisted hip extension.

Knee Joint

Tables 14-17 provide details of the muscles of the lower leg, and figure 87a–h illustrates the bones and muscles. Figure 88a,b shows anteroposterior and lateral radiographs of the normal knee and figure 88c,d shows the details that can be obtained of bone and soft tissue with MRI images; they are particularly valuable in identifying abnormalities of the menisci and cruciate ligaments.

The neutral position of the knee is in extension and a painful knee is often held in a few degrees of flexion. **Compare** the two sides. Note skin changes, swellings, deformity, and other changes of contour (figure 89a,b). Pre- and infrapatellar bursae, popliteal cysts, and cartilaginous protrusions along the joint line are common pathologies. Quadriceps **wasting** is most easily seen by hollows on either side of, and just above, the patella (particularly medially, due to loss of bulk of the lower fibers of the vastus medialis muscle). General or local muscle wasting is assessed by **measurement** of leg circumference and comparing with the opposite side (page 349).

Palpate the circumference of the patella, the femoral and tibial condyles and the joint margins. Look for warmth, tenderness, and synovial thickening, the latter particularly on either side of the patella, and note any of the lumps mentioned in the previous paragraph.

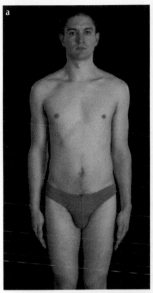

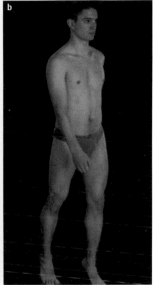

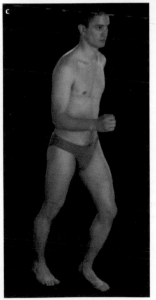

Figure 85 a,b,c. Observing lower limb on standing, walking and running.

157

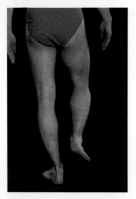

Figure 86 Trendelenburg test – normal tilting of pelvis on raising leg off ground.

Table 14 **MUSCLES OF ANTERIOR (EXTENSOR) COMPARTMENT OF THE LEG**

MUSCLE	PROXIMAL ATTACHMENT	DISTAL ATTACHMENT	FUNCTION	NERVE SUPPLY
Tibialis anterior	Lateral condyle and upper half of the lateral surface of the tibia	Medial aspect of the medial cuneiform and adjacent base of the first metatarsal	Dorsiflexion and inversion of foot	Deep peroneal (fibular) (L4,5)
Extensor hallucis longus	Middle of the medial surface of the fibula and adjacent interosseous membrane	Base of the distal phalanx of the hallux	Extension of the hallux and dorsiflexion of the ankle	Deep peroneal (fibular) (L5,S1)
Extensor digitorum longus	Lateral condyle and upper three-quarters of the anterior surface of the tibia and adjacent interosseous membrane	Middle and distal phalanges of the lateral four toes, through the dorsal digital expansions	Extension of the toes and dorsiflexion of the ankle	Deep peroneal (fibular) (L5,S1)
Peroneus (fibularis) tertius	Lower medial surface of the fibula and adjacent interosseous membrane	Dorsal surface of the base of the fifth metatarsal	Dorsiflexion of the ankle and weak eversion of the foot	Deep peroneal (fibular) (L5,S1)

Table 15 **MUSCLES OF THE LATERAL (PERONEAL/FIBULAR) COMPARTMENT OF THE LEG**

MUSCLE	PROXIMAL ATTACHMENT	DISTAL ATTACHMENT	FUNCTION	NERVE SUPPLY
Peroneus (fibularis) longus	Head and upper two-thirds of the lateral surface of the fibula	Base of the third, fourth and fifth metatarsals	Eversion of the foot and weak plantar flexion of the ankle	Peroneal (fibular) (L5,S,1,2)
Peroneus (fibularis) brevis	Lower two-thirds of the lateral surface of the fibula	Lateral aspect of the base of the fifth metatarsal	Eversion of the foot and weak plantar flexion of the ankle	Peroneal (fibular) (L5,S1,2)

Table 16 **SUPERFICIAL MUSCLES OF THE POSTERIOR (FLEXOR) COMPARTMENT OF THE LEG**

MUSCLE	PROXIMAL ATTACHMENT	DISTAL ATTACHMENT	FUNCTION	NERVE SUPPLY
Gastroc-nemius	Two heads. Lateral: lateral condyle and lateral supra-condylar line of the femur Medial: just above and on the medial condyle of the femur	Middle of the posterior surface of the calcaneus by the tendo-calcaneus (Achilles – the thickest and strongest tendon in the body)	Flexion of the knee and plantar flexion of the ankle	Tibial (S1,2)
Soleus	Head and upper quarter of the fibula, soleal line and upper third of the tibia and a fibrous band between (arching over the popliteal vessels and tibial nerve)	Tendo-calcaneus (Achilles)	Plantar flexion of the ankle	Tibial (S1,2)
Plantaris	Lateral supra-condylar line of the femur	Tendo-calcaneus (Achilles)	Weak accessory to gastrocnemius	Tibial (S1,2)

Table 17 **DEEP MUSCLES OF THE POSTERIOR (FLEXOR) COMPARTMENT OF THE LEG**

MUSCLE	PROXIMAL ATTACHMENT	DISTAL ATTACHMENT	FUNCTION	NERVE SUPPLY
Popliteus	Lateral aspect of the lateral condyle of the femur and the lateral meniscus	Posterior surface of tibia above the soleal line	Weak flexion of the knee, and unlocking by rotation and retraction of the lateral meniscus	Tibial (L4,5,S1)
Flexor hallucis longus	Lower two-thirds of the posterior surface of the fibula	Base of the distal phalanx of the hallux	Flexion of the hallux, plantar flexion of the ankle, support to the medial longitudinal arch	Tibial (S2,3)
Tibialis posterior	Upper half of the interosseous membrane and the adjacent tibia and fibula	Tuberosity of the navicular, the medial cuneiform and a variable number of metatarsals	Plantar flexion of the ankle and inversion of the foot	Tibial (L4,5)
Flexor digitorum longus	Posterior surface of the tibia below the soleal line	Base of the distal phalanges of the lateral four toes	Flexion of the lateral four toes, plantar flexion of the ankle and support to the longitudinal arches of the foot	Tibial (S2,3)

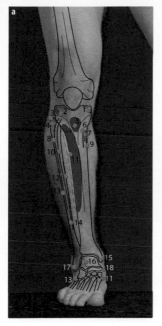

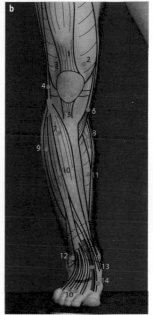

Figure 87

a. Bones and b. muscle of right lower leg: anterior.

a.
1. Semimembranosus
2. Iliotibial tract
3. Lateral collateral ligament, passing to head of fibula
4. Biceps tendon: attached around collateral ligament
5. Patellar tendon
6. Sartorius
7. Gracilis
8. Peroneus longus
9. Semitendinosus
10. Extensor digitorum longus
11. Tibialis anterior: to medial cuneiform and first metatarsal
13. Peroneus brevis: to styloid process of fifth metatarsal
14. Peroneus tertius
15. Medial malleolus
16. Talus
17. Lateral malleolus
18. Tibialis posterior

b.
1. Quadriceps tendon
2. Vastus medialis
3. Vastus lateralis
4. Iliotibial tract
5. Patellar tendon
6. Sartorius
7. Tibialis anterior
8. Gastrocnemius
9. Peroneus longus
10. Extensor digitorum longus: passing to distal phalanx
11. Soleus
12. Perforating peroneal artery: palpate on lateral maleolus
13. Dorsalis pedis artery: palpated lateral to flexor hallucis tendon, on metatarsal
14. Extensor hallucis longus

161

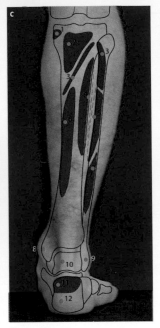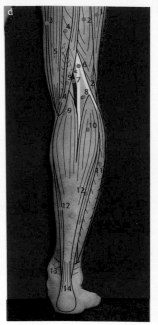

Figure 87

c. Bones and d. muscles of right lower leg: posterior.

c.
1. Semimembranosus
2. Popliteus
3. Soleus
4. Tibialis posterior
5. Flexor hallucis longus
6. Flexor digitorum longus
7. Peroneus brevis
8. Medial malleolus
9. Lateral malleolus
10. Talus
11. Tendo Achilles (tendocalcaneus)
12. Calcaneus

d.
1. Vastus lateralis
2. Biceps
3. Gracilis
4. Semitendinosus
5. Semimembranosus: on either side of semitendinosus
6. Low division of sciatic nerve
7. Popliteal artery
8. Poplietal vein (divided)
9. Medial head of gastrocnemius
10. Lateral head of gastrocnemius
11. Peroneus longus and brevis
12. Soleus; bulging on either side of gastrocnemius
13. Extensor retinaculum
14. Tendo Achilles (tendocalcaneus)

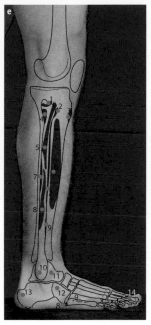
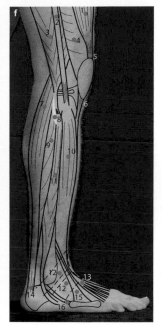

Figure 87

e. Bones and f. muscle of right lower leg: lateral.

e.
1. Biceps
2. Extensor digitorum longus
3. Patellar tendon
4. Soleus
5. Peroneus longus
6. Tibialis anterior
7. Flexor hallucis longus
8. Peroneus brevis
9. Peroneus tertius
10. Lateral malleolus
11. Talus
12. Cuboid
13. Calcaneus
14. Extensor hallucis longus

f.
1. Rectus femoris
2. Iliotibial tract
3. Biceps femoris
4. Vastus lateralis
5. Quadriceps tendon
6. Patellar tendon
7. Gastrocnemius, lateral head
8. Common peroneal nerve
9. Soleus
10. Muscles of anterior compartment
11. Peroneus longus
12. Dotted lines: upper and lower extensor retinaculi
13. Extensor digitorum longus tendons
14. Tendo Achilles (tendocalcaneus)
15. Expanded tendon of peroneus tertius
16. Peroneus brevis

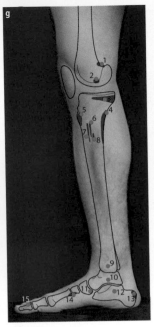 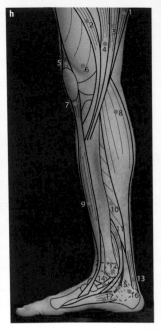

Figure 87

g. Bones and h. muscle of right lower leg: medial.

g.
1. Gastrocnemius
2. Femoral attachment of medial collateral ligament
3. Semimembranosus
4. Popliteus
5. Patellar tendon
6. Gracilis
7. Sartorius
8. Semitendinosus
9. Medial malleolus
10. Talus
11. Tibialis posterior: to navicular tuberosity
12. Calcaneus
13. Tendo Achilles (tendocalcaneus)
14. Tibialis anterior: to medial cuneiform and first metatarsal
15. Extensor hallucis longus

h.
1. Semimembranosus
2. Sartorius
3. Semitendinosus
4. Gracilis
5. Quadriceps tendon
6. Vastus medialis
7. Patellar tendon
8. Medial head of gastrocnemius
9. Tibialis anterior
10. Soleus
11. Flexor digitorum longus
12. Medial malleolus
13. Tendo Achilles (tendocalcaneus)
14. Tibialis posterior
15. Posterior tibial artery
16. Flexor retinaculum: passing from the calcaneus
17. Abductor hallucis

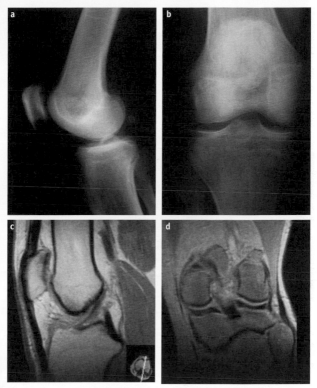

Figure 88 a,b. Anteroposterior and lateral radiographs of normal knee; c,d. coronal and sagittal MRI of normal knee, note the sections of cruciate ligaments and menisci demonstrable with this technique.

Tears of the medial or lateral ligament produce tenderness at their proximal and distal attachments to the femoral and tibial condyles, and the upper end of the fibula (figure 90a,b). Cartilage (**meniscal**) tenderness is along the joint line (figure 91a–d).

Injection and aspiration of the joint is through an anterior approach, and the needle is placed behind the patella. However, this may be achieved from a number of directions: from above (figure 92a); laterally (figure 92b); medially (figure 92c); or inferiorly, on the lateral or medial side of the patellar tendon (figure 92d,e). Injection may also be undertaken of the prepatellar bursa (figure 93a), and the infrapatellar bursa (figure 93b) and tibial tendon sheath.

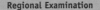

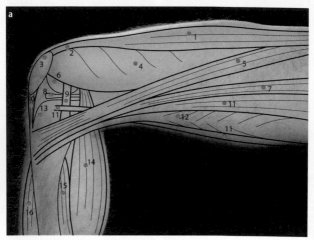

Figure 89
a. Surface anatomy of medial aspect of right knee.

1. Rectus femoris
2. Quadriceps tendon
3. Patella
4. Vastus medialis
5. Sartorius
6. Medial condyle of femur
7. Gracilis
8. Medial meniscus
9. Medial collateral ligament
10. Patellar tendon
11. Semimembranosus: deep to and on either side of 12
12. Semitendinosus
13. Medial condyle of tibia
14. Gastrocnemius
15. Soleus
16. Muscles of anterior compartment of leg

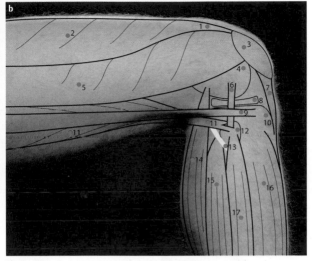

Figure 89
b. Surface anatomy of lateral aspect of right knee.

1. Quadriceps tendon
2. Rectus femoris
3. Patella
4. Lateral femoral condyle
5. Vastus lateralis
6. Lateral collateral ligament
7. Patellar tendon
8. Lateral meniscus
9. Iliotibial tract
10. Lateral tibial condyle
11. Biceps
12. Head of fibula
13. Common peroneal nerve
14. Gastrocnemius, lateral head
15. Soleus
16. Muscles of anterior compartment
17. Peroneus longus

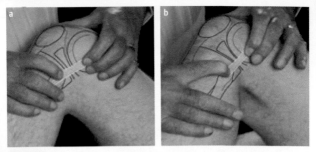

Figure 90
a. Medial aspect right knee: index fingers on medial collateral ligament (medial femoral to medial tibial condyle); b. lateral aspect: index fingers on lateral collateral ligament (lateral femoral condyle to head of fibula).

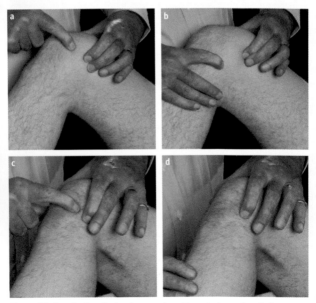

Figure 91 Examination for tenderness along the anterior and posterior aspects of: a,b. medial (right index finger) and b,c. lateral knee joint.

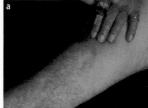
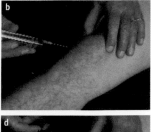
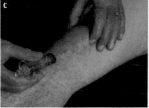
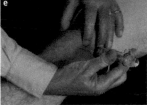
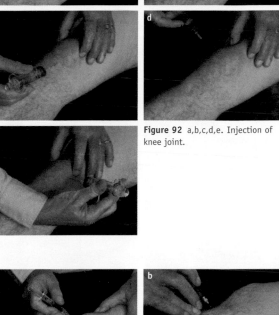

Figure 92 a,b,c,d,e. Injection of knee joint.

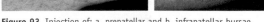

Figure 93 Injection of: a. prepatellar and b. infrapatellar bursae.

Tests for effusion

The classical test for fluid is the **patellar tap** (figure 94a,b). With your left hand, compress the lower thigh and slide the hand down toward the patella, pushing fluid out of the suprapatellar pouch. Maintain this hand in position above the patella and use your right hand to push the patella back onto the femoral condyle. If fluid is present, the patella is separated from the condyle and the pressure produces a bony tap as the patella hits the underlying femur.

If only a small amount of fluid is present, empty the medial side of the joint by gently sweeping the fluid upward into the suprapatellar pouch. Use one hand to press above the medial side of the patella to prevent backflow on this side, and, with the other hand, sweep down the lateral side of the patella (figure 94c,d). Small amounts of fluid pass back into

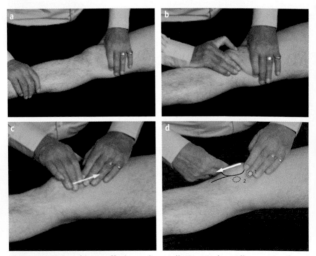

Figure 94 Tests of knee effusion: a,b. patellar tap; c,d. small amounts of fluid are swept into and retained in the suprapatellar pouch. Two hands used sequentially to compress fluid from medial compartment of knee to suprapatellar pouch – left hand used to retain fluid in this position by pressure on 1. tip of middle finger; right hand drawn down along lateral aspect of knee. Small quantities of fluid are compressed back into medial compartment, and produce a bulge 2. behind middle of patella

the medial side of the joint, producing a bulge behind the patella. If the joint is tensely swollen, pressure on one side behind the patella can be felt transmitted to the other.

Active knee **flexion** is 0–135 degrees; a few extra degrees can be obtained by passively compressing the calf against the thigh muscles (figure 95a,b). Up to 5 degrees of passive **extension** may be present (figure 95c,d). Look for hyperextension (figure 96); this may indicate ligament abnormality, as in injury or Marfan syndrome. Listen for clicks and creaks. Place your left hand on the patella to feel for **crepitus** during passive movements produced with your right hand (figure 97).

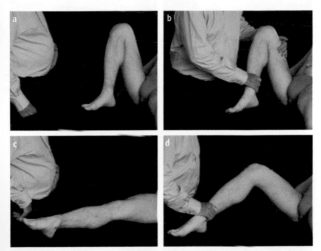

Figure 95 a,b. Active and resisted knee flexion and c,d. extension.

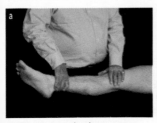

Figure 96 Assessing knee hyperextension.

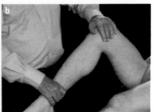

Figure 97 Palpating for patellofemoral crepitus.

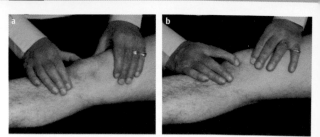

Figure 98 a,b. Testing for patellar mobility and crepitus.

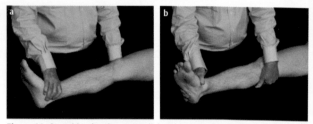

Figure 99 Stretching/testing: a. medial and b. lateral knee ligaments.

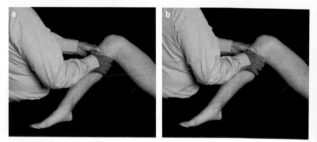

Figure 100 a,b. Drawer test of cruciate function.

This may also be detected by sliding the patella from side to side across the femoral condyles (figure 98a,b).

The **medial** ligament is tested for pain and laxity by placing your left fist on the lateral side of the extended knee. Grip the ankle with your right hand and attempt to abduct the tibia on the femur (figure 99a). The **lateral** ligament is tested similarly by placing your fist against the medial side of the joint and attempting adduction (figure 99b). In the normal knee, neither of these movements should be present and the test should be pain free.

Cruciate ligament function is assessed by the **drawer test**. Flex the knee to 90 degrees, with the foot resting on the couch. Sit on the forefoot and grip the upper end of the calf with both hands and pull forward and push backward (figure 100a,b). There should be no gliding movement. Anterior movement suggests laxity of the anterior cruciate ligament; the reverse, laxity of the posterior.

Loose bodies within the knee, and damage to the **menisci**, can cause locking of the joint. This can be assessed by sitting, squatting and standing movements, and by the **McMurray test**. In the latter, hold the ankle with your right hand and the flexed knee with your left. Use the right hand to rotate the foot, first in one direction and then the other. In each case use both hands to apply abduction across the knee and gradually extend the knee from the flexed position (figure101a–d). In the presence of an abnormal cartilage this maneuver may produce pain, a click or the protrusion of a lump along the joint margin.

Complete the examination of the knee by asking the patient to stand; look for valgus (knock knees) and varus (bow legs) deformities, and observe the gait.

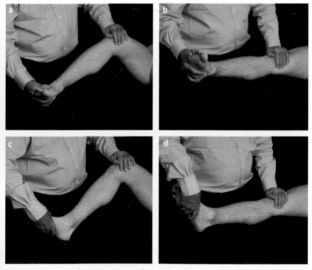

Figure 101 a,b,c,d. McMurray test for medial and lateral meniscal damage.

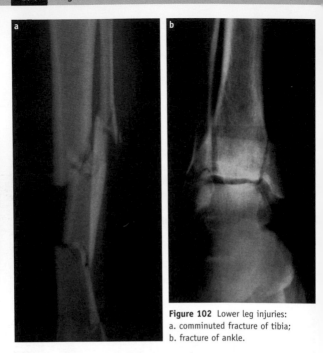

Figure 102 Lower leg injuries:
a. comminuted fracture of tibia;
b. fracture of ankle.

Ankle and Foot

The ankle and lower leg are common sites of injury in all walks of life; figure 102a,b shows fractures resulting from more severe forms of trauma. The natural position of the ankle is in slight plantar flexion and slight inversion. The lateral malleolus is a little more prominent and its tip is just distal to that of the medial; the joint line is 1 cm above the latter (figure 103). There may be color changes, scars, swelling, and deformity of all joints. Examine the sole for callosities. A small amount of fluid in the ankle joint presents as puffiness just in front of each malleolus. Larger amounts of fluid fill in the hollow on either side of the tendo Achilles (figure 104). Other common findings in the foot are: fixed lateral deviation of the main axis of the great toe (hallux valgus), clawing of the toes (fixed flexion deformities), and abnormalities of the transverse and longitudinal arches.

Palpate the medial (figure 105a–d) and lateral (figure 106a–d) malleoli and collateral ligaments of the ankle joint, for tenderness and swelling.

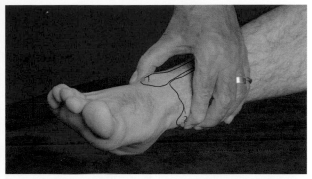

Figure 103 Relative positions of medial (index finger) and lateral (thumb) malleoli: lateral is approximately 1 cm distal.
1. Lateral malleolus
2. Medial malleolus

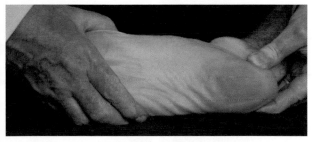

Figure 104 Examining for fluid anterior to tendo Achilles.

A transmitted pulse may be obtained between the two sides of the tendo Achilles if sufficient fluid is present. Any tender areas of the medial and lateral ligaments can be injected, and the tendon sheaths of: tibialis anterior (figure 107a); tibialis posterior (figure 107b); the peroneal tendons over the calcaneus (figure 107c); and the tendon of peroneus brevis, as it is attached to the styloid process of the fifth metatarsal (figure 107d). The ankle joint can be approached anteriorly, medial to the tendon of tibialis anterior (figure 108).

Dorsiflexion (figure 109a,b) and **plantar flexion** (figure 110a,b) occur primarily at the ankle joint. The former, raising the toes toward the knee, is to 20 degrees and the latter to 50 degrees. The ligaments of the

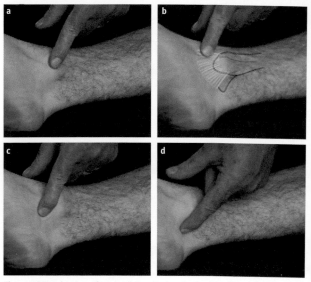

Figure 105 Palpation of: a. medial malleolus; b. the anterior, c. inferior and d. posterior parts of the deltoid ligament fan out onto navicular tuberosity, calcaneonavicular ligament, and sustentaculum tali; posterior fibers pass to the lateral aspect of the talus.

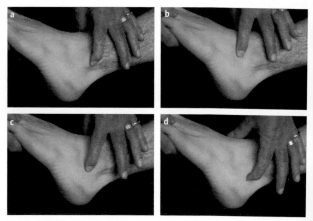

Figure 106 Palpation of: a. lateral malleolus; b. anterior, c. inferior and d. posterior aspect of the lateral ankle ligament.

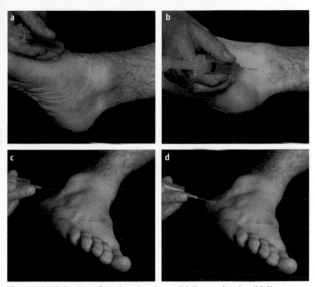

Figure 107 Injection of tendon sheath: a. tibialis anterior, b. tibialis posterior, c. peronei over calcaneus, d. peroneus brevis at attachment to styloid process.

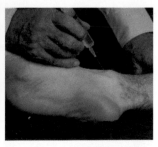

Figure 108 Injection of ankle joint, medial to tendon of tibialis anterior.

ankle joint are more lax in plantar flexion, when a few degrees of passive abduction and adduction can be obtained. Flex the knee to reduce the calf tension when assessing the degree of fixed flexion deformity of an ankle.

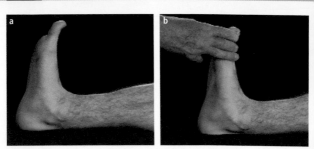

Figure 109 a,b. Active and resisted dorsiflexion of ankle.

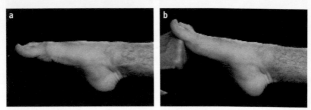

Figure 110 a,b. Active and resisted plantar flexion.

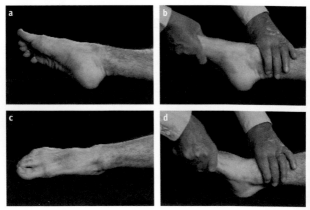

Figure 111 Active and passive: a,b. inversion and c,d. eversion of ankle.

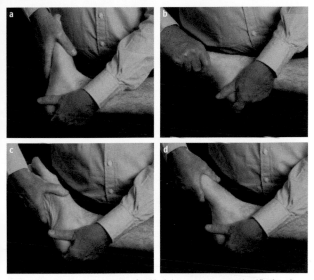

Figure 112 Passive assessment of ankle joint movement: a. dorsiflexion, b. plantar flexion, c. inversion, and d. eversion.

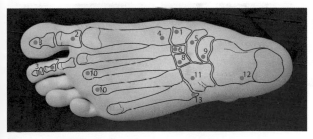

Figure 113 Anatomy of sole.

1. Medial cuneiform
2. Proximal phalanx
3. Distal phalanx
4. Base of first metatarsal
5. Navicular
6. Intermediate cuneiform
7. Middle phalanx

8. Lateral cuneiform
9. Head of talus
10. Head of metatarsal
11. Cuboid
12. Calcaneus
13. Styloid process of fifth metatarsal

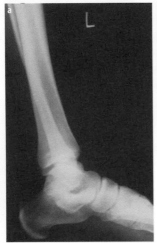

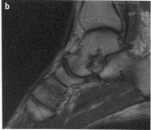

Figure 114 a. Lateral radiograph of foot; b. MRI of foot.

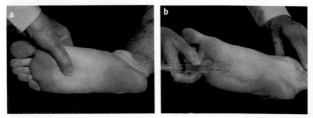

Figure 115 a,b. Palpation of and injection for deep tenderness of sole.

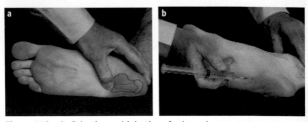

Figure 116 a,b. Palpation and injection of calcaneal spur; pressure over distal calcaneus causes pain and discomfort.

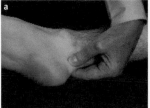

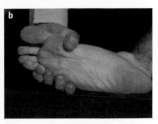

Figure 117 Pressure across: a. tendo Achilles, b. metatarsophalangeal and, c. interphalangeal joints.

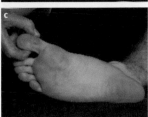

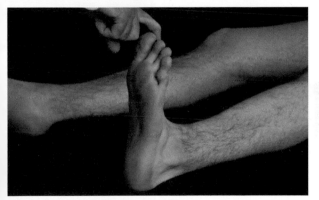

Figure 118 Resisted dorsiflexion of great toe.

Inversion (figure 111a,b) and **eversion** (figure 111c,d) take place mainly at the subtalar and talocalcaneonavicular joints. The calcaneum and navicular bones carry the front part of the foot.

In passive assessment, hold the ankle in your left hand and the forefoot in your right. Assess: dorsiflexion (figure 112a) and plantar flexion (figure 112b); inversion (figure 112c), when the sole turns inwards, is to 30 degrees and eversion (figure 112d) is to 5 degrees.

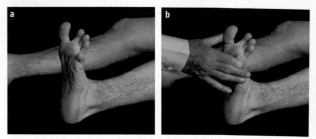

Figure 119 a,b. Active and resisted plantar flexion of metacarpophalangeal and interphalangeal joints.

Figure 120 a,b. Active and resisted toe abduction.

Figure 113 illustrates the bones of the sole of the foot; information obtained from clinical examination is supplemented by radiographs and MRI (figure 114a,b).

Palpation of the sole may identify deep tenderness, and this may be injected (figure 115a.b). Common complications are a calcaneal spur that may require injection (figure 116a,b), and injuries of the muscles, bones, and ligaments of the sole and heel.

Squeezing across the tendo Achilles, and the metatarsophalangeal and interphalangeal joints (figure 117a–c) may reveal tenderness, suggestive of injury or inflammatory disorders.

Dorsiflexion of the metacarpophalangeal joints is to 60 degrees (figure 118). Plantar flexion of the metacarpophalangeal and interphalangeal joints (figure 119a,b) is to 40 and 60 degrees respectively.

A variable small degree of fanning (abduction) of the toes is possible (figure 120a,b).

Thorax

The chest wall is formed from the **sternum** anteriorly, 12 pairs of **ribs**, costal cartilages and intercostal muscles laterally, and the **thoracic vertebrae** posteriorly. The palpable midline sternum is variable in size and shape; it is made up of the **manubrium** superiorly, the **body** and the **xiphisternum** (figure 1). The manubrium has an upper central

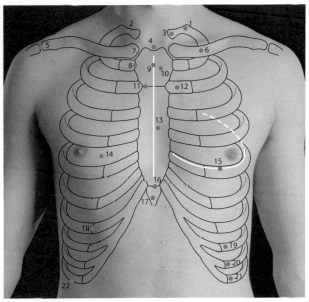

Figure 1 Surface anatomy of anterior chest wall.

1. Tubercle of first rib
2. Neck of first rib
3. Head of first rib
4. Suprasternal notch
5. Acromioclavicular joint
6. Clavicle
7. Sternoclavicular joint
8. Costosternal junction of first rib
9. Sternal split; approach to mediastinum
10. Manubrium
11. Manubriosternal joint
12. Second costal cartilage (an important landmark)
13. Body of sternum
14. Fourth interspace
15. Anterolateral thoracotomy incision
16. Xiphisternal joint
17. Xiphisternum
18. Seventh costal cartilage (lowest of true ribs)
19. 20. 21. Eighth, ninth and tenth (floating) ribs
22. Lower costal margin

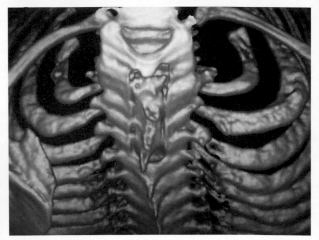

Figure 2 Spiral CT of thoracic inlet: three-dimensional picture viewed from above, showing cervical and upper thoracic vertebrae.

depression, the **suprasternal notch**. This has the attachments of the sternomastoid muscles and articulations of the medial ends of the clavicles on each side. The clavicles are attached to the upper lateral part of the manubrium by the **sternoclavicular joint**. This is a synovial joint, its bony surfaces are covered by fibrocartilage and it has a fibrocartilaginous disc. The first costal cartilage is attached to the manubrium just below this joint. The entry from the neck to the thorax (thoracic inlet – figure 2) is surrounded by the first thoracic vertebra, the first ribs and the manubrium.

The joint between the manubrium and body of the sternum (manubriosternal joint) is a symphysis and has slight mobility. The two bones are joined at a slight angle that protrudes anteriorly (**sternal angle**, angle of Louis). This is an important landmark, as the **second costal cartilage** is attached to it laterally, and from here the ribs can be easily seen and counted in thin subjects. This is more difficult in the female, on account of the breasts, and is also a problem with generalized obesity.

The **manubriosternal joint** is at the level of the lower border of the body of the fourth thoracic vertebra and the xiphisternal joint at the level of the ninth. The **xiphisternum** is of variable length and covered by the attachments of the rectus muscles. It is important to feel the xiphisternum of patients, and be aware of its variations, as not infrequently a patient needs reassurance that the xiphisternum they have just felt is not an abdominal tumor. The first seven ribs are attached directly by their costal cartilages to the sides of the sternum and are termed **true ribs**. The eighth to tenth (**false**) ribs are attached via their costal cartilages to the costal cartilage of the rib above. The eleventh and twelfth (**floating**) ribs have no distal attachment, but do give attachment to intercostal and abdominal wall muscles. In the male the nipples lie approximately in the fourth intercostal space and the liver rises to this level underneath the central dome on the right side of the diaphragm.

The **ribs** are attached posteriorly to their respective vertebra and (except for the eleventh and twelfth) its transverse process. The heads of the second to the ninth ribs also articulate with the intervertebral disc and the body of the vertebra above. The shape of these articulations contributes to respiratory expansion of the chest: the upper part of the chest expands primarily in an anteroposterior direction and the lower half from side to side; in the latter, the ribs moving in a "bucket handle" fashion. These different directions of rib movement are reflected in the shape of their articular surfaces.

Posteriorly, the thorax merges with the neck and lumbar regions (figure 3). The vertebra prominens (C7) and the spine of the first thoracic vertebra are easily palpable. The remaining thoracic spines lie subcutaneously, but the downward angled spines are less easily defined. The upper ribs are covered by the powerful muscles of the shoulder girdles. The scapulae overlie the second to the seventh ribs. The eleventh and twelfth ribs are usually palpable inferiorly; they overlie the kidneys. On the left side the tenth rib overlies the longitudinal axis of the spleen. With the arms abducted to 180 degrees, the lower medial border of the scapula approximates to the line of the oblique fissure of the lung on each side.

THE RESPIRATORY SYSTEM

Respiration is gas exchange at both a tissue level (through the blood-stream) and with the external environment (by the mechanical act of breathing). Diaphragmatic contraction, expanding the capacity of the thoracic cavity, is essential for **inspiration**. The upper ribs are fixed by the scalene muscles, and the intercostals and levator costae muscles approximate and elevate the ribs, further increasing the chest capacity (table 1).

By fixing the upper limbs, e.g., by gripping the head of the bed, the muscles of the neck and shoulder girdle can become accessory muscles of respiration.

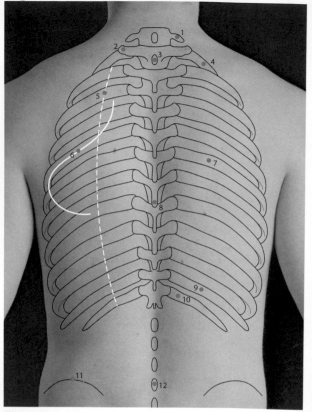

Figure 3 Surface anatomy of posterior chest wall.

1. Transverse process of seventh cervical vertebra (angled downward)
2. Transverse process of first thoracic vertebra (angled upward)
3. Spine of first thoracic vertebra
4. First rib
5. Line of angle of ribs; also lateral limit of erector spinae muscles
6. Posterolateral thoracotomy incision
8. Spinous process of seventh thoracic vertebra (angled downward for more than a vertebra in depth)
9.
10. Eleventh and twelfth (floating) ribs
11. Iliac crest
12. Spine of fourth lumbar vertebra (supracristal plane – through the two iliac crests)

Table 1 MUSCLES OF THE THORAX

MUSCLE	UPPER/OUTER ATTACHMENT	LOWER/CENTRAL ATTACHMENT	FUNCTION	NERVE SUPPLY
External intercostals	Pass between all adjacent rib borders, from the tubercle to the costal cartilage (space completed anteriorly by the anterior intercostal membrane)	Fibers pass obliquely downward: posterior-laterally, lateral-medially, anteriorly, anterior-medially	Together approximate the ribs, and prevent bulging or drawing in of the intercostal space during respiration	All three muscles supplied by the adjacent intercostal nerves
Internal intercostals	Pass obliquely downward from the subcostal groove, from the sternal edge to the angle of each rib (space completed posteriorly by the posterior intercostal membrane)	Upper edge of each rib, fibers pass at right angles to the external intercostals that lie outside them		
Transversus thoracis	Lower border of the second to sixth costal cartilages	Back of the sternum: body and xiphoid process	Draw down the rib cage	
Levator costarum	Tip of transverse processes, C7-T11, fibers pass downward and laterally to the rib below, with an extra slip to the second rib below in the lowest four muscles	Upper edge and outer surface, between the tubercle and the angle of each rib	Elevation of the ribs	Dorsal rami of adjacent thoracic nerves
Diaphragm	Peripherally: two slips from the back of the xiphoid process; the lower six ribs and costal cartilages that form the costal margin; the lateral and medial arcuate ligaments (over the quadratus lumborum and psoas muscles); the right crus (containing the esophageal opening) from the bodies of the first three and the left crus from the first two lumbar vertebrae; the two crura arch over the aortic opening	Centrally: forms a musculofibrous domed sheet between the thoracic and abdominal cavities. The thin, strong trifoliate-shaped central tendon lies beneath the pericardium and contains the inferior vena caval opening	The essential muscle of inspiration	Phrenic C3,4,5 Some peripheral sensation from the lower intercostal nerves

Expiration is by diaphragmatic relaxation, and recoil of the lungs and rib cage. It can be accentuated by contraction of the abdominal wall muscles, as in coughing and straining.

The **upper airway** is usually through the nose (page 27) and the naso- and oropharynx, into the larynx and trachea, but breathing may also be through an open mouth, particularly if the nose is blocked, and in deep breathing, as in severe exercise or in pulmonary disease. Mouth breathing is also required when you are listening to the chest, to allow the rapid intake of large breaths.

The **larynx** is a tube between the pharynx and the trachea. It protects the tracheal inlet in swallowing and contains the vocal cords for vocalization. It is surrounded by a number of cartilages; the lowest, the **cricoid**, is the only complete cartilaginous ring in the respiratory passage, adding stability and maintaining an open airway. The **thyroid** cartilage has two laminae that meet anteriorly in V-shaped fashion, the apex producing the prominent **Adam's apple** of the male (page 65). The **vocal folds** are attached behind the apex. The posterior end of each fold is attached to the muscular process of an **arytenoid** cartilage; the two arytenoids rest on either side of the posterosuperior border of the cricoid. Movement at the joints, between the arytenoid and cricoid cartilages, allows widening of the opening between the vocal folds (rima glottides), in either a V or a diamond shape, thus adjusting the airflow between them. The joints between the inferior horns, at the back of the thyroid laminae, and the cricoid cartilage allow adjustment of the length and tension in the vocal folds, altering the pitch of the emitted sound.

The **epiglottis** is also attached to the back of the V of the thyroid cartilage and extends upward. The laryngeal opening is closed during swallowing, by a combination of raising the larynx and pulling down the epiglottis towards it. This upward movement of the larynx can be observed by asking a subject to swallow (page 65), or watching your own larynx in a mirror; it is easier to see in the male because of the Adam's apple.

The **trachea** descends from the larynx through the lower neck into the thorax. It divides at the level of the manubriosternal joint into right and left **main bronchi**; these enter the hilum of each lung, together with a pulmonary artery, two pulmonary veins, and surrounding lymphatics.

In development, the **pleural cavity** on each side starts as an empty epithelial lined space, but the lung pushes into it from the medial side, like a fist into a balloon (letting out most of the air in the process!). The lining on the outside remains attached to the chest wall as the **parietal pleura**. The evaginated medial wall remains, separating the pleural cavity from the mediastinum, but the expanding lung takes with it a covering of **visceral pleura** that is continuous with the mediastinal pleura around the lung root (**hilum**). The cavity remains only as a potential space; the parietal and visceral pleura are in contact, a little fluid lubricating the surfaces to aid movement of the expanding and collapsing lung during respiration.

The **surface markings** of the parietal pleura can be remembered from what happens on the even-numbered ribs (figure 4). The apex of the lung domes upward within the circumference of the first rib, to about

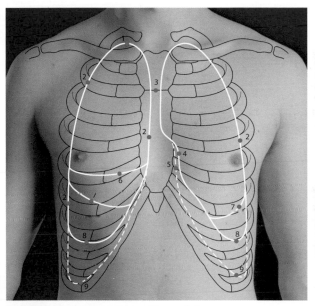

Figure 4 Anterior surface markings of lung and pleura.

1. Dome of pleura/apex of lung
2. Lung and pleural markings
3. Pleural layers coming together at manubriosternal joint
4. Cardiac notch of left lung
5. Costomediastinal pleural recess
6. Transverse fissure of right lung
7. Oblique fissure of lungs
8. Lower border of lungs
9. Lower limit of pleural cavities

2 cm above the level of the clavicle. From here the **pleura** on the two sides pass medially and they meet opposite the **second** costal cartilage. At the **fourth**, the pleura on the left is pushed laterally by the developing heart (**costomediastinal pleural recess**). At the level of the **sixth** costal cartilage, the pleura on both sides pass laterally crossing the midclavicular line at the **eighth** costal cartilage and reaching the midaxillary line at the **tenth**. Posteriorly (figure 5) the pleura follows the

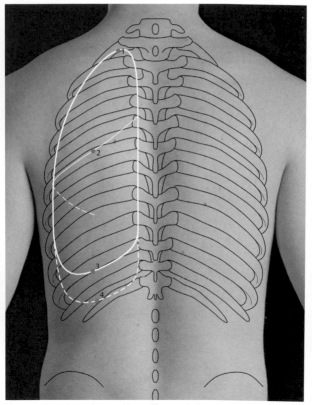

Figure 5 Posterior surface markings of lung and pleura.

1. Dome of pleura
2. Oblique fissure
3. Lower border of lung
4. Lower limit on pleural cavity

twelfth rib before ascending along the line of the transverse processes.

Inferiorly, the **diaphragm** bulges into the pleural cavity on each side, reaching, during expiration, the fourth interspace on the right and the fifth on the left. The outer gutter, between the diaphragm and ribs, is known as the **costodiaphragmatic recess**. Radiological examination is routinely used to screen for unsuspected, as well as suspected, disease (figure 6a,b).

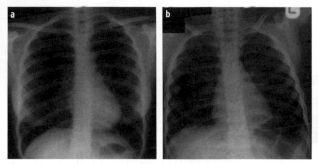

Figure 6 a. Normal adult and b. child chest radiographs.

Each **lung** has an **upper** and **lower lobe** divided by the **oblique fissure**, which follows the line of the sixth rib posteriorly, running obliquely downward and forward. On the right side, the **transverse fissure**, at the horizontal level of the fourth costal cartilages, produces a separate **middle lobe**. On the left, the ventricles bulge into the lung and the middle lobe is represented as the **lingula**, a part of the lower lobe.

The bronchial division follows that of the lobes, with further division into functional **bronchopulmonary segments**, each with its own major vessels. The upper lobes have three (apical, anterior, and posterior); the middle lobe, two (medial and lateral); the lingula, two (superior and inferior); and the lower lobe on the right, five (apical, anterior, posterior, median, and lateral). The left lung has no medial bronchopulmonary segment of the lower lobe, on account of the space taken by the heart. This lobe has a **cardiac notch** over the heart, corresponding to the costomediastinal recess of the pleural cavity.

The **surface markings** of the lungs follow those of the pleura, except inferiorly, where the base is approximately two rib spaces higher. Needles and drains can be introduced in the pleural cavity to inject or withdraw fluid, gasses, and drugs; a needle can be passed directly into

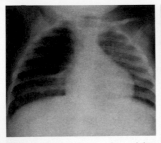

Figure 7 Pneumothorax – large right upper lobe congenital lung cyst has leaked, but not collapsed. Associated pneumothorax in lower lateral aspect of right pleural cavity has collapsed underlying lung.

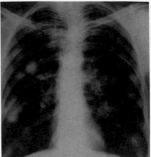

Figure 8 Pulmonary metastases: these "cannon ball" deposits are typical of renal carcinoma.

the pericardial cavity and heart, below the cardiac notch of the left lung, although in an emergency it is inserted at a lower level (page 233).

Abnormalities of the larynx, such as **inflammation** and **neoplasia**, may interfere with the airway and/or produce voice changes. Damage to the **recurrent laryngeal nerve** may be produced by cancers of the thyroid, cervical esophagus or the apex of the lung. The interior of the larynx may be observed by laryngoscopy or endoscopy.

Pulmonary diseases present with dyspnea, cough, cyanosis, chest pain, clubbing, and the signs of cardiac failure. Common chest diseases encountered are **asthma**, **chronic bronchitis**, **emphysema**, **pneumonia**, **pneumothorax** (figure 7) and **cancer of the bronchus**. The latter produces local respiratory problems and its **metastases** may also produce symptoms in the bone, brain, and liver. The lung is also a common site for metastases from other sites (figure 8).

Pulmonary infection may progress to a **pulmonary abscess** and, in the pleural cavity, to an **empyema**. Blocking of a bronchus may produce collapse of part or all of a lung (**atelectasis** – figure 9); this can occur postoperatively as well as with infection and malignancy. Chronic infection of the bronchi can lead to destruction of their lining and abscess formation of the wall (**bronchiectasis**). **Pulmonary embolus** (figure 10) is also a postoperative problem, following lower limb deep venous thrombosis.

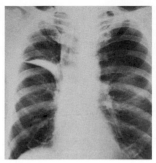

Figure 9 Atelectasis: collapse of right upper lobe has produced linear white shadow; lower lobe expanded to fill upper pleural cavity. Linear shadows are a common finding in segmental and lobar pulmonary collapse.

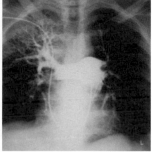

Figure 10 Left pulmonary artery embolus: from lower limb venous thrombosis, completely blocked upper lobe artery, with only a trickle passing to the left lower lobe.

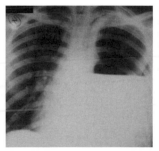

Figure 11 Pneumohemothorax: combination of fluid and air in pleural cavity produces the distinctive horizontal level. Fractured ribs, from trauma to lower left chest, are not visible.

Severe trauma may produce a palpable **sternal fracture**, but also consider associated myocardial contusion and spinal injury. Similarly, with **rib fractures**, look for a **pneumothorax**, **hemothorax** (figure 11) a **flail chest**, and damage to the liver and spleen.

NB Pulmonary disease may give rise to abdominal pain; abdominal disease may produce a pleural effusion; diaphragmatic pain may be referred to the tip of the shoulder (phrenic nerve C3,4,5); and remember, "pus somewhere, pus nowhere, pus under the diaphragm."

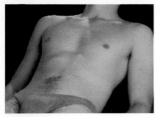

Figure 12 Exposure of anterior chest.

Examination

Inspection

The patient should be undressed to the waist – in the case of a female, explain the need to expose the front of the chest to examine the heart and lungs (figure 12). A patient may be lying semirecumbant, or seated with their feet hanging over the side of the bed. Initially stand back and observe the patient for evidence of **dyspnea** (difficulty with breathing), **tachypnea** (count the respiratory rate), and note the depth and regularity of respiration, the use of the accessory muscles of respiration, intercostal indrawing of the lower ribs, cyanosis, and evidence of cachexia. The jugular veins may be distended and empty rapidly with changes of intrathoracic pressure, and the larynx may move forcibly up and down.

Inspect the back (at this stage if sitting up or later when the posterior aspect of the chest is examined) for evidence of **scoliosis**, **kyphosis** and other deformities, such as **thoracotomy** scars and prominent veins. Deformities of the anterior chest wall include **pectus excavatum** (indrawn sternum) and **pectus carinatum** (pigeon chest).

Note the position of the nipples, and whether the thoracic cavity is expanded, such as in the barrel chest of **emphysema**. Measure the chest expansion from inspiration to expiration, using a tape measure (figure 13a,b).

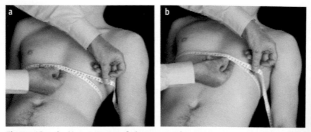

Figure 13 a,b. Measurement of chest expansion.

Several types of abnormal breathing patterns may be diagnosed at the bedside. In **Cheyne-Stokes** breathing, periods of **apnea** (cessation of breathing movements) alternate with periods of **hyperpnea** (deep inspirations). This is due to a delay in the medullary chemoreceptor response to blood gas changes, and can occur in left ventricular failure, brain damage, chronic hypoxemia, and at high altitudes.

In **Kussmaul** breathing (air hunger), there is deep, rapid breathing due to stimulation of the respiratory center. This typically occurs in diabetic ketoacidosis and lactic acidosis. **Ataxic** breathing (irregular in timing and depth) occurs in brainstem damage.

Listen carefully for abnormalities in breathing, such as noise, wheezing, and coughing. **Stridor** is a continuous rasping or croaking noise, caused by obstruction to the larynx; this is accentuated in inspiration. It may signify the presence of a foreign body, tumor or inflammatory process in the trachea.

Listen to the **voice**: hoarseness may signify recurrent laryngeal nerve palsy. Ask the patient to **cough**, to check whether there is a loose cough, a dry cough or a bovine cough. The latter occurs in recurrent laryngeal nerve palsy, when a vocal cord is paralyzed and the vocal cords cannot be approximated. Ask the patient to take a maximum inspiration and blow out as rapidly and as forcefully as possible. Listen carefully, as it may be possible to hear a wheeze and prolongation of the expiration phase, suggesting chronic airflow limitation.

Next, pick up the patient's **hands**, note **clubbing** and evidence of peripheral **cyanosis**, **nicotine staining**, and **anemia**. Causes of clubbing in the respiratory system include: chronic suppurative lung disease, bronchiectasis, lung abscess, empyema, bronchial carcinoma, and pleural and mediastinal tumors.

Wasting of the muscles of the hand may signify a first thoracic nerve lesion, such as caused by an apical lung tumor. It may be accompanied by damage to the cervical sympathetic chain, over the neck of the first rib, giving a **Horner's** syndrome; this combination of symptoms is termed a **Pancoast** syndrome.

The wrist should be palpated for tenderness (caused by the symmetrical periostitis of **hypertrophic pulmonary osteoarthropathy**) and the radial pulse for **pulsus paradoxus** (page 219). Look at the face, observing the pupils for evidence of a Horner's syndrome, anemia of the conjunctivae, and central cyanosis (tip of the tongue).

The **sputum** should be examined as a matter of routine. The volume and type should be noted (purulent, mucoid or mucopurulent). In infection, it varies from green to yellow and rusty colored, depending on the

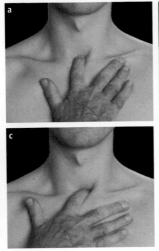

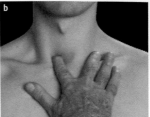

Figure 14 a,b,c. Determining position of trachea, palpating centrally and then to each side.

organism; a large purulent volume suggests bronchiectasis. Pink frothy sputum occurs in pulmonary edema and eosinophilic sputum in asthma. Evidence of **hemoptysis** (coughing blood) should be sought; it can occur in pulmonary embolism and pulmonary malignancy.

Palpation

Note the position of the trachea in the suprasternal region. Ask the patient to relax the sternomastoid muscles by dropping their chin, and to lean slightly forward. Rest your middle finger on the suprasternal notch and pass it on either side of the trachea as deeply and inferiorly as possibly (figure 14a,b). The latter is important because even gross tracheal deviation may be missed if the examining finger comes into contact with the trachea at too high a level. The trachea may be displaced by tumors in the neck or upper mediastinum, by a mediastinal shift due to a pneumothorax, a massive pleural effusion or a collapsed lung.

A **tracheal tug** (figure 15) indicates the presence of significant lung fibrosis or severe airflow obstruction. Rest your fingers on the trachea to feel it move inferiorly during inspiration.

Palpate the supraclavicular fossae for **lymphadenopathy** (figure 16). This can be undertaken from the front, but the pulps of the fingers can be inserted deep to the clavicle more easily from behind. Supraclavicular

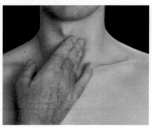

Figure 15 Examining for tracheal tug.

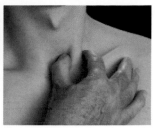

Figure 16 Palpating for scalene node behind lower attachment of left sternomastoid muscle.

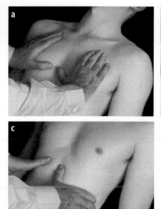

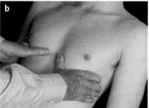

Figure 17 a,b,c. Examining for anterior chest expansion.

nodes of interest in pulmonary disease include the scalene lymph nodes that lie deep to the sternomastoid muscle insertion (page 267).

Anterior Chest

Expansion of the chest is tested with the palms of your hands resting symmetrically, first superiorly, then on the middle and finally on the lower chest wall, with the thumbs pointing toward the midline (figure 17a–c). This is to pick up possible asymmetry of expansion; this is highly suggestive of underlying pulmonary disease.

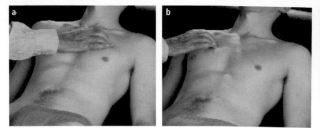

Figure 18 a,b. Coarse percussion of anterior upper chest.

Percussion

Coarse percussion, using three or four fingers to lightly tap on the chest, can compare the two sides, and pick up stony dullness, this is then precisely mapped by more careful percussion (figure 18).

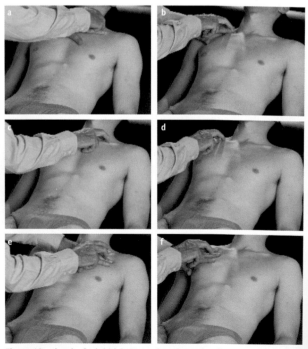

Figure 19 a,b,c,d,e,f,g,h,i,j,k,l. Percussion of anterior chest.

Percussion requires considerable practice, and the ability to percuss well is obvious to an observer; it usually denotes that you have spent a reasonable amount of time on the wards. Start percussion at the apex, bearing in mind that there is 1 or 2 cm of lung above the clavicle. The clavicle is percussed directly by your finger. Percuss the rest of the lung initially anteriorly, then within the axillae. Percuss the same area on the two sides consecutively, for comparison (figure 19a–l).

The percussion may be resonant, dull or stony dull. A hyper-resonant tone may indicate an underlying pneumothorax although in practice this is difficult to detect. The axillae are best percussed by asking the patient to raise their arms above the head, and placing your fingers as high up in the axilla as possible. Failure to do so may miss vital physical signs.

Your percussion of the anterior chest also defines the cardiac borders (page 223): right border (figure 20a–c), left border (figure 21a–c) and the upper border of the liver (figure 22a–c). Place your percussed finger

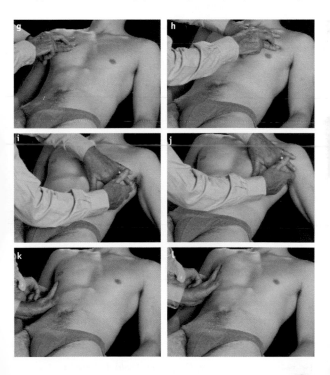

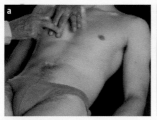

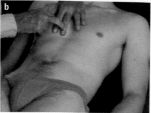

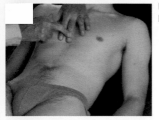

Figure 20 a,b,c. Defining right border of heart.

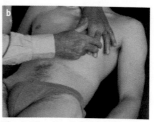

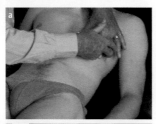

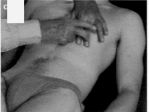

Figure 21 a,b,c. Defining left border of heart.

parallel to the edge you are seeking, and percuss from resonant (hollow lung) to dull (the solid organ).

Tactile vocal fremitus may be found by placing the side of your hand over each lung during enunciation (figure 23a,b). However, it is less

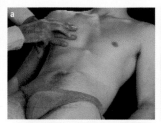

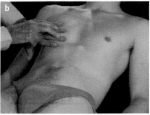

Figure 22 a,b,c. Defining upper border of liver.

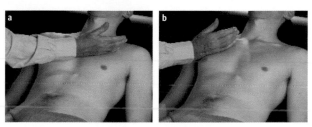

Figure 23 a,b. Examining for tactile vocal fremitus.

effective in assessing the lung's ability to transmit sound than vocal resonance (see below).

Auscultation

Use the diaphragm of the stethoscope to assess the breath sounds (figure 24a–l). Ask the patient to take moderately deep breaths and to breathe in and out through their open mouth; excessive inspiration and too complete an expiration may precipitate the symptoms and signs of hypocarbia, the patient feeling faint.

Normal breath sounds are produced by the airways rather than the alveoli. They have been likened to wind rustling in leaves, and are called vesicular sounds. **Vesicular sounds** are louder and longer on inspiration

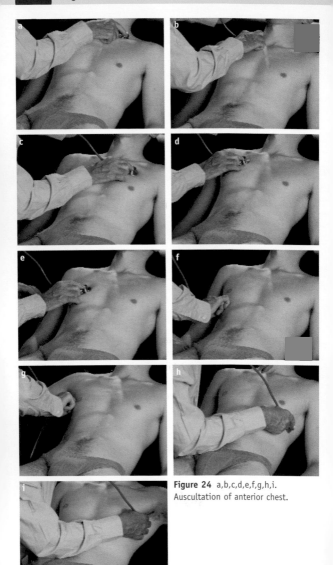

Figure 24 a,b,c,d,e,f,g,h,i.
Auscultation of anterior chest.

than expiration; there is no gap between inspiration and expiration. These sounds are generated by the turbulence of air in the large airways filtering through the normal lung to the chest wall.

Bronchial breath sounds have a more hollow and blowing nature. They are audible throughout expiration and there is often a gap between inspiration and expiration. The expiratory sound has a higher intensity than the inspiratory sound. They are normally audible over the trachea and the main bronchi, as well as over areas of **consolidation**.

Breath sounds are described as normal or reduced in quality. Causes of reduced breath sounds include emphysema, pleural effusion, pneumothorax, and pleural thickening.

Adventitious sounds are either **wheezes** (**rhonchi**) or **crackles** (**râles**). Wheezes have a musical quality and may be heard both on inspiration and expiration. They are caused by continuous oscillation of opposing airway walls and imply airway narrowing. The pitch depends on the speed of airway flow.

Auscultation over the chest while the patient utters some words (e.g., ninety-nine), **vocal resonance**, gives further information about the lung's ability to transmit sound. Over the normal lung, the low-pitched components of speech are heard with a booming quality and high-pitched sounds are attenuated. In consolidation, high-pitched sounds are preferentially transmitted and the speech heard through the stethoscope has a bleating or **egophonic** quality. When the vocal resonance is increased to a great extent, even whispered speech may become audible, a sign known as **whispering pectoriloquy**.

Posterior Chest

When examining the back of the chest, sit the patient upright, on a chair or a bed, so that you can sit or stand behind them (figure 25).

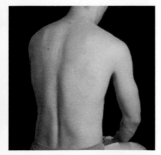

Figure 25 Exposure of posterior chest wall.

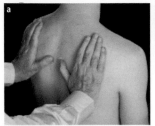

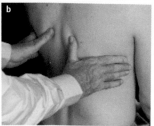

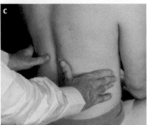

Figure 26 a,b,c. Chest expansion.

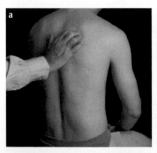

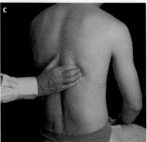

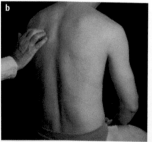

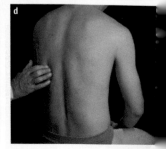

Figure 27 a,b,c,d. Coarse percussion.

The procedure follows the same order already described: inspection, palpation, percussion and auscultation, using identical techniques. Again examine equivalent sites on the two sides consecutively.

Start with expansion (figure 26a–c), followed by course percussion (figure 27a–d).

On percussion posteriorly, ask the patient to move their elbows forward, which rotates the scapulae anteriorly (figure 28a–m). Tactile vocal fremitus is assessed superiorly and inferiorly (figure 29a–d).

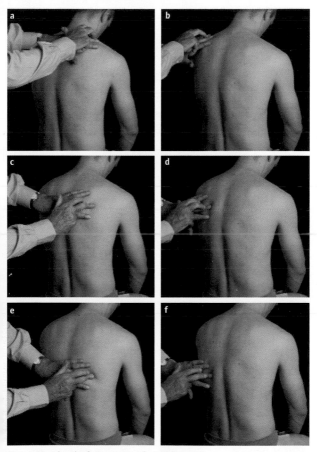

Figure 28 a,b,c,d,e,f. Percussion of posterior chest.

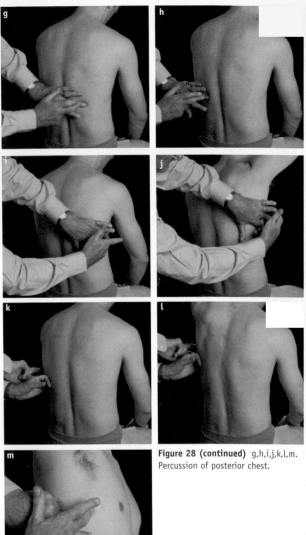

Figure 28 (continued) g,h,i,j,k,l,m. Percussion of posterior chest.

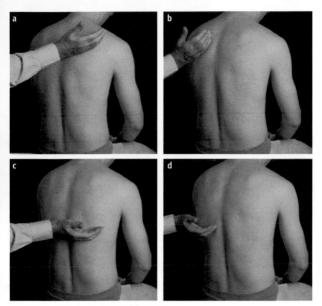

Figure 29 a,b,c,d. Tactile vocal fremitus.

Listen at first in the apices and then in the upper, middle and lower zones, and anteriorly within the axillae (figure 30a–m).

Examining for Vertebral Tenderness

Tenderness may occur with metastatic bone deposits or cervical spondylosis. When assessing vertebral tenderness, start with light pressure over the cervical and thoracic spines. If no tenderness is found, progress to heavier percussion by tapping your fist onto the back of your hand, over each area in turn (figure 31a–e).

Percuss (see above) and palpate for evidence of liver enlargement (figure 32) from metastases, in known or suspected pulmonary malignancy.

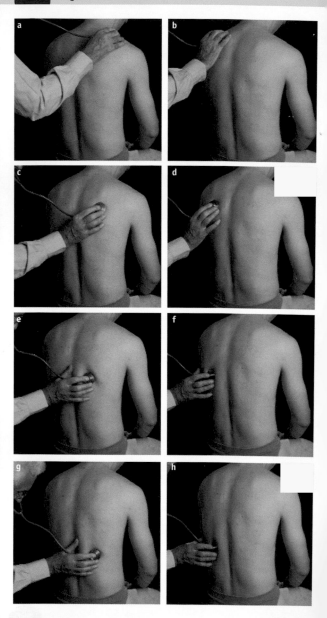

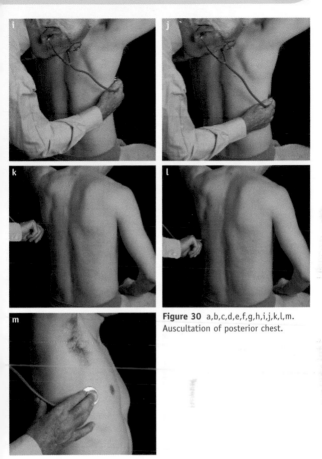

Figure 30 a,b,c,d,e,f,g,h,i,j,k,l,m.
Auscultation of posterior chest.

Chest Aspiration

Needle biopsy of pleural and pulmonary lesions is usually undertaken using image guidance. However, every doctor should be able to aspirate a chest.

This is particularly so for a **tension pneumothorax:** use a syringe and insert the needle through the second intercostal space, in the midclavicular line (figure 33a). If formal drainage is required, insert a

209

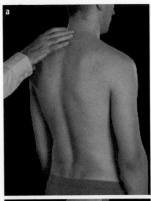

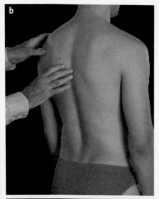

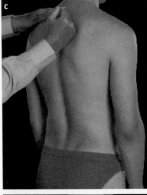

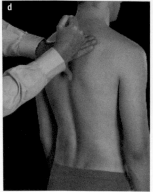

Figure 31 a,b,c,d,e. Examining for vertebral tenderness.

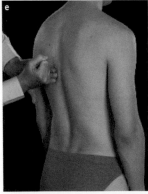

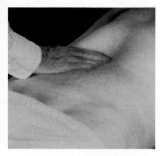

Figure 32 Palpating for liver enlargement.

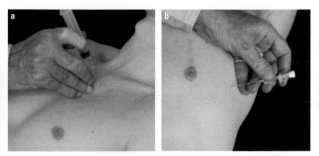

Figure 33 a,b. Aspiration of pneumothorax.

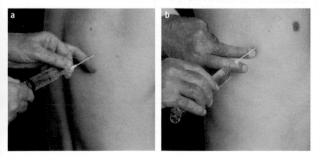

Figure 34 a,b. Drainage of pleural effusion.

cannula through the fourth intercostal space, in the midaxillary line (figure 33b).

When time allows, the procedures should use sterile techniques and local anesthesia down to the parietal pleura; a two-way tap is needed for the needle. The main neurovascular bundle passes just under the lower border of each rib, insertion is therefore above or between the ribs. An under-water seal is required for continued drainage.

Fluid drainage, such as for an **effusion** or a **hematoma**, is usually undertaken posteriorly, through the seventh intercostal space (the level of the lower border of the scapula), but it may also be in the midaxillary line, through the fourth or fifth intercostal space (figure 34a,b). Access is improved posteriorly by placing the elbows forwards, and in the axilla by raising the patient's arm.

CARDIOVASCULAR SYSTEM

Heart

The **thoracic cavity** is divided into the right and left pleural cavities, and, centrally, the mediastinum (situated between the sternum anteriorly and the vertebral column posteriorly). For descriptive purposes, the **mediastinum** is divided by a horizontal plane through the manubriosternal joint. This crosses the lower border of the body of the fourth thoracic vertebra posteriorly. The **superior mediastinum** containing the great vessels lies above this plane. The cavity below the plane contains the heart, within its pericardial sac. The potential space in front of the heart is the **anterior mediastinum** and the **posterior mediastinum** lies behind the heart; it contains the tracheal bifurcation, the hila of the lungs, the esophagus, and the descending thoracic aorta.

The heart is a muscular pump that maintains blood flow through the systemic and pulmonary circulations. It is about the size of a fist. The complex coiling and division of the primitive cardiac tube produces four cavities, **two atria** and **two ventricles**, separated by **interatrial** and **interventricular septa** that divide the heart into **right** and **left** sides: the axis of the heart comes to lie downward and to the left.

The **right atrium** receives deoxygenated blood from the upper and lower halves of the body through the **superior** and **inferior venae cavae**, and from the cardiac muscle via the **coronary sinus**, and pumps it through the **tricuspid valve** to the **right ventricle**. This in turn pumps the blood through the **pulmonary valve** to the **pulmonary trunk** and **pulmonary arteries**, into the lungs. Oxygenated blood is returned to the **left atrium** via **four pulmonary veins** and is pumped through the **mitral valve** to the **left ventricle**, and from there through the **aortic valve** into the **aorta** to be distributed throughout the body.

The synchronous activity of the two atria and the two ventricles, and the sequential contraction of the atria followed by the ventricles, is maintained by cyclical electrical activity passing through the **conducting system** of the heart. The **valves** ensure unidirectional flow without regurgitation.

The **base** of the heart faces posteriorly and is formed of the left atrium. The pulmonary veins enter at each side forming a rough rectangular shape that lies in front of the tracheal bifurcation (carina) and the esophagus. The right atrium, and superior and inferior venae cavae form the **right border** and side of the heart; the apex projects to the left and is formed of the ventricles. The left ventricle is larger and forms most of the **apex** and the **inferior** and **posterior surfaces**. The right ventricle forms the **anterior** and most of the **superior surface** of the heart. The pulmonary trunk and aorta leave the heart superiorly to the right enclosed in a common pericardial sheath.

The **pericardial sac** is attached around the base and right side of the heart around the great vessels, which leaves the rest of the heart free for its pump action. Figure 35 shows the anterior surface marking of the cavities, valves, and great vessels; the lower border of the heart is at the level of the xiphisternal joint. The heart and great vessels are well demonstrated with CT transverse sections of the thorax (figure 36a–c). The **heart sounds**, produced by opening and closing of the valves, radiate to specific sites on the chest wall, as do sounds of abnormalities of the valves and heart muscle.

The heart is subject to a wide variety of **congenital defects**, some of which are incompatible with life. Those encountered in clinical practice include **atrial** and **ventricular septal defects**, **patent ductus arteriosus**, various components of **Fallot's tetralogy** and **coarctation** of the aorta. These conditions give rise to characteristic changes of heart sounds with additional sounds, murmurs, and alteration in rhythm. They may produce **cardiac failure** with the symptoms of dyspnea, palpitations, and peripheral edema. In some cardiac abnormalities there is a mixing of venous and arterial blood producing cyanosis.

The **cardiac valves** may be congenitally abnormal or damaged after **rheumatic fever**. These abnormalities may be detected on clinical examination as well as by tests of cardiac function. **Ischemic** damage to the myocardium, due to **coronary artery disease**, gives rise to **angina** (cardiac pain on exercise), abnormal cardiac rhythms, and cardiac failure.

The clinical assessment of cardiac function is an essential part of the general as well as the cardiac examination. The pulse provides information on cardiac output. Enlargement of the heart and signs of excess fluid in the tissues and body cavities indicate pump failure, and

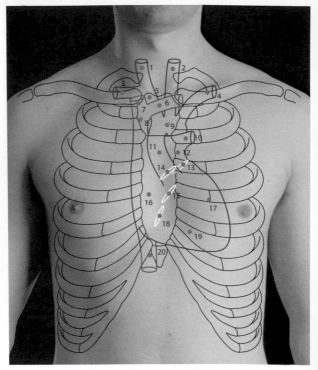

Figure 35 Surface markings of heart and its cavities.

1. Right common carotid artery
2. Left common carotid artery
3. Right subclavian artery
4. Left subclavian artery
5. Brachiocephalic (innominate) artery
6. Brachiocephalic vein, left
7. Brachiocephalic vein, right
8. Superior vena cava
9. Aortic arch
10. Left pulmonary artery
11. Ascending aorta
12. Pulmonary trunk
13. Pulmonary valve
14. Aortic valve
15. Mitral valve
16. Right atrium
17. Left ventricle
18. Tricuspid valve
19. Right ventricle
20. Inferior vena cava

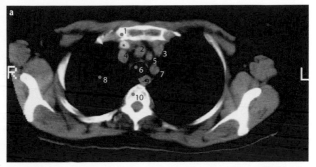

Figure 36 a,b,c. CT through the chest at thoracic vertebral levels 3, 5 and 7.

CT through T3

1. Manubrium sternum
2. Brachiocephalic (innominate) artery
3. Left brachiocephalic vein
4. Right brachiocephalic vein
5. Left common carotid artery
6. Trachea
7. Right subclavian artery
8. Right lung
9. Esophagus
10. Vertebral body T3

*Calcified structure (probably related to sternoclavicular joint)

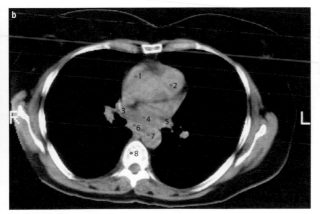

CT through T5

1. Right atrium
2. Right ventricle
3. Right pulmonary vein
4. Left atrium
5. Left pulmonary vein
6. Esophagus
7. Descending thoracic aorta
8. Vertebral body T5

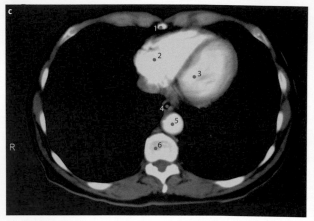

Figure 36 *continued*
CT through T8

1. Xiphisternum
2. Right ventricle
3. Left ventricle

4. Esophagus
5. Descending thoracic aorta
6. Vertebral body T8

the heart sounds provide evidence of valvular and other cardiac abnormalities. The examination of the chest includes both the heart and lungs, but in this section the heart is considered separately. The pulse provides an indication of cardiac activity, but examination of the vascular system includes all peripheral pulses and the venous and lymphatic systems. These are usually examined separately and this practice is followed below.

The cardiac history and examination (page 407) play a key role in assessment, as investigations only record function at a specific moment in time. In the cardiac history, consider chest pain, dyspnea, syncope, palpitations, fatigue, hemoptysis, and edema. Check the past history for **rheumatic fever**, **bacterial endocarditis**, **congenital valvular anomalies**, and tissue disorders such as **Marfan syndrome** and **Ehlers-Danlos syndrome** that may lead to heart valve abnormalities. Note previous cardiac problems and operations, and question for cardiac risk factors, such as **diabetes**, **hypercholesterolemia**, **hypertension**, **smoking**, and a **family history** of coronary artery disease.

Assessment of cardiac function is an important preoperative measure and valuable in long-term follow-up. A number of **grading systems** have been developed but that of the New York Heart Association (NYHA) is a useful monitor:

NYHA 1: No limitation of ordinary physical activity
NYHA 2: Ordinary physical activity causes discomfort
NYHA 3: Moderate to great limitation of ordinary physical activity
NYHA 4: Unable to perform any physical activity without discomfort

Examination

Ensure the patient is lying comfortably in a semirecumbent position at 45 degrees, with the upper half of the body exposed. In the female patient, cover the breast with a loose garment. The cardiac examination begins with a general examination of the patient. The respiratory rate should be noted, the normal resting rate is between 12 and 16 breaths per minute. Patients in heart failure are likely to have **tachypnea** (increased respiration rate) with often shallow, rapid breathing exceeding 20 breaths per minute. The presence of a reduced cardiac output leads to stagnant hypoxia, with evidence of peripheral and possibly central cyanosis. Look for cyanosis of the hands and lips, and for central cyanosis (mucous membrane of the mouth and tongue). Note **clubbing** (figure 37) of the fingers or toes, and examine the extensor tendons of the hands and later the tendo Achilles for **xanthoma**. In the **hands** also look for splinter hemorrhages (figure 38) and Osler's nodes, which are features of bacterial endocarditis.

Pulse

First examine the radial pulse: note the **rate**, the **volume**, the **character**, the **rhythm**, and the **vessel wall**; if the right side is difficult to detect, check and compare it with the left (figure 39a,b). The rate is between 60 and 80 beats per minute in fit individuals. In healthy young subjects the rate varies with the breathing cycle (**sinus arrhythmia**); this becomes less noticeable with age.

A low volume pulse may indicate low stroke volume. A **bounding pulse** suggests a large pulse pressure, as seen in a number of conditions, such

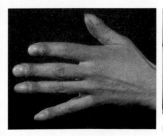

Figure 37 Clubbing.

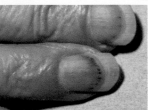

Figure 38 Splinter haemorrhages.

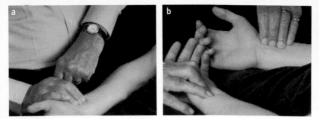

Figure 39 a,b. Assessment of pulse.

as pregnancy, thyrotoxicosis, anemia, ateriovenous fistulae, Paget disease and chronic respiratory failure.

The **rhythm** in health is **sinus rhythm**, and beat-to-beat variation is not usually detectable. Irregular rhythms may be caused by the presence of **atrial fibrillation** (irregularly irregular pulse, usually obvious when the pulse is rapid), or may be caused by the presence of atrial or ventricular premature beats. With ventricular premature beats, there is usually a compensatory pause immediately after the premature beat, and the very next beat is likely to be a larger pulse volume. When these variations occur in health they can be eliminated by exercise.

The **character** of the pulse is best determined by examining the carotid pulse (figure 40). This enables you to see and analyze the waveform. A slow rising pulse suggests aortic outflow obstruction due to either aortic stenosis or subvalvular aortic stenosis.

The **anacrotic** pulse (due to slow ejection of blood from the left ventricle in aortic stenosis) can be combined with a collapsing pulse to produce the bisferiens pulse.

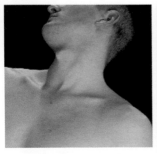

Figure 40 Observing character of carotid pulse

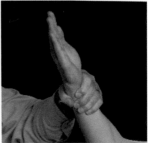

Figure 41 Assessment of collapsing pulse.

A **collapsing** pulse (figure 41), characterized by a rapid up and down stroke, may occur when there is significant aortic regurgitation, a patent ductus arteriosus or an arteriovenous malformation. This "water-hammer" pulse is felt by your palm placed around the wrist.

In **pulsus paradoxus**, deep inspiration lowers the pulse volume (rather than the normal increase) and this may occur with **constrictive pericarditis**, **pericardial tamponade**, and **severe asthma**. The latter is caused by abnormal movement of the septum, occluding the cavity of the left ventricle during systole.

In assessment of the **jugular venous pulse**, remember that the surface marking of the internal jugular vein is a line passing from just behind the angle of the jaw to the depression between the sternal and clavicular heads of the sternomastoid muscle. The patient should be at an angle of 45 degrees, with their head turned slightly away from the midline. Look just deep to the sternomastoid muscle: in health, the pulsation is barely visible. In heart failure or pericardial constriction, the jugular venous pulse is elevated.

It can be difficult to distinguish between a venous and arterial pulsation in the root of the neck. Press lightly over the internal jugular vein, in the root of the neck, to obliterate the venous pulse; the arterial pulsation can then be observed independently (figure 42).

Another technique to identify the jugular pulse is to apply light pressure over the liver, which expels more blood into the right side of the heart. The maneuver exaggerates a raised jugular venous pulse (**hepatojugular reflex** – figure 43). Non-pulsatile elevation of venous pressure is suggestive of superior vena caval obstruction.

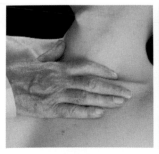

Figure 42 Distinguishing arterial from venous pulsation.

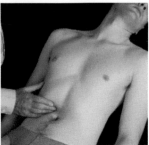

Figure 43 Demonstrating hepatojugular reflex.

When there is an abnormality of the venous pulse, try to synchronize it with the arterial pulse by compressing the contralateral carotid pulse. In this way, you can time the systolic waves of **tricuspid regurgitation** and the occasional cannon wave, typical of complete **heart block**.

Occasionally flutter waves may be seen and, if there is a 2:1 block, the venous wave moves twice as fast as the carotid rate. The ACXVY components of a normal venous pulse are a textbook rather than a clinical phenomenon.

Blood Pressure

The blood pressure should be taken at a set point in the cardiovascular or general examination, so that it is not forgotten (figure 44). The upper limb is exposed up to the axilla. The patient sits or lies on a couch. The cuff should not impinge on the axilla or the cubital fossa and should be wrapped closely and evenly around the upper arm. Smaller cuffs are available for children. Too small a cuff can give a falsely high reading, while too large a cuff prevents access to the brachial artery. The manometer should be at your eye level.

Palpate the radial pulse as the cuff is inflated – raise the pressure to 30 mm of mercury above the level at which the pulse disappears. Apply your stethoscope lightly over the brachial artery on the medial aspect of the cubital fossa. Lower the cuff pressure 5 mm of mercury at a time. The systolic blood pressure is the level at which you first hear the sound. The diastolic is the point at which the sound becomes suddenly faint or inaudible (**Korotkoff sounds**: I – appearance; IV – muffling; V – disappears).

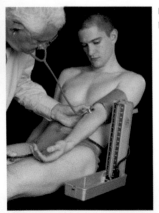

Figure 44 Measurement of blood pressure.

In cardiovascular disease, take the blood pressure in both arms and, in hypertensive patients, in lying and standing positions. An initial falsely high reading may be obtained, together with an increased pulse rate. Repeat any reading that is abnormal, but allow the cuff pressure to drop to zero between measurements.

In peripheral vascular disease the blood pressure may also be measured in the lower limbs. A wider cuff is required for thigh compression and a Doppler probe is used to detect the presence or absence of a distal pulse. The systolic blood pressure is the point of detectable sound when letting down the cuff.

Examination of the Chest
Examination of the heart is subdivided into inspection, palpation, percussion and auscultation.

Inspection and Palpation
Observe the shape of the anterior chest wall, noting any abnormality or scars (figure 45). Asymmetry of the parasternal costal areas may indicate underlying right ventricular or left ventricular hypertrophy. The **apex beat** is the lowest and outermost point at which the cardiac pulse may be felt; it may be visible in thin subjects.

The normal apex is located in the fifth intercostal space, in the midclavicular line. In order to locate it, place the flat of your hand just below the nipple in both males and females (figure 46). In the female, lift the breast to observe and palpate the appropriate area: a **mitral valvotomy** scar is easily missed if this observation is not made. Note the position of the apex beat, by counting down from the second costal cartilage (opposite the manubriosternal joint).

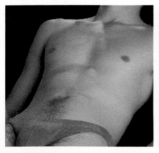 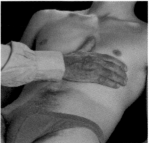

Figure 45 Observing anterior chest in cardiac examination. **Figure 46** Palpation of apex beat.

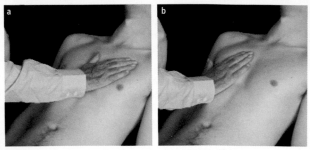

Figure 47 a,b. Palpation for abnormal pulsation across chest.

Displacement of the apex beat may be due to movement of the mediastinum (check for the position of the trachea if this is suspected) or true **cardiac enlargement**. The left ventricle normally produces the apex beat and, when the ventricle is hypertrophied, the beat is forceful and may extend outwards towards the axilla. This **hyperdynamic pulse** of left ventricular hypertrophy is in contrast to the hyperkinetic and rather sustained impulse characteristic of volume overload. The latter may occur in heart failure, and mitral and aortic regurgitation.

Palpation across the chest may reveal an abnormal pulsation due, for example, to an aneurysm of the left ventricle or, more rarely, of the ascending aorta (figure 47a,b). A very rare anomaly is right/left transposition of the viscera (situs inversus), where the heart and apex beat project to the right side.

A tapping apex beat is suggestive of **mitral stenosis**. A dyskinetic impulse may be due to transmission of a powerful atrial contraction and this typically occurs in hypertrophic obstructive cardiomyopathy (**HOCM**) and in systemic **hypertension**. A dyskinetic impulse may also result from a left ventricular aneurysm.

When your hand is placed firmly over the chest, just lateral to the sternum on the left, abnormal impulses from the right ventricle may be felt, as for example in right ventricular hypertrophy due to pulmonary hypertension. If the pulmonary artery is dilated, an impulse may be felt in the second left intercostal space during expiration.

An arterial impulse in the suprasternal notch may indicate an unfolded aorta and abnormal arterial pulses in the neck may result from the **tortuosity** and hardening of the carotid arteries. A prominent pulsation just above the right sternoclavicular joint is usually due to hardening, lengthening, and rotation of the bifurcation of the brachiocephalic

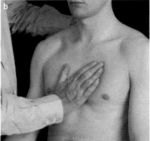

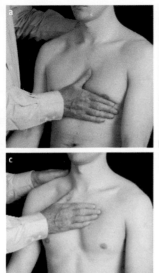

Figure 48 a,b,c. Palpating for fluid thrill.

artery, rather than an aneurysm. The subject is hypertensive, with some wasting of the overlying sternomastoid muscle. In thin patients, especially if affected by chronic airways obstruction, it is not unusual for a pulsation to be detected in the epigastrium.

The presence of a palpable **thrill** almost always indicates an organic lesion (figure 48a–c). It indicates turbulent flow, usually through a small orifice, such as a narrowed valve or a ventricular septal defect. Thrills are usually systolic, i.e., coincident with the apex beat, but may occur in diastole. In order to detect a thrill, it may be necessary to lean the patient forward during expiration and apply the palm of your hand to the base of the heart (central sternum). The pulmonary component of the second sound may also be palpable. In this position also palpate for thrills over the apex.

Percussion
Percussion is useful to define the **right** and **left borders** of the heart; the technique is considered in more detail with the respiratory system.

To define the right heart border, start percussion in the right midclavicular line, at the level of the fourth costal cartilage, and percuss horizontally toward and across the sternal border (figure 49a–c).

223

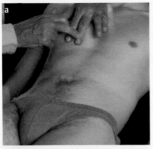

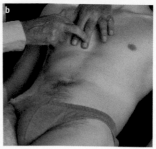

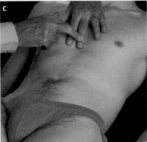

Figure 49 a,b,c. Defining right border of heart.

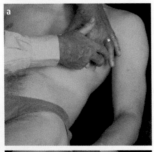

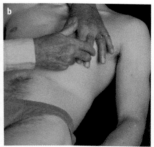

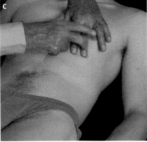

Figure 50 a,b,c. Defining left border of heart.

An indication of the position of the apex of the heart is obtained from palpation. To define the left border, start percussion lateral to this point, or in the midaxillary line, and percuss medially along the line of the fifth rib (figure 50a–c).

Auscultation

Note the quality of the first and second heart sounds at each site, and whether there are any additional sounds. The first heart sound has two components, caused by mitral and tricuspid valve closure. Mitral closure occurs slightly before tricuspid but this does not normally cause splitting of the sound. The second heart sound is a slightly lower pitch than the first; it occurs at the end of systole. It comprises both aortic and pulmonary valve closure. A useful mnemonic is that the valves close in alphabetical order, i.e., aortic before pulmonary and mitral before tricuspid.

During inspiration, splitting of the second sound may be detected over the pulmonary area: this is due to the increased venous return to the right ventricle, leading to more prolonged systole on the right side of the heart. Splitting of the first heart sound may indicate complete right bundle branch block, whereas increase of the normal splitting of the second heart sound occurs if there is delay in right ventricular emptying, as in right bundle branch block, pulmonary stenosis, ventricular septal defects, and mitral incompetence.

Atrial septal defects typically cause a fixed splitting of the second sound. Reverse splitting of the second sound (i.e., splitting occurring in expiration, as opposed to inspiration) is due to delayed left ventricle depolarization (e.g., left bundle branch block) and delayed left ventricular emptying (e.g., aortic stenosis, coarctation of the aorta, and patent ductus arteriosus).

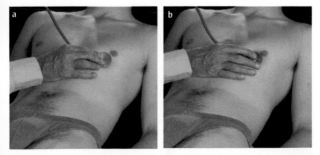

Figure 51 a,b. Auscultating apex with bell and diaphragm.

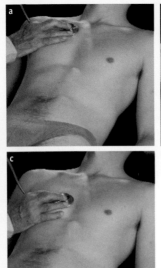

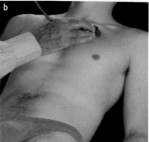

Figure 52 Auscultating: a. aortic, b. pulmonary, and c. tricuspid areas.

Auscultation starts over the apex, where the mitral valve is assessed. In this **mitral area**, apply the bell of the stethoscope (figure 51a). It produces a resonating chamber that is particularly efficient in amplifying the low pitched sounds that may occur with mitral diastolic murmurs and a fourth heart sound.

Next change to the diaphragm (figure 51b). This is appropriate for detecting high pitched sounds, such as those generated by systolic murmurs.

Follow this by applying the stethoscope systematically over the **aortic area** (second right intercostal space), the **pulmonary area** (second left intercostal space), and finally the **tricuspid areas** (fifth left intercostal space). At each site use both the bell and the diaphragm (figure 52a–c).

The above order of auscultation links the mitral and aortic valves, and the pulmonary with the tricuspid, i.e., the valves on the respective sides of the heart. Auscultation must not be limited to these four sites. When abnormalities are found or suspected, move the stethoscope over each area to identify the positions of optimal sound, and also to follow the radiation of sound: typical sites are along the left sternal border, radiation from the apex into the left axilla, and from the aortic area into the right side of the neck (figure 53).

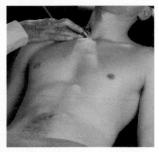

Figure 53 Auscultating neck for radiation of aortic murmurs.

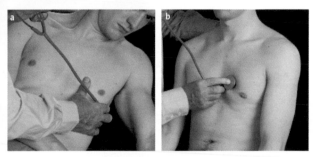

Figure 54 a,b. Repositioning to accentuate abnormal sounds.

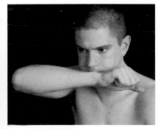

Figure 55 Production of Valsalva response. This is combined with auscultation of the cardiac area of interest.

Repositioning a patient may accentuate sounds, such as turning to the left lateral position or sitting upright (figure 54a,b); sounds may be further accentuated by deep inspiration, deep expiration or a Valsalva manoeuver. A **Valsalva** maneuver is performed by asking the patient to blow hard on the back of their hand or forearm, without releasing air (figure 55).

227

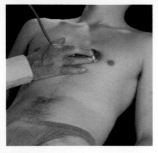

Figure 56 Auscultating opening snap over left sternal edge.

Additional Heart Sounds

The third heart sound is a low pitched diastolic sound usually best heard over the apex. It is probably caused by tautening of the mitral and tricuspid capillary muscles at the end of rapid diastolic filling. It usually indicates left ventricular dysfunction.

A fourth heart sound is a late diastolic sound, more high pitched than the third. It is never physiological, and usually reflects poor ventricular function (e.g., aortic stenosis, systemic hypertension, HOCM).

Characteristic sounds occur with some lesions, such as the opening snap of mitral stenosis, heard over the left sternal border in the fourth interspace (figure 56).

Cardiac Murmurs

Murmurs must be fully assessed. Note their timing (i.e., systolic or diastolic), the area of greatest intensity, their loudness and the effect of various maneuvers, such as inspiration and a Valsalva.

Systolic murmurs can be pansystolic, ejection systolic or late systolic. Pansystolic murmurs extend throughout systole beginning with the first heart sound and going right up to the second heart sound. The loudness of pitch may vary during systole and common causes include mitral regurgitation. The intensity of midsystolic murmurs (or ejection murmurs) is greatest in midsystole. The usual cause is turbulent flow through a narrow aortic or pulmonary valve. Late systolic murmurs typically occur with mitral valve prolapse or papillary muscle dysfunction.

Diastolic murmurs may be either early, where they usually have a deep crescendo quality (e.g., caused by pulmonary or aortic regurgitation), or mid-diastolic. The latter begin later in diastole, and are usually short, extending up to the first sound; they have a low-pitched quality. Their usual cause is impairment of blood flow in ventricular filling, such as caused by mitral or tricuspid stenosis. Presystolic murmurs are caused by atrial systole across a narrow valve. Continuous murmurs are caused by a patent ductus arteriosus, arteriovenous shunts, and congenital aortopulmonary windows. Rare causes include a ruptured sinus of Valsalva and a coronary artery fistula.

The area of intensity of a murmur is important. For example, mitral regurgitation is best heard at the apex and radiates towards the axilla, while others may be heard over the entire chest wall. Conduction of an ejection systolic murmur into the carotid artery suggests an aortic valvular origin for the lesion. Loudness of atrial murmurs is not clinically relevant and, paradoxically, more severe lesions may produce quieter murmurs.

Dynamic maneuvers, such as inspiration, should be employed to evaluate murmurs. Inspiration increases venous return and therefore blood flow through the right side of the heart, usually accentuating right-sided murmurs. A Valsalva maneuver changes the murmurs of HOCM and mitral valve prolapse.

The site of maximum intensity and any radiation provide information on the underlying disease. Low pitched sounds are best heard with the bell of the stethoscope and high pitched sounds with the diaphragm. Grades are from I to VI. I: very soft; II: soft but easily audible; III: moderately loud; IV: loud with associated thrill; V: very loud plus thrill; VI: maximum loudness with thrill, heard without a stethoscope.

Figure 57 summarizes the relation of murmurs to the heart sounds, and ventricular systole and diastole: the murmurs are classified by their timing, position, pitch, and grade. Figure 57 also shows the typical combination of heart sounds and murmurs of some common disorders.

A **pericardial friction rub** may be audible over the base of the heart with the patient leaning forward; it is caused by the movement of inflamed pericardial surfaces rubbing against each other. Once fluid accumulates (figure 58), it may separate the surfaces, with the disappearance of the rub.

If the clinical features suggest tricuspid regurgitation, an attempt should be made to elicit **pulsatility of the liver** (figure 59). This is best done during deep inspiration with the patient supine and the examiner's hands sandwiching the liver, accentuating the abnormal pulsation. This is an extremely useful sign, together with the systolic waves in the jugular venous pulse of tricuspid regurgitation.

The cardiac examination is completed by searching for the excess tissue fluid produced in **cardiac failure**. Listen over the bases of the lungs for evidence of crepitations caused by pulmonary edema (figure 60a,b).

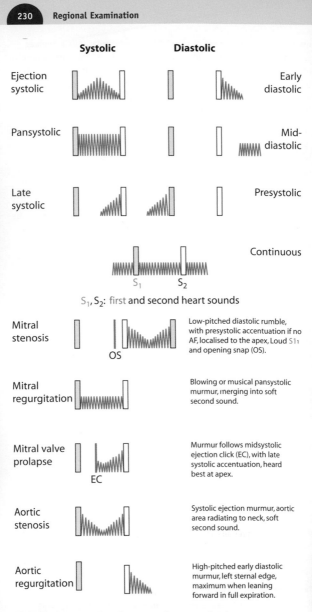

Figure 57 Heart sounds and murmurs of common disorders.

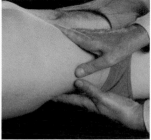

Figure 59 Palpating for liver pulsation.

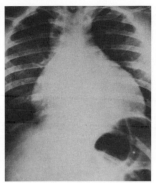

Figure 58 Pericardial effusion.

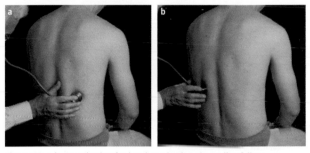

Figure 60 a,b. Auscultating for basal crepitations in cardiac failure.

Liver enlargement is detected by downward percussion in the chest, and upward percussion and palpation in the abdomen (figure 61a–e): **ascites** is detected by shifting abdominal dullness (figure 62 a,b). Pitting **edema** is best sought below the knee and in the **sacral** area (figure 63a). When extensive, it may involve the thighs and creep up the anterior abdominal wall. The critical sign is pitting, which occurs when applying light pressure to the skin. This can be demonstrated by pressure in front of the tendo Achilles or over the **shins** (figure 63b–d). The latter may cause discomfort so watch the patient's face.

Emergency management of cardiac arrest includes cardiac massage and defibrillation. Another important technique, used usually in hospital, is inserting a needle into the pericardium and the heart, to drain a

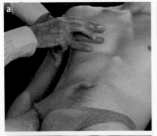

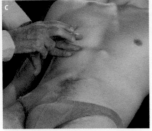

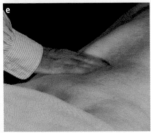

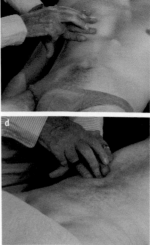

Figure 61 a,b,c,d,e. Assessment of liver enlargement in cardiac failure by percussion and palpation.

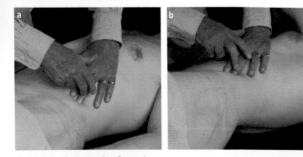

Figure 62 a,b. Percussing for ascites.

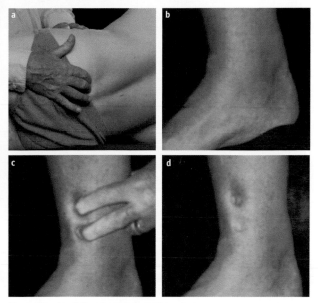

Figure 63 a,b,c,d. Examinating for peripheral edema.

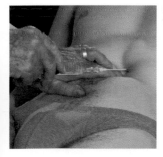

Figure 64 Aspiration of pericardium in cardiac tamponade.

pericardial effusion (**pericardiocentesis**) and insert drugs (usually adrenalin) into the heart in asystole.

The needle is inserted in the angle between the xiphisternum and the left costal margin, and directed at the inferior angle of the left scapula. This direction is at approximately 45 degrees to the sagittal, coronal, and transverse planes (figure 64).

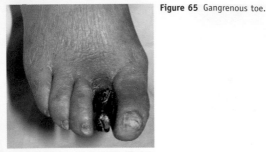

Figure 65 Gangrenous toe.

ARTERIES

Arteries may bleed or block. The former is usually due to **trauma**, but may be from rupture of an **aneurysm** or from an **arteriovenous malformation**. **Arteriosclerosis** produces arterial stenosis and occlusion. In the **coronary** and **cerebral** vessels this gives rise to myocardial infarction and stroke respectively, and these effects are currently the commonest cause of death in the Western world. Reduction in blood flow to the lower limb gives rise to **claudication** (pain on exercise) and, when more severe, **rest pain**, nutritional changes to the skin, and ultimately **gangrene** (figure 65).

Examination of the pulses is usually undertaken regionally, but in patients with arterial disease, a more systematic approach is required, as followed in this section. Figure 66 shows the main arteries in the body.

Figure 66 Arteries of body.

1. Right common carotid bifurcation
2. Left common carotid
3. Left subclavian
4. Brachiocephalic (innominate)
5. Right axillary
6. Aortic arch
7. Ascending aorta
8. Left profunda brachii
9. Left brachial
10. Cubital anastomosis
11. Left ulnar
12. Left radial
13. Right deep palmar arch
14. Right superficial palmar arch
15. Descending thoracic aorta
16. Abdominal aorta
17. Right common iliac
18. Left internal iliac
19. Right external iliac
20. Left common femoral
21. Left profunda femoris
22. Right superficial femoral
23. Geniculate anastomosis
24. Left popliteal
25. Left anterior tibial
26. Right peroneal
27. Left posterior tibial
28. Right dorsalis pedis
29. Right plantar arch

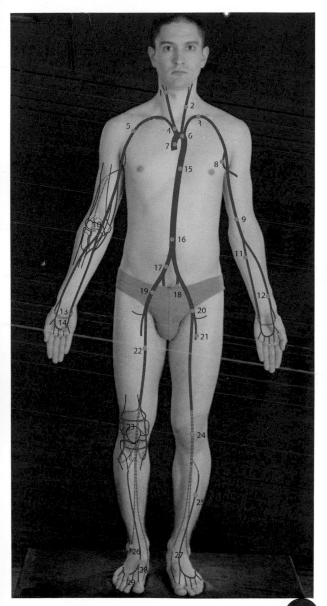

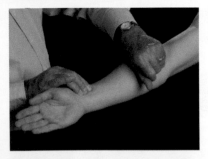

Figure 67 Palpating pulse.

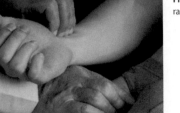

Figure 68 Measuring radio-femoral delay.

To feel a pulse effectively it is compressed on a firm adjacent structure, usually a bone (figure 67). The distal of three fingers is used to compress the vessel while the proximal two assess the rate, rhythm, volume, and character of the pulse: rolling the vessel indicates a normal or thickened vessel wall. Commence by examining the radial pulses at the wrist, compressing the vessels on the lower end of each radius.

Radial and femoral pulses are compared for the **radio-femoral delay** of coarctation of the aorta (figure 68).

It is useful to **compare** the two sides of the body and also to compare the apical rate with an upper limb or cervical pulse, to look for missed beats, as for instance in atrial fibrillation (figure 69a,b).

The ulnar artery passes superficial to the lateral aspect of the flexor retinaculum and is prominent in some individuals (figure 70). The distal arteries may be occluded by emboli due to proximal disease, such as a cervical rib (figure 71).

If a subject first clenches their fist firmly, while you compress both the radial and ulnar arteries, when the fist is released return of the capillary

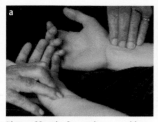

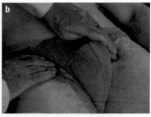

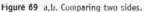

Figure 69 a,b. Comparing two sides.

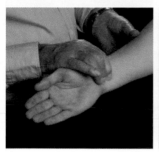

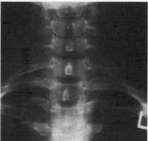

Figure 70 Palpating ulnar artery.

Figure 71 Cervical rib. Note downward angulation of cervical (particularly seventh) transverse processes, compared to the upward angulation of the first thoracic transverse process.

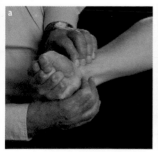

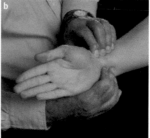

Figure 72 a,b. Allen's test.

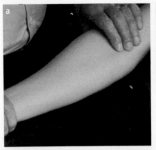

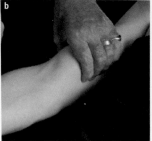

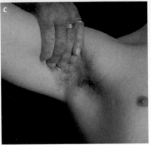

Figure 73 a,b,c. Palpating brachial and axillary arteries.

circulation is slow. The relative contribution of these two vessels to the circulation of the hand can be assessed by the effect of individual compression (**Allen's** test – figure 72a,b).

The brachial artery lies superficial at the level of the elbow joint, medial to the tendon of biceps, partly covered by the bicipital aponeurosis. To facilitate palpation, ask the subject to fully extend the elbow, to allow compression of the artery against the lower end of the humerus. It is at this site that the pulse is usually auscultated when measuring the blood pressure (figure 73a). You can also palpate the brachial artery against the midshaft of the humerus (figure 73b), in the groove between brachialis and biceps muscles. The axillary artery is palpated against the head of the humerus, by deep lateral palpation in the depths of the axilla (figure 73c). Palpate the subclavian artery by compression against the first rib. This is in the posterior triangle of the neck just behind the middle of the clavicle (figure 74).

The common carotid arteries can be palpated in the midcervical region, pressing backwards on the transverse processes of the cervical vertebrae (figure 75).

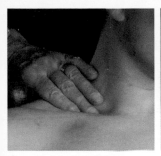

Figure 74 Palpating subclavian artery.

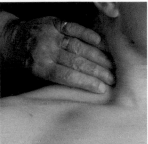

Figure 75 Palpating common carotid artery.

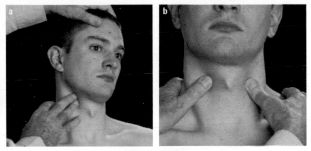

Figure 76 a,b. Unilateral and bilateral carotid compression.

Unilateral or bilateral carotid compression is undertaken in this region (figure 76a,b). The common carotid bifurcation can be felt more distally, at the upper border of the thyroid cartilage; the external and internal branches are difficult to define independently.

Palpate the facial artery on the inferior margin of the mandible, just anterior to the masseter muscle (figure 77a). The border of the muscle can be identified by asking the subject to clench their teeth.

Palpate the superficial temporal artery at a preauricular level or its anterior division as it crosses the temple (figure 77b).

Soft bruits are commonly found over major arteries, even in normal individuals. However, stenotic disease often produces high pitched and prominent sounds. These signs, together with other symptoms and signs of stroke or lower leg ischemia, prompt more detailed investigation of the vascular tree.

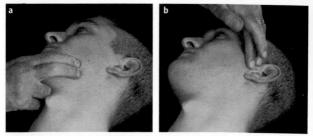

Figure 77 a,b. Palpating facial and superficial temporal arteries.

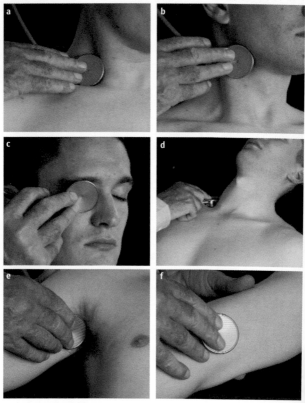

Figure 78 Auscultating a,b,c. carotid (lower cervical, bifurcation and orbit), d. subclavian, e. axillary, and f. brachial arteries.

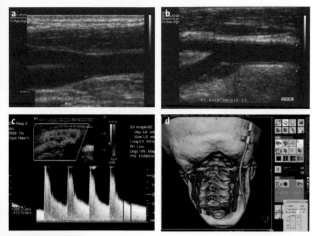

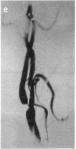

Figure 79 Assessment of carotid vessels: a. ultrasound of normal carotid bifurcation; b. atheromatous stenosis of internal carotid artery; c. scan and wave form analysis of carotid bifurcation; d. spiral CT of carotid and vertebral arteries (a shunt is draining a hydrocephalus); e. arteriogram of internal carotid stenosis.

Listen to the carotid arteries in the lower cervical region, over the carotid bifurcation and the orbit, the subclavian over the first rib, the axillary in the lateral axilla and the brachial in the arm and cubital fossa (figure 78a–f). The relation of carotid artery disease to stroke has led to the refinement of a number of measurement techniques to be used in this area (figure 79a–e).

Palpate the abdominal aorta above and below the umbilicus (figure 80a,b). It is easily felt in thin individuals and, when you first notice this, it can be mistaken for enlargement.

The aorta is difficult to feel in the obese, and when looking for aneurysms, press backwards with two hands, one on either side of the aorta, to obtain an estimate of its diameter (figure 81a,b). Abdominal ultrasound, or another imaging modality, is required to exclude or

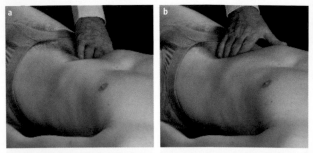

Figure 80 a,b. Palpating abdominal aorta.

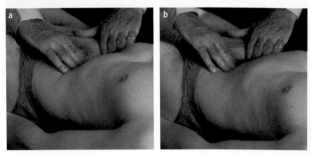

Figure 81 a,b. Palpation of outer limit of abdominal aortic aneurysms.

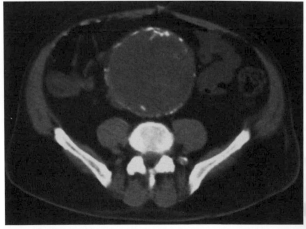

Figure 82 MRI of abdominal aortic aneurysm in transverse section.

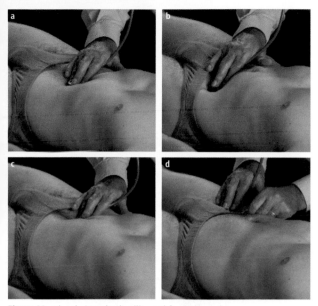

Figure 83 a,b,c,d. Auscultating iliac and femoral vessels.

confirm the presence of a suspected aneurysm, and determine its size. If your hand can palpate the top of an abdominal aortic aneurysm, it is infrarenal (even when you cannot, it usually is). MRI provides good imaging and information of the surrounding structures (figure 82).

Listen to the aorta at the level of the umbilicus, and the iliac vessels from the aortic bifurcation (just to the left of the umbilicus, at the level of the L4 vertebral body) to the midinguinal point (midway between the anterior superior iliac spine and the symphysis pubis – figure 83a–d).

Epigastric bruits are common in the young, but may represent aortic branch disease in the elderly (figure 84a). Bruits in either loin are an important diagnostic sign in suspected renal artery disease (figure 84b). The aorta and iliac vessels are common sites for arteriosclerotic disease (figure 85a,b).

Palpate the femoral arteries over the midinguinal point, compressing them backwards onto the head of the femur (figure 86). Compare the two sides for volume; they may differ in lower limb vascular disease,

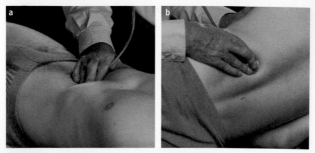

Figure 84 a,b. Checking for epigastric and renal bruits.

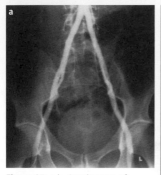

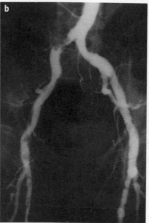

Figure 85 a,b. Arteriograms of normal and diseased abdominal aorta and branches.

when bruits are also common (figure 87a–c). The superficial position of the femoral arteries facilitates their ultrasound assessment, and their value for vascular access (figure 88a,b). Anatomically, the femoral artery extends from its formation at the inguinal ligament to where it becomes the popliteal, at the adductor hiatus. In clinical practice, the femoral is referred to as the common femoral, down to its profunda branch, and the superficial femoral artery beyond. This is in keeping with the way arterial disease often differs at these two sites.

Palpate the popliteal artery against the upper end of the tibia, with the knee slightly flexed and the muscles relaxed. Use the pulps of all eight

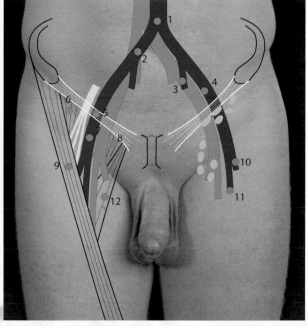

Figure 86 Diagram of femoral artery.

1. Aortic bifurcation
2. Right common iliac artery
3. Left internal iliac artery
4. Left external iliac artery
5. Midinguinal point
6. Iliopsoas muscle
7. Right common femoral artery
8. Pectineus muscle
9. Sartorius muscle
10. Left profunda femoris artery
11. Left superficial femoral artery
12. Adductor longus muscle

fingers to compress the artery onto the tibia, between the heads of gastrocnemius (figure 89a). The popliteal artery is deeply situated in the popliteal fossa, but you can palpate it against the lower end of the femur, with the patient supine or prone (figure 89b,c). This is particularly useful if the distal popliteal artery is occluded.

Listen to the superficial femoral and popliteal arteries at the level of the adductor canal and over the popliteal fossa (figure 90a,b).

The anterior tibial artery crosses the ankle joint midway between the two malleoli, becoming the dorsalis pedis at this point. It then passes

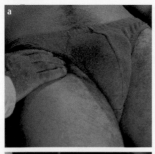

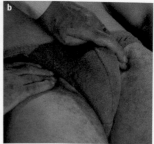

Figure 87 a,b,c. Palpation and auscultation of femoral arteries.

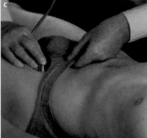

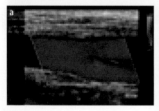

Figure 88 Ultrasound of normal femoral artery; a. arteriogram: b. false aneurysm of femoral artery.

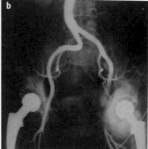

toward the first interdigital web. Palpate the latter over the heads of the metatarsals, just lateral to the extensor hallucis longus tendon (figure 91a–c).

The posterior tibial artery passes under the foot. You can palpate it behind the lower tibia or over the talus, midway between the medial malleolus and the medial prominence of the heel, before it passes into the sole (figure 92a,b).

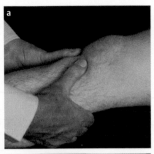

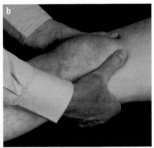

Figure 89 a,b,c. Palpating popliteal artery.

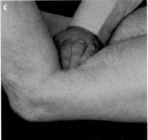

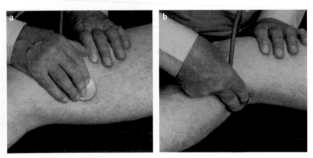

Figure 90 a,b. Auscultating superficial femoral and popliteal arteries.

The anterior perforating branch from the peroneal artery can be palpated just in front of the lateral malleolus. The vessel may be palpable in the normal individual or may become prominent with occlusion of other foot vessels (figure 93).

Foot pulses can be difficult to feel and you can be confused by feeling pulsation in your own fingers. If in doubt, palpate an easily palpable wrist or femoral pulse at the same time, or count out the beats of the

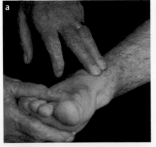
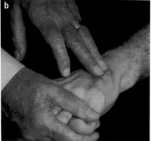

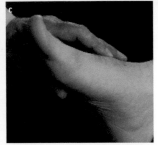

Figure 91 a. Palpating anterior tibial and b,c. dorsalis pedis arteries.

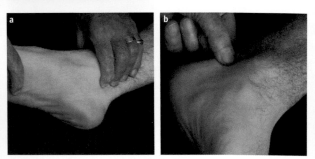

Figure 92 a,b. Palpating posterior tibial artery.

palpated pulse, while another observer compares this with the pulse rate taken at another site.

In severe **ischemia**, the blood pressure at the ankle is markedly reduced and, as this approaches zero, the foot blanches and the veins empty if you raise the foot. In extreme cases, a gutter replaces the line of the vein. When you subsequent lower the ischemic limb, venous refilling can

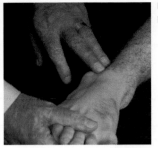

Figure 93 Palpating perforating peroneal artery.

take over a minute, compared to the normal few seconds, and this is followed by a distal reactive hyperemia.

In severe ischemia there may be **trophic changes**. Observe the lateral side of the foot and the heel for evidence of fissuring or infection, and examine between the toes for **ulceration** and **gangrene**. Diabetic patients are prone to foot ischemia, and these problems are accentuated by the associated **neuropathy** and infection.

VEINS

Most venous disorders occur in the lower limb. Here the **superficial veins** are prone to cosmetically unsatisfactory, dilated tortuous (**varicose**) veins, and the **deep veins** are a common site of **thrombosis**, following inactivity, as with postoperative state, and in pregnancy, autoimmune disorders and malignancy. Figure 94 is a normal venogram, and figure 95 demonstrates a vein using ultrasound. Complications of thrombosis are swelling (which in extremes cases may produce **venous gangrene**) and **pulmonary emboli**. Late sequelae are secondary varicose veins and **leg ulceration** (figure 96). (See table 2 for the differential diagnosis of leg ulceration, and table 3 (page 262) for the causes of a swollen leg.)

Superficial venous thrombosis (**thrombophlebitis migrans**; over the breast, this is termed **Mondor disease**) is usually a manifestation of deep malignancy that may be difficult to locate. It also occurs after local trauma.

Varicose veins are usually assessed with a hand held **Doppler instrument**, but a good deal of information can be obtained from clinical examination. Palpation of the lower leg can often define the sites where large perforating veins have produced palpable **defects** in the deep fascia

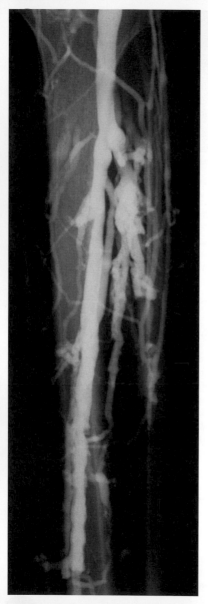

Figure 94 Normal venogram.

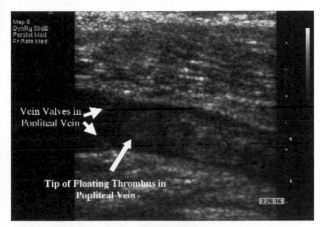

Figure 95 Ultrasound of deep venous thrombosis.

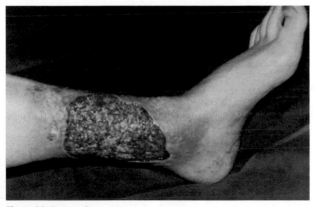

Figure 96 Venous ulcer.

(figure 97a). The normal **impulse** felt proximally along a vein, following a distal **tap**, may also be felt passing distally, through defective valves (figure 97b); there is usually a **cough impulse** demonstrating incompetence at the saphenofemoral junction (figure 97c).

Place a venous tourniquet (i.e., occluding the superficial but not the deep veins or arterial flow) around a leg sequentially from above downward (after first emptying the superficial veins by raising the leg

251

Table 2 LEG ULCERS

VASCULAR	NEURO-PATHY	HAEMATO-LOGICAL	MALIG-NANCIES	MISCELL-ANEOUS
Primary and secondary venous insufficiency	Diabetes mellitus	Sickle cell disease	Kaposi's sarcoma	Infection
	Alcohol	Leukemia	Melanoma	Syphilis
	Syringomyelia	Hemolytic jaundice	Basal cell carcinoma	Tropical pyoderma gangrenosa
Arterial obstructive disease	Paralysis		Epithelioma	
Arteriovenous malformations				Skin diseases
				Rheumatoid arthritis
Vasculitis				Pressure sores
				Trauma/burns
				Artifactual

Note: flat sloping (venous, septic, often with transparent healing edge along part of its circumference); punched out (syphilitic, trophic, diabetic, leprosy, ischemic); undermined (tuberculous, pressure necrosis, particularly over the buttocks, carbuncles); raised (rodent ulcer, often a slightly rolled appearance); raised and everted (carcinoma)

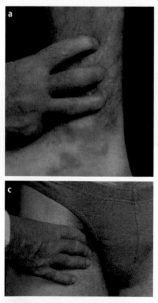

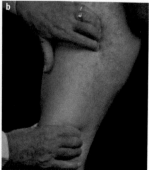

Figure 97 Assessment of varicose veins: a. palpating fascial defects, b. tap test (tapping with left hand, palpating with right); c. groin cough impulse.

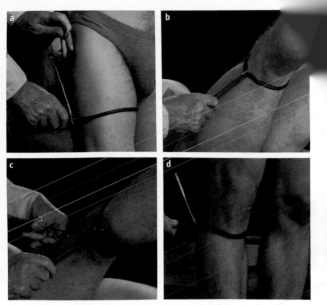

Figure 98 a,b,c,d. Use of venous tourniquet to identify levels of venous incompetence.

Figure 99 Perthe test.

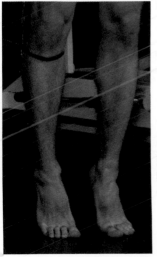

...he horizontal), and ask the patient to stand up (figure 98a–d). ...echnique can be used to define the level of greatest **leakage** from ...deep to the superficial system (**Trendelenburg test**).

...ace a venous tourniquet below the knee in a patient with varicose ...eins, and ask them to stand on their toes ten times (**Perthe test** – figure 99). This is usually sufficient for the muscle pump to empty engorged superficial veins into the deep system. However, if there is **gross incompetence** or **thrombosis** in the deep system, emptying is prevented: the superficial veins become more rather than less engorged with activity.

VASCULAR ACCESS

Vascular access is a requirement for most branches of medicine. The commonest need is for **venepuncture**; blood is routinely taken from the veins crossing the cubital fossa, alternatively from veins over the dorsum of the hand or the cephalic vein at the wrist. Larger volumes, and in cases of difficult access, the femoral and internal jugular veins may be used. The same veins may be used for administration of drugs and fluid, e.g., for anesthetic agents, and delivery of perioperative blood, and fluid support and replacement. Repeated access, e.g., for delivering **chemotherapy** and for **hemodialysis**, usually requires some permanent arrangement. A common example is the **Hickman line** introduced using ultrasonic guidance into the subclavian vein, or surgically into the subclavian vein through the terminal cephalic vein; alternatively, access is gained via the internal jugular. Another method is to produce an arterialized vein by means of a surgically fashioned **arteriovenous fistula**, preferably in the non-dominant forearm. **Arteries** may be stabbed, e.g., for blood gas analysis and for monitoring arterial pressure. In all these situations, you need to know the normal anatomy of common access sites and possible complications of the proposed procedure.

For a **venepuncture** you will need a sterile syringe (usually 10 ml) and needle, a spirit swab to clean the skin just before skin puncture, a bottle to receive withdrawn blood, or a prepared giving set (set up in an aseptic fashion) capped with a two- or three-way tap, a pledget of cotton wool to press on the skin puncture site and a skin plaster, to cover this site when the bleeding has stopped. If the syringe nozzle is off center, keep this lowermost, and attach the needle with the bevel facing upward. Tell the patient what you are going to do at each stage.

For venepuncture of an antecubital vein, examine both arms, and other sites if these veins are known to be inappropriate from previous attempts or when preserving certain sites for dialysis. The median cubital vein joins the cephalic and basilic veins in front of the elbow and may have a median forearm tributary.

Once chosen, use some form of proximal compression to encourage venous filling. Gripping the upper arm by the patient or an assistant may suffice, but it is advisable to carry a quick release venous tourniquet or a length of rubber tubing for this application. It is applied tightly enough to compress the veins but not arteries. Once applied, it may be easier to feel rather than see a superficial vein in a fat arm. Clenching the fist four to eight times aids venous filling and gentle tapping over the vein also encourages dilatation. When access problems are anticipated, preheating the arm in warm water helps vasodilatation.

Once a dilated vein has been identified and its direction noted, choose a 1- to 2-cm segment and clean the skin over it with a spirit swab. Pick up the syringe and pierce the skin over the distal end of this segment, keeping the needle in line with the target segment (figure 100). The angle of venous entry and passing the needle along the vein is 10–20 degrees to the surface, but it may be easier to pierce the skin with an entry angle of 30–40 degrees, and then lower your hand once the subcutaneous level is reached. Watch the point of the needle pushing into and entering the superficial wall of the vein, and then advance it for 5–10 mm along the lumen.

Hold the syringe firmly in this position and use your other hand to withdraw the plunger. Once the required amount of blood has been obtained, use the withdrawing hand to release the tourniquet and place the pledget of cotton wool over the skin puncture site. Withdraw the needle and at the same time apply pressure over the puncture site. Ask the patient to take over this pressure and to bend their elbow, while you

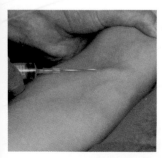

Figure 100 Venepuncture of antecubital vein.

end to the blood sample and ensure that the needle and syringe are appropriately disposed of. Maintain pressure for at least 2 minutes (longer if there is a history of oozing) and check that bleeding has stopped before applying the plaster.

If the needle is being used for infusion, release the tourniquet once it is in place and inject the prepared contents of the syringe, or hold the hub of the needle firmly, twist off the syringe and attach the giving set that you have prepared. Make sure the tubing is secured and the puncture site covered before attending to the infusion. The complications of antecubital puncture include stabbing a nerve (painful but not usually a long-term problem) and entering the brachial artery; this passes along the medial aspect of the cubital fossa. Puncture is not usually a serious problem if recognized, but firm pressure must be applied on needle withdrawal. However, if the problem is not recognized, intra-arterial injection of certain compounds can be harmful, so carefully note the depth of your needle, the ease of withdrawal, the color of the blood aspirated into the syringe and any associated pulsation of the blood column or the needle. If in doubt, apply pressure and start again later or at another site.

Bruising is a common complication and due to trauma to the vein wall, lack of adequate post-withdrawal pressure, and any bleeding tendency. Make sure you can withdraw blood through the needle before injection, as extravasation of injected/infused material is painful and may harm subcutaneous tissues. For the same reason, ensure stability of any infusion line, and note the ease of the infusion and monitor all subsequent changes. Blockage of peripheral lines is common and it is essential, if you need to flush the system, to establish that the needle has not come out of the target vein. A later complication is thrombosis of the vein; this is usually painful. All pain associated with a line must immediately be investigated, to establish why and to stop any harmful infusion. An aseptic technique is essential, as infection in a line may not only produce a local inflammatory response but also has the potential of systemic spread of an infection.

The above steps can equally be used for other sites in the upper limb, notably the cephalic vein as it passes over the anatomical snuffbox at the wrist (figure 101) and the veins over the dorsum of the hand (figure 102a). For longer periods of infusion, a cannula is used (figure 102b). This is mounted on a central needle. Techniques follow the same principles described but the needle is withdrawn once the cannula is housed within the vein; the tourniquet is first released and the infusion set attached, using full aseptic precautions.

More proximally in the upper limb, the subclavian vein is used for access, either from above or below the clavicle. The subclavian artery

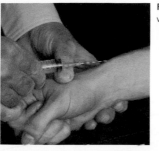

Figure 101 Venepuncture of cephalic vein.

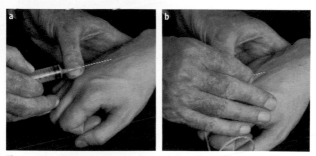

Figure 102 a,b. Venepuncture and cannulation of vein on dorsum of hand.

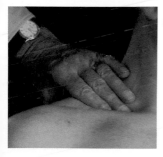

Figure 103 Palpation of the subclavian artery over the first rib.

(figure 103) can be palpated as it crosses the first rib, behind the junction of the middle and medial thirds of the clavicle; the vein passes anterior and inferior to this point. The skin entry is just above the middle of the clavicle and directed at the suprasternal notch (figure 104a). The inferior access point is below the middle of the clavicle, directed at the same target (figure 104b). Problems of bruising are more

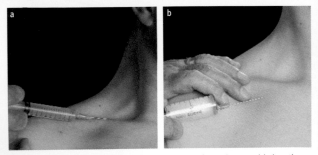

Figure 104 a,b. Venepucture of subclavian vein, from above and below the clavicle.

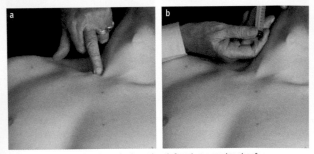

Figure 105 a,b. Palpation of triangular defect between heads of sternomastoid muscle; this overlies the internal jugular vein, where it can be accessed by venepucture or open surgery.

severe because pressure cannot be applied to the subclavian vein, and one is usually inserting larger catheters in these larger proximal veins. Unwanted entry into the subclavian artery or the innominate artery bifurcation are possible, and must be recognized before any infusion. Ensure that the needle is kept close to the clavicle, to avoid damage to the pleura or the apex of the lung.

The internal jugular vein has a consistent surface marking deep to the triangle formed by the clavicular and sternal heads of the sternomastoid muscle, and the upper border of the clavicle. This can be palpated when turning the chin to the opposite side (figure 105a). The patient lies supine, with their feet slightly raised, to engorge the internal jugular system. The needle is passed caudally in the parasagittal plane, at an angle of 30 degrees to the skin; it enters the internal jugular vein or its

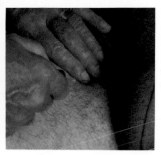

Figure 106 The femoral artery is palpated over the midinguinal point (midway between anterior superior iliac spine and midline). The vein is medial to the artery. If nonpulsatile, the firm cylinder of the occluded artery is usually still palpable.

junction with the subclavian vein (figure 105b). Problems of bruising and intra-arterial injection are again present. Venous access in the internal jugular and subclavian veins is facilitated by using ultrasonic guidance. The internal jugular site defined is also appropriate for surgical access. Another common surgical approach is through the terminal cephalic vein, as it passes along the medial border of the deltoid, over the clavicular head or pectoralis major, before it passes under the clavicle. A Hickman line is commonly inserted through both the internal jugular and cephalic vein approaches.

In the lower limb, rapid access to a large vein is through the femoral. The femoral artery is palpated with one hand and, after skin preparation, the needle is introduced a centimeter medial to this point and pointed cranially, at an angle of 30–40 degrees to the surface (figure 106). If the upper limb is inappropriate for long-term access, the great saphenous vein at the ankle has a consistent site, as it ascends over the anterior surface of the medial malleolus of the lower tibia. It is first palpated, by rolling from side to side, and proximal compression is applied before access with a needle or a cannula (figure 107a,b). Complications are again bruising, and local infection and thrombosis of the line; the approach restricts mobility. The saphenous nerve is closely applied to the vein and should be avoided.

Intra-arterial injections are usually the concern of experienced clinicians, such as radiologists, cardiologists or anesthetists. Aseptic precautions and preparation are again essential. The main difference is the direction of needle access. This is usually at 30–45 degrees to the skin surface, puncturing both anterior and posterior walls of the artery in a single movement, to transfix and stabilize the vessel; the needle is slowly withdrawn, while applying suction, until the lumen is reached. On withdrawal of arterial blood, lower your hand and advance the needle or cannula along the lumen and apply suitable equipment.

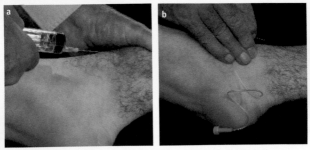

Figure 107 a,b. Venepuncture and cannulation of great saphenous vein.

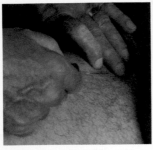

Figure 108 Puncture of femoral artery just below midinguinal point.

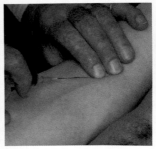

Figure 109 Puncture of brachial artery.

Figure 110 Puncture of radial artery over lower end of radius.

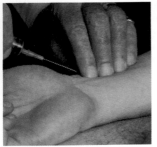

The commonest radiological approach is through the femoral artery (figure 108). This is palpated over the midinguinal point, i.e., midway between the anterior superior iliac spine and the midline, just below the inguinal ligament; this lies above the groin crease. The brachial artery is a common approach for the cardiologist, either by direct stab or a small cut down. With the extended arm, the brachial artery can be palpated against the lower humerus at the upper border of the cubital fossa, the median nerve crosses it above this level and lies on its medial side (figure 109). The radial artery is easily accessible but requires sound technique. It is palpated over the anterior lower radius, just before it passes underneath abductor pollicis longus, to enter the anatomical snuffbox (figure 110). In all arterial punctures, a constant firm pressure must be applied for four to five minutes on withdrawal of the needle or cannula.

LYMPHATIC SYSTEM

The lymphatic system collects excess tissue fluid and large particles, particularly proteins and protein debris, and returns them to the blood-stream. The extensive **lymphatic plexuses** that cover the surface of the body, and all organs except the brain, are not usually visible unless they become inflamed (**lymphangitis**). The **lymph nodes** placed along the lymphatic collecting pathways are palpable, and become enlarged in certain diseases. The final common pathways back to the venous system are through the thoracic duct and the right lymphatic duct, respectively passing to the left and right subclavian veins.

Maldevelopment of lymphatics (**aplasia**, **hypoplasia**, and **hyperplasia**) may lead to an accumulation of tissue fluid (**primary lymphedema** – figure 111), and this may also occur with occlusion of the lymphatic

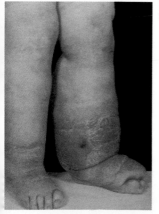

Figure 111 Primary lower limb lymphedema.

Table 3 **SWOLLEN LEG**

LOCAL	SYSTEMIC
Venous thrombosis and venous insufficiency	Cardiac failure
Arteriovenous fistula	Constrictive pericarditis
Neurofibromatosis	Renal failure
Lipidemia	Hepatic failure
	Hypoproteinemia – malnutrition, beri beri
LYMPHEDEMA	Myxedema
Primary:	Cushing's syndrome
Congenital malformation: onset at birth, puberty or late in life	
Secondary:	
Chronic infection	
Cellulitis	
Abscess formation	
Pyomyositis	
Chronic ulceration	
Trauma: including sunburn, insect and animal bites	
Radiation fibrosis	
Surgical lymphadenectomy	
Metastatic and local malignancy (notably Kaposi sarcoma, lymphosarcoma, malignant melanoma)	
Artifactual: edema bleu	
Tropical infection:	
Filariasis	
Onchocerciasis	
Mycetoma	
Dracunculiasis	
Lymphogranuloma venereum	
Cutaneous larva migrans	

vessels and nodes, as with chronic inflammatory and metastatic disease, radiotherapy, and after surgical removal (**secondary lymphedema**). The causes of a swollen leg are considered in table 3.

Lymph node enlargement (**lymphadenopathy**) may be primary, due to lymphoid disease (**Hodgkin** and **non-Hodgkin lymphoma**) or secondary. The latter is usually due to inflammatory or metastatic disease (table 4). Lymph node enlargement secondary to acute inflammation is very

Table 4 **LYMPHADENOPATHY**

ACUTE INFECTION		CHRONIC INFECTION	PRIMARY MALIGNANCY	SECONDARY MALIGNANCY
Local: Inflammation, infection adjacent skin, mucous membrane, glandular epithelium Cervical nodes typically upper respiratory tract infection Inguinal nodes include infections listed under leg swelling (table 3)	**Generalized:** Measles Rubella Varicella Glandular fever Toxoplasmosis Cytomegalo-virus Cat scratch fever	**Local:** Tuberculosis Sarcoid Histiocytosis Syphilis	Hodgkin, non-Hodgkin lymphoma	Almost any malignancy can pass to any nodal group, but usually from local disease, e.g., cervical from the upper aerodigestive tracts (exceptions e.g., scalene node from abdominal malignancy) Inguinal nodes primarily from lower limb, anal canal and perineum. Marked nodal enlargement; Kaposi, lympho-sarcoma, malignant melanoma

common, e.g., lymph nodes are the commonest lump in the neck (figure 112). Lymphadenopathy often occurs at specific sites and this can be a useful diagnostic feature, e.g., the **jugulodigastric** node is commonly involved with disease of the anterior two-thirds of the tongue, and all lymph from the tongue drains via the **jugulo-omohyoid** node.

When examining the lymphatic system, start with the head and neck, proceed to examine the axillae and, if enlarged nodes are located, examine for inguinal, epitrochlear and popliteal node enlargement, and for hepatosplenomegaly. In practice, in the absence of demonstrable or suspected lymphadenopathy, examine the axillae with the breasts in the

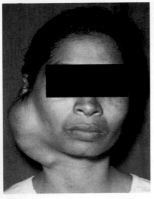

Figure 112 Cervical lyphadenopathy of tuberculous origin.

female and with the thorax in the male. The inguinal nodes are then palpated when you examine the inguinal, scrotal, and perineal regions.

Cervical Nodes

The lateral view of the head and neck in figure 113 demonstrates lymph nodes, salivary and thyroid glands, the common carotid artery bifurcation, and the internal jugular vein.

The cervical lymph nodes are commonly enlarged, secondary to infective conditions of the tonsil, throat, ear and nose, and are the commonest lumps in the neck. They may occasionally undergo suppuration with abscess formation, which is most common with tuberculous infections. Cervical node enlargement may also be the first sign of generalized lymphatic disease or of metastases. The latter may be from anywhere in the head and neck, but also elsewhere in the body and it may require extensive investigation to find the primary lesion: particular attention must be given to the breast and lung.

The **submental**, **submandibular**, **parotid**, **postauricular**, and **occipital** nodes are examined in their circle around the base of the skull (figure 114a–e).

The **deep cervical lymph chain** lies around the internal jugular vein; commence your examination in the submandibular triangle. The chain passes deep to the sternomastoid muscle and, in the lower neck, extends laterally into the supraclavicular region (figure 115a–c).

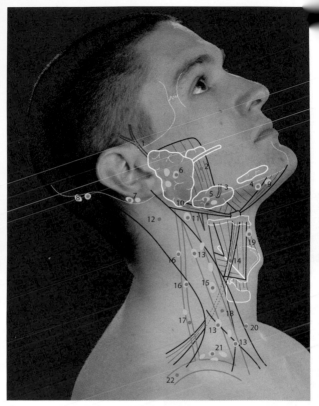

Figure 113 Anatomy of cervical lymphatic chains.

1. Superficial temporal artery
2. Masseter muscle
3. Facial artery
4. Submental
5. Submandibular gland
6. Superfical and deep parotid
7. Posterior auricular
8. Occipital
9. Anterior belly of digastric muscle
10. Posterior belly of digastric muscle
11. Jugulodiagastric
12. Sternomastoid muscle
13. Deep cervical lymph chain
14. Omohyoid muscle
15. Jugulo-omohyoid
16. Superficial cervical lymph chain
17. External jugular vein
18. Internal jugular vein
19. Prelaryngeal
20. Pretracheal
21. Supraclavicular
22. Subclavian vein

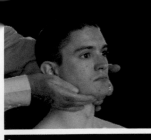

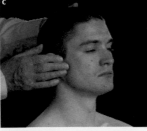

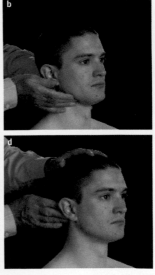

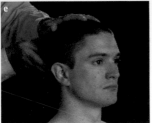

Figure 114 a,b,c,d,e. Examination of lymphatic groups around skull base: submental; submandibular; parotid; postauricular; occipital.

Although the vast majority of cervical lymphadenopathy is related to head and neck disease, the **scalene** nodes are an exception. This group of **supraclavicular** nodes is situated behind the lower end of the sternomastoid muscle. They are a common site for metastases from breast, lung, gastrointestinal, and genitourinary malignancies, particularly on the left side.

The scalene nodes can easily be missed if you do not palpate deep to the sternomastoid. To assess whether a mass is deep, fixed to, or superficial to the sternomastoid muscle, ask the subject to turn their chin away from the side being examined, pressing against your hand. This allows the demonstration of mobility of superficial or deep masses in relation to the tensed muscle (figure 116a–c).

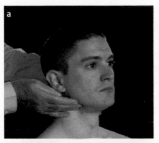

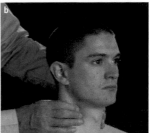

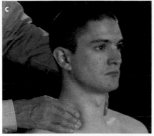

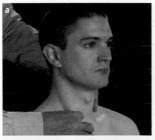

Figure 115 a,b,c. Examination of deep cervical lymph chain: submandibular triangle; along the internal jugular vein.

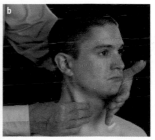

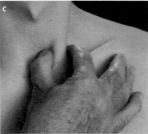

Figure 116 a,b,c. Palpation deep to lateral head of sternomastoid muscle for scalene node enlargement. Tension in the muscle determines whether the lump is superficial or deep to its fibers.

Smaller **superficial cervical** nodes are frequently palpable along the line of the external (figure 117), and to a lesser extent the anterior, jugular veins.

Palpate the superficial lymph chain along the length of the external jugular vein completing the examination by palpation along the borders of the trachea and larynx for nodes along the anterior jugular vein. Occasionally nodes are encountered on the isthmus of the thyroid gland

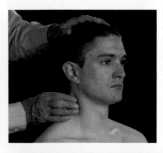

Figure 117 Superficial chains lie along external and anterior jugular veins, with occasional pretracheal and prelaryngeal nodes.

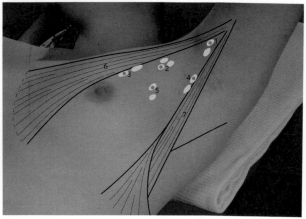

Figure 118 Axillary node anatomy.

1. Lateral
2. Apical
3. Anterior
4. Posterior
5. Medial
6. Anterior axillary fold (pectoralis major)
7. Posterior axillary fold (teres major and tendon of latissimus dorsi)

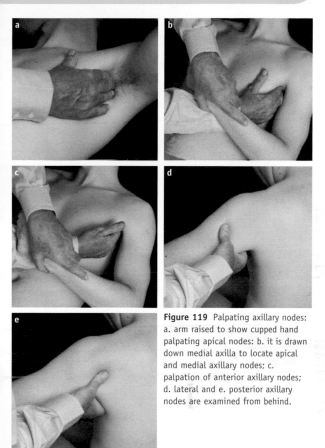

Figure 119 Palpating axillary nodes: a. arm raised to show cupped hand palpating apical nodes: b. it is drawn down medial axilla to locate apical and medial axillary nodes; c. palpation of anterior axillary nodes; d. lateral and e. posterior axillary nodes are examined from behind.

and over the larynx; these small "delphium" nodes are related to thyroid and other superficial malignancies.

Axillary Nodes

Figure 118 illustrates the anatomy of the axillary nodes.

When examining axillary nodes, take the weight of the subject's arm in your non-palpating hand.

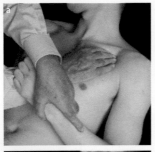

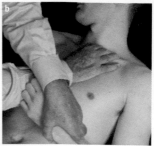

Figure 120 a,b,c. Examination of infraclavicular and supraclavicular nodes.

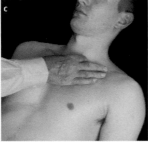

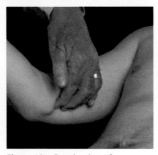

Figure 121 Examination of epitrochlear nodes.

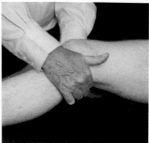

Figure 122 Popliteal nodes lie deep in popliteal fossa.

In the illustrations, the arm is raised to demonstrate the position of the cupped hand palpating the apical nodes. In practice, the arm lies by the subject's side as your hand is drawn down over the medial wall, searching for **apical** and **medial** axillary nodes (figure 119a,b). The **anterior** nodes are compressed against the anterior wall of the axilla

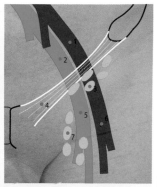

Figure 123 Inguinal nodes are horizontal, parallel to the inguinal ligament, and vertical, along the femoral vein.

1.2. External iliac artery and vein
3. Horizontal and 7. vertical groups of inguinal nodes
4. Inguinal ligament
5.6. Femoral vessels

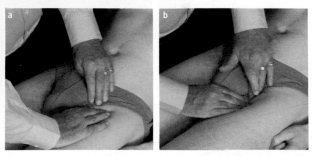

Figure 124 Examination of a. horizontal and b. vertical groin nodes.

(figure 119c), and the **lateral** and **posterior** axillary nodes are examined from behind (figure 119d,e).

This is followed by examination of the **infraclavicular** and **supraclavicular** lymphatic drainage sites (figure 120a–c).

Other lymphatic sites: epitrochlear nodes are palpated just above the medial epicondyle of the humerus (figure 121).

Popliteal nodes may be palpable deeply placed over the popliteal vein in the lower aspect of the popliteal fossa (figure 122).

The **horizontal** group of **inguinal** nodes lies below and parallel to the inguinal ligament, and the **vertical** group along the femoral vein, in the femoral triangle (figure 123). Inguinal nodes are commonly palpable in normal subjects (figure 124a,b), but are the site of a number of specific diseases, particularly related to anal pathology (table 11, page 339).

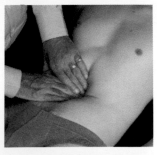

Figure 125 Examination of preaortic and para-aortic nodes.

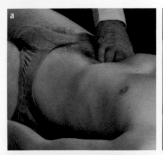

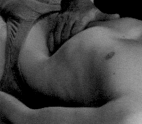

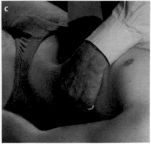

Figure 126 a,b,c. Examining for hepatomegaly and splenomegaly.

Lymphatic drainage of the lower limb and perineum is to the iliac and **para-aortic** nodes, and that of the alimentary tract to the **preaortic** nodes; the testis drains to both aortic groups. Palpate deeply along the midline when looking for these **para-aortic** groups (figure 125).

When searching for evidence of abdominal and other malignancy, make sure you also examine the **liver** and **spleen** (figure 126a–c).

Female Breast and Axilla

The female breast is formed of 15–20 **lobules** of glandular tissue embedded in a variable amount of **fat**. The lobules are separated by **fascial septa** (ligaments of **Cooper**) that blend deeply with the investing layer of superficial fascia and, superficially, are attached to the overlying skin. The **ducts** from each lobule join to form a lactiferous duct that opens onto the nipple. The skin of the nipple and the surrounding areola is thin and pigmented, and contains a number of modified sebaceous glands (glands of **Montgomery**) and smooth muscle.

The **base** of the breast extends vertically from the second to the sixth ribs, and horizontally from the sternal edge to the midaxillary line (figure 1). It rests mainly on the pectoralis major muscle, but also laterally on the external oblique and serratus anterior muscles. An extension of breast tissue from the upper outer quadrant extends into the axilla (**axillary tail**).

The breast has subcutaneous and submammary **lymphatic plexuses** that drain mainly to the **axillary lymph nodes**. It may also drain directly to the infraclavicular nodes, nodes around the internal thoracic artery, lymphatics over the abdominal wall, and to the opposite breast.

The female breast undergoes extensive changes during life, particularly at the menarche and during parturition, and undergoes cyclical variation with menstruation; **nodularity** and **cystic changes** are therefore frequently encountered. Most lumps are benign and nodularity, discomfort and tenderness are common symptoms, and often bilateral. However,

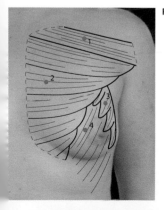

Figure 1 Anatomy of left breast.

1. Clavicular and
2. sternal heads of pectoralis major
3. Serratus anterior
4. External oblique

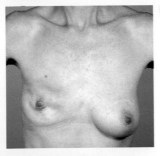

Figure 2 Carcinoma of right breast.

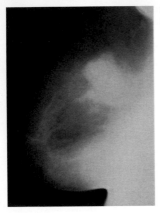

Figure 3 Mammogram of malignant lesion of breast.

cancer of the breast may present with similar signs, and it is essential to ensure early diagnosis and treatment of this common female malignancy. A rise in public awareness of the need to treat early breast malignancy has prompted self-examination and attendance at screening programmes. Patients with breast cancer usually present with a **lump** (figure 2), but **pain** and **nipple discharge** are important symptoms to fully investigate.

Take a full menstrual history, noting pregnancies, breast feeding, use of the pill, and hormone replacement. Ask about previous lumps, their management and any family history of breast malignancy. The most important genetic link is premenstrual malignancy in a first-degree relative. A persistent or progressive lump requires further investigation, possibly with **mammography** or **needle aspiration**. Mammography can be diagnostic of benign or malignant disease, while aspiration may remove both the cyst and the accompanying anxiety (figure 3). A fine needle aspirate from solid lesions is examined histologically. A subsequent diagnosis of malignancy allows patient involvement in the planned intervention.

Progression of local malignancy gives rise to skin and deep tethering, nipple inversion and, when more extensive, skin ulceration. There may also be spread to local lymph nodes and **metastases**, particularly to bone, liver, and lungs; these areas are a routine part of the physical examination of breast disease.

The commonest nipple **discharge** is milk and this may persist after pregnancy or present at other times (**galactorrhea**), such as with endocrine abnormalities. Green or yellow discharge is often associated with **cystic disease** of the breast, blood staining may accompany benign or malignant lesions and the cause must always be identified.

Other abnormalities include breast **infection**, and **supernumerary breasts** and **nipples** along the milk line (from the axilla to the symphysis pubis). Although the male breast is rudimentary, it is subject to the same range of diseases as the female.

EXAMINATION

Seclusion and warmth are particularly important for examination of the breasts, to avoid discomfort and embarrassment to a patient; a good light is essential to detect minor abnormalities.

There is wide variation in the size, shape and consistency of the female breast, not only between individuals, but also in each subject, during development, the menstrual cycle, pregnancy, and in later life. If the breasts are asymmetrical establish if this is recent or longstanding.

The nipple usually points forward; unilateral or bilateral nipple retraction may be congenital, but recent changes and nipple deviation suggest underlying disease, as do a discharge or surrounding eczema (**Paget disease**). The initial pink-colored areolar becomes darker with age and brownish after pregnancy. The glands of Montgomery may stand out as tubercles, especially in pregnancy.

Start the examination with **inspection** (figure 4); this must always precede palpation. The subject is undressed to the waist and sits upright on the side of the couch. Observe from the front. Look for lumps in the breasts and axillae, flattening of the breast contour and skin dimpling.

Abnormal features are accentuated during arm movements and fixation. At first, ask the subject to rest her hands on the couch, on each side (figure 5a–c). This is followed by raising her arms above her head and leaning forward, and then by pressing the hands together, or on the

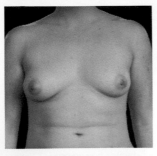

Figure 4 Observation in the sitting position, looking for symmetry and abnormality.

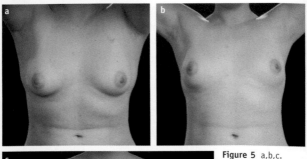

Figure 5 a,b,c. Asymmetry accentuated by arm raising, leaning forward and backward, and pressing down on hips.

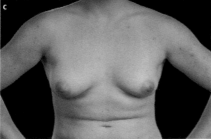

hips. To assess tethering to the serratus anterior muscles, the subject leans forward with outstretched hands against resistance.

During these movements, observe the breasts for symmetry, compare the two sides and note the mobility of the breast on the chest wall. Elevation may produce unequal ascent in the presence of underlying abnormalities; it also allows examination of the skin under the breasts. Note any redness, edema, peau d'orange, ulceration, skin nodularity, or abnormal venous patterns that could indicate associated pathology.

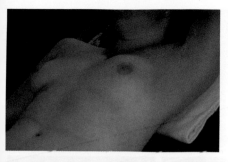

Figure 6 Position of breast for clinical and self-examination.

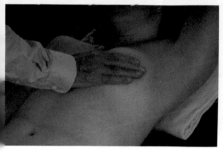

Figure 7 Palpation over central breast.

Palpate the breast with the subject lying flat on the couch with the hand of the same side placed behind her head, and a pillow behind her shoulder (figure 6). This position serves to relax the pectoral muscles and allow the breast to spread evenly, "floating" on the chest wall. If an abnormality has been reported on one side, begin with the other. On coming to the abnormal side, ask the patient to point out the area of abnormality, if it is not obvious.

Begin palpation with gentle pressure and rotation of the flat of the hand over the central part of the breast (figure 7).

Examine every part of the breast systematically. A possible technique is to start with the upper inner quadrant and progress anticlockwise (on the left; clockwise on the right) to the upper outer quadrant and the axillary tail (figure 8a–d). Palpate with the flat of the outstretched fingers with rotatory and to-and-fro movements, gently pressing the breast tissue onto the chest wall.

Be sure to gently palpate the nipple area and retroareolar tissues between the fingers and thumb, to detect any nodularity within this region (figure 9). In the case of nipple discharge, particularly in

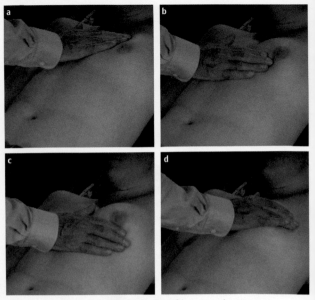

Figure 8 a,b,c,d. Systematic examination of breast quadrants.

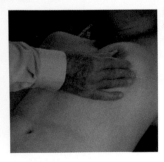

Figure 9 Gentle palpation of nipple, for local abnormality and expression of any discharge.

galactorrhea, gently **express** fluid from the breast by mediolateral and superoinferior expression, followed by expression from the nipple, and spread any discharge on a slide for microscopy.

Abnormal areas are further palpated between finger and thumb: pendulous breasts may have to be examined bimanually (figure 10). The axillary tail requires particular attention to define lumps.

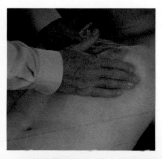

Figure 10 Bimanual examination is useful in the larger breast.

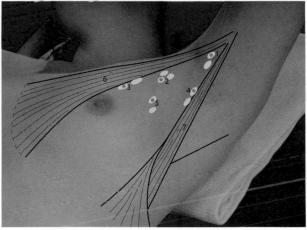

Figure 11 Anatomy of axillary nodes.

1. Lateral
2. Apical
3. Anterior
4. Posterior

5. Medial
6. Anterior axillary fold (pectoralis major)
7. Posterior axillary fold (teres major and tendon of latissimus dorsi)

Measure and record the size, shape, consistency, and mobility of any abnormal areas. **Tethering** to the underlying fascia and muscles is defined by asking the subject to press her hands on her hips, and then moving the abnormal area to-and-fro in different directions. Superficial tethering is demonstrated by gently squeezing the overlying skin to assess whether it is free of the underlying abnormality. Normal breast

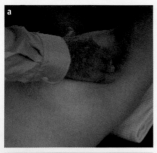

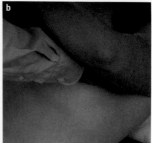

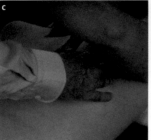

Figure 12 a,b,c. Examination of apical and medial axillary nodes.

tissue is commonly nodular and becomes engorged premenstrually. In doubtful cases, repeat the examination at a different time in the menstrual cycle.

AXILLA

Examination of the axilla is a routine part of the general examination of the lymphatic system. It is of particular importance in examination of the female breast, as much of the lymphatic drainage from the organ is to this group of nodes (figure 11). For the left axilla, take the weight of the subject's left arm in your left hand. Now use your right hand to examine the axilla.

Cup your fingers and press them upwards and inwards into the apex of the axilla. Lower the subject's arm onto your hand, and draw your fingers downwards over the medial wall, to palpate the **apical** and **medial** nodes (figure 12a–c). During this maneuver explain what you are doing and that pressure is being applied. Watch the subject's face to ensure that it does not cause any marked discomfort.

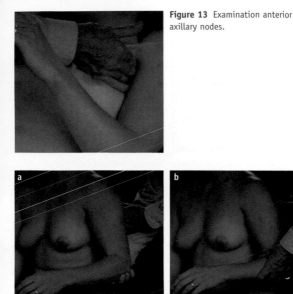

Figure 13 Examination anterior axillary nodes.

Figure 14 a,b. Examination from behind: posterior and lateral axillary nodes.

Examine the **anterior** group (figure 13) of lymph nodes against the muscles and the fascia of the anterior wall of the axilla, and between the pectoralis major and minor muscles.

The **posterior** and **lateral** groups of axillary lymph nodes are more easily palpated from behind; apply pressure respectively to the posterior wall of the axilla, and the medial aspects of the humeral neck and shaft (figure 14a,b).

In examination of the right axilla the procedure is repeated, using your right hand to support the subject's right arm and palpating with your left hand. It is common to find small palpable axillary nodes in the normal subject and these are often termed "shotty nodes." They can be found on self-examination. Note any swelling of the arm that could be indicative of lymphatic obstruction.

On completion of examination of the axilla on each side, palpate the **infraclavicular** and **supraclavicular** fossae for their respective groups of

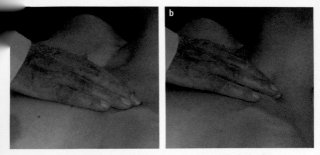

Figure 15 a,b. Assessment of infraclavicular and supraclavicular fossae.

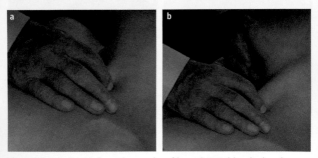

Figure 16 a,b. Search for scalene nodes of lower internal jugular lymph chain.

nodes (figure 15a,b). In the latter, look particularly for the scalene node behind the lower attachment of the sternomastoid muscle.

Enlarged **scalene** nodes should be specifically looked for, not only in breast, but also lung and abdominal malignancies. Ask the subject to turn their head to the other side, against your hand, to define the sternal head and the relationship of any lump to the muscle (figure 16a,b).

Complete the examination of the breast by examining for **hepatomegaly** (figure 17), and tenderness along the length of the spine. **Spinal tenderness** is first explored by digital pressure and, if no tenderness is found, progress to more vigorous percussion of a fist on the back of the other hand (figure 18a,b).

Patients should also be instructed in self-examination, observing for symmetry in front of a mirror with arms at their sides, raised, and

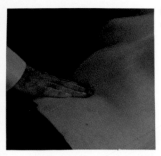

Figure 17 Examining for hepatomegaly.

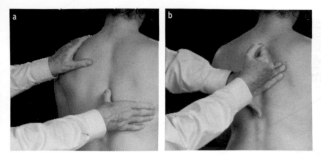

Figure 18 a,b. Palpating for spinal tenderness.

pressed on hips. They should then lie with their hand behind their head and the shoulder supported on a pillow, as already described, palpating with the opposite hand.

Explain the technique of examination of the breast described, and cupping the fingers into the axilla. Medical advice should be sought for new symptoms or changing signs.

Abdomen

ALIMENTARY TRACT

The alimentary tract starts at the mouth and extends to the anus. Thus, examination includes these areas as well as the abdomen. Disease of the alimentary tract may also produce systemic effects and alimentary examination commences with the:

a) **hands**
b) **conjunctivae and sclera**, for subconjunctival pallor and jaundice (page 16)
c) **root of the neck**, for supraclavicular lymphadenopathy (page 267)
d) **mouth**, tongue, teeth, gums, and salivary glands.

Hands (page 7)

In the hands (figure 1), the nails may show pallor and/or **koilonychia**. **Clubbing** may be present in chronic liver and bowel disease. Liver damage may also produce **palmar erythema** and **spider nevi**.

Examination of the mouth

Halitosis (bad breath – figure 2) may be due to bad teeth, and infection and ulceration of the gums or oral mucosa. Other causes include infection, and degenerative tumors of the nose and paranasal air sinuses, bronchiectasis and intestinal obstruction. Ketoacidosis, uremia

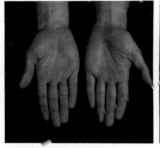

Figure 1 Hands.

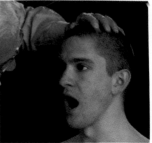

Figure 2 Examining for halitosis.

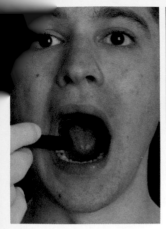

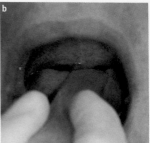

Figure 3 a,b. Use of torch and spatula.

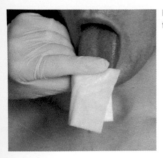

Figure 4 Tongue drawn forward to facilitate examination of oropharynx.

and hepatic failure have specific fetors, as do alcohol and certain drugs, such as paraldehyde.

The lips may be dry and fissured, and fissuring of the angles of the mouth may accompany nutritional problems and **anemia**.

Examination of the mouth requires a good light. This may be provided by daylight, but usually a torch (figure 3a) or lamp is necessary. A torch, tongue depressor, and disposable gloves are useful accessories for detailed inspection and palpation of the mouth. A spatula (figure 3b) allows movement of the lips, cheek, and tongue to observe these areas; this may be aided by a dental mirror. Palpation is with a gloved finger, while your other hand, placed externally, is used for bimanual

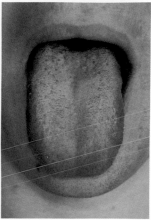

Figure 5 Examination of tongue.

exploration of the floor of the mouth and the cheeks. The tongue can be pulled forward and held with a swab (figure 4), to examine its sides and adjacent structures.

The tongue (figure 5) is a good indicator of **systemic disease**, as well as being prone to specific disorders, such as **congenital abnormalities**, **glossitis**, and benign and malignant **tumors**. There is a good deal of variation of ethnic **pigmentation** and capillary pattern, such as geographic tongue. The pallor of **anemia**, central cyanosis, and the yellow tinge of jaundice may be recognized in all races.

Note any **furring** of the tongue; many tongue coatings have no clinical significance or may reflect a recent meal, or a specific dietary habit. **Dietary deficiencies**, such as vitamin C and D, may produce an abnormally smooth tongue; coating is increased in heavy smokers and mouth breathers. Oral **candidiasis** produces a white fungal coating; it occurs in debilitating disease, prolonged antibiotic or steroid therapy, immunological diseases (e.g., sarcoidosis), immunodeficiency (e.g., HIV) and with immunosuppressive drugs.

Mouth breathing may dehydrate the surface of the tongue; however, when this is accompanied by the loss of **skin turgor** and **sunken eyes**, it is a valuable indicator of the general state of dehydration, such as postoperatively, in fevers and with reduced fluid intake. There may be tongue atrophy in the Plumber-Vincent syndrome, associated with **angular stomatitis** and abnormalities of the gastric mucous membrane.

Ulcerated tongue

Ulceration of the tongue is common and is usually due to dental trauma and **aphthous ulcers**. In the former there may be sharp teeth or poorly fitting dentures and the gums must be carefully checked for any associated damage. Falls, fits and sports or other injuries may be associated with tongue biting, and fish bones may lodge anywhere in the tongue or alimentary tract producing trauma and infection.

Aphthous ulcers may be associated with generalized disease but are usually of unknown etiology. Ulcers may also be associated with inflammatory changes of the tongue and this **glossitis** may be due to generalized disease. Examples are drug reactions, such as Stevens-Johnson and Magic syndromes. Sexually transmitted diseases causing glossitis and inflammation include HIV, syphilis and gonorrhea, and may be part of Reiter syndrome. **Autoimmune** connective tissue disorders and occasionally gut abnormalities (such as ulcerative colitis and Crohn's disease) have associated mouth ulceration. White patches are associated with **candida** but also with **lichen planus**, a disorder of unknown etiology. It has a number of characteristic patterns usually involving the edges of the tongue associated with mucosal atrophy and erosions. An important differential diagnosis of a white coating is **leukoplakia**, a premalignant condition (figure 6); note that this cannot be removed by scratching the mucosal surface.

Large tongues are seen in **hypothyroidism** and **acromegaly**, in developmental abnormalities and associated with some **congenital disorders**, such as Down syndrome.

The tongue receives bilateral cortical innervation, therefore wasting only occurs with bilateral upper motor neuron lesions (**pseudobulbar palsy**). However, the twelfth nerve nucleus may be affected by motor neuron disease and nerve damage from surgical or other trauma. With lower motor neuron paralysis the tongue deviates towards the side of the lesion (page 61). Tongue weakness and difficulty in swallowing may be present in **myasthenia gravis** and **Parkinson** disease. Thus disease can often be well demonstrated by asking the patient to stick their tongue out.

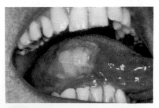

Figure 6 Extensive white area of leukoplakia, it cannot be scraped off and is premalignant.

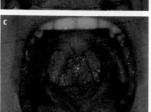

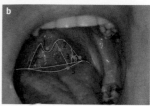

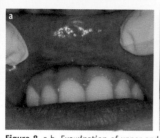

Figure 7 a,b,c. Floor of mouth; tonsillar bed; oropharynx.

1. Uvula
2. Posterior (palatopharyngeus) and
4. anterior (palatoglossus) pillars of fauces
3. Tonsil
5. Sulcus terminalis

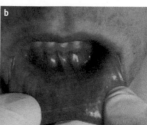

Figure 8 a,b Examination of upper and lower lips.

The features described in the examination of the tongue apply equally to the mucous membrane of the rest of the **mouth** and **pharynx** (figure 7a–c). Observe the inside of the upper and lower lip (figure 8a,b) and sulci passing on to the gums. Inspect the tonsillar bed and the oropharynx for **erythema** and nodularity. The **tonsils** and the lymphoid follicles on the back of the oropharynx are often prominent in young subjects and may become infected (figure 9). Note the mucosa over the hard and soft palate (figure 10), and the movement of the soft palate when asked to say "ah."

Teeth, Gums

The average eruption times of each half of the upper and lower jaws are:

	Eruption of deciduous (months)		
	I	C	M
Upper jaw	7 8	18	12 24
Lower jaw	6 9	18	12 24

	Eruption of permanent (years)			
	I	C	P	M
Upper jaw	7 8	12	9 12	6 12 18+
Lower jaw	7 8	12	9 10	6 12 18+

The first deciduous tooth is a lower central incisor; the first permanent tooth is a first molar. The lower permanent teeth appear slightly earlier than the upper. The wisdom teeth (third molars) appear between the 17th and 25th years and are usually the first to be shed.

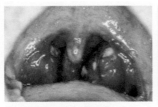

Figure 9 Tonsils frequently enlarge and suppurate, with occasional abscess (quinsy) formation.

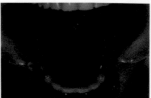

Figure 10 Palate: photographed through mirror; a dental mirror is a valuable tool for palatal examination.

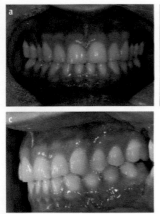

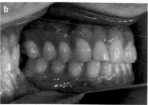

Figure 11 a,b,c. Views of teeth.

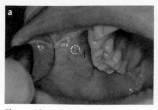

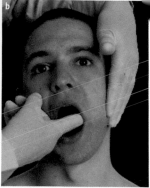

Figure 12 a. Opening of parotid duct opposite second upper molar tooth; b. bimanual examination of gland.

1. Opening of duct opposite crown of second upper molar

Note the number and the state of the teeth (figure 11). Normal gums are closely applied to the teeth but may recede and become infected or, in some conditions, **hypertrophic**. In edentulous subjects examine the gums for evidence of damage from dentures.

Salivary Glands

The large paired salivary glands (parotid, submandibular, submaxillary) are subject to generalized **enlargement**: this may be symmetrical, as in mumps, or variable as in sarcoid, and Sjögren and Mikulicz syndromes. Like all glands, they are subject to **inflammation** and **neoplasia**, while blocking of a duct, by a **stone** or inspissated debris, may produce intermittent swelling on eating, and progress to retrograde infection and **abscess** formation. Swellings of the submandibular and parotid glands are easily mistaken for enlargement of the overlying lymph nodes.

The **parotid duct** opens opposite the crown of the second upper molar tooth (figure 12a). The **parotid gland** is palpated mainly externally but also bimanually around the anterior border of the ramus of the mandible (figure 12b). The gland extends below and behind the angle of the jaw and parotid lumps in this region may be difficult to differentiate from lymph nodes or submandibular gland enlargement. Abscess formation (figure 13) is less common, and is in children or debilitated adults.

The **submandibular ducts** open on the sublingual papillae on either side of the midline, adjacent to the frenulum of the tongue (figure 14a). Saliva can be seen to exude from the papillae and occasionally a submandibular calculus becomes lodged at this site. The **sublingual** and **submandibular glands** can be palpated bimanually throughout their lengths in the floor of the mouth (figure 14b).

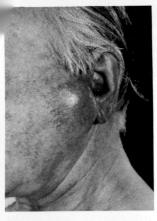

Figure 13 Parotid abscess is usually in children or a debilitated adult.

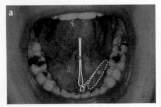

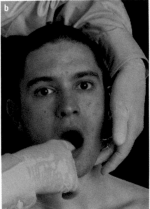

Figure 14 a. Submandibular duct opening (the sublingual gland is outlined); b. bimanual examination of gland.

1. Frenulum
2. Sublinguinal gland
3. Submandibular papilla, containing opening of submandibular duct

ABDOMEN

The **anterior abdominal wall** extends from the lower costal margin down to the **iliac crests**, **inguinal ligaments**, and the **symphysis pubis**. However, the abdominal cavity passes up behind the rib cage under the diaphragm, to the level of the fourth intercostal space, and down into the pelvis to the pelvic diaphragm, formed by the levator ani muscles. The anterior and lateral aspects of the abdominal wall are formed of the

Table 1 MUSCLES OF THE ANTERIOR ABDOMINAL WALL

MUSCLE	SUPERIOR/ LATERAL ATTACHMENT	INFERIOR/ MEDIAL ATTACHMENT	FUNCTION	NERVE SUPPLY
External oblique	Outer surface of the lower eight ribs	Linea alba, pubic tubercle, forms the inguinal ligament with the opening of the superficial inguinal ring, anterior half of the iliac crest	All these muscles support and compress the abdominal contents, partake in respiratory movement and, to a variable extent, flex and rotate the trunk	T6-T12
Internal oblique	Thoracolumbar fascia, iliac crest and lateral two-thirds of the inguinal ligament	Costal margin, linea alba and pubic crest via the conjoint tendon (arching over the inguinal canal)		T6-T12, L1
Transversus abdominis	Internal surface of the lower six costal cartilages, thoracolumbar fascia, iliac crest, and lateral third of the inguinal ligament	Jointly, with internal oblique, to the linea alba, pubic crest via the conjoint tendon; with the oblique muscles, forms the rectus sheath		T7-T12, L1
Rectus abdominis	Xiphoid process, anterior aspect of the fifth to the seventh costal cartilages	Pubic symphysis, pubic crest		T7-T12

three layers of flat **abdominal wall muscles** (table 1) that contain and compress the abdominal contents (defecation, micturition, coughing, and parturition) and participate in respiratory movements, and flexion and rotation of the trunk. Posteriorly, the wall is formed by the **erector**

Table 2 **MUSCLES OF THE POSTERIOR ABDOMINAL WALL**

MUSCLE	SUPERIOR ATTACHMENT	INFERIOR ATTACHMENT	FUNCTION	NERVE SUPPLY
Psoas major	Fibrous arches across the bodies and the transverse processes of the lumbar vertebrae, and the T12 and lumbar intervertebral discs	Psoas and iliacus have a common attachment to the lesser trochanter of the femur	Psoas and iliacus act together as a powerful flexor and weak medial rotator of the femur, and raise the trunk from the sitting position	L1,2,3
Iliacus	Concavity of the iliac fossa, and adjacent iliac crest, iliolumbar ligament and sacrum			L2,3
Quadratus lumborum	Medial half of the lower border of the twelfth rib	Iliolumbar ligament and adjacent iliac crest	Fixes the twelfth rib in trunk movement and respiration	T12,L1,2,3

spinae muscles, with the psoas and quadratus lumborum lying within the cavity (page 86; table 2).

The abdominal cavity is lined by **parietal peritoneum**, which is reflected from the posterior wall around the gut and abdominal organs as the visceral peritoneum. Sensation from the parietal peritoneum (usually due to inflammation) is appreciated directly over it, whereas that of the **visceral peritoneum** may be referred to its dermatome of derivation (e.g., sensation from under the diaphragm is referred to the tip of the shoulder and that of the small gut to the umbilicus).

For descriptive and recording purposes, the anterior abdominal wall is divided by two horizontal and two vertical lines, into nine regions (figure 15). The horizontal lines are the **subcostal** and **transtubercular** and the vertical lines pass through the **midinguinal** point and cross the

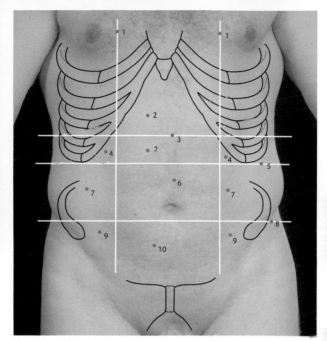

Figure 15 Abdominal planes.

1. Vertical line through midinguinal point
2. Epigastrium
3. Transpyloric plane
4. Right and left hypochondria
5. Subcostal line
6. Umbilical
7. Lumbar regions
8. Transtubercular line
9. Right and left iliac fossae
10. Suprapubic

costal margin at the ninth costal cartilage. From above downwards, the nine regions are: centrally, the **epigastric**, **umbilical**, and **suprapubic**, and, on each side, the **hypochondral**, **lumbar**, and **iliac**. Each lumbar region extends laterally and posteriorly into the loin.

Another useful landmark is the horizontal **transpyloric plane**, midway between the suprasternal notch and the symphysis pubis. It crosses the body of the second lumbar vertebra, passes through the pylorus, just above the hilum of the right kidney and just below the hilum of the left kidney (figure 16). In clinical practice it is also common to refer to the

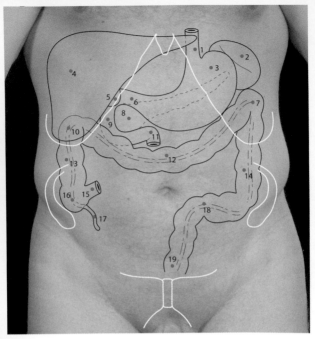

Figure 16 Abdominal viscera.

1. Esophagus
2. Spleen
3. Stomach
4. Liver
5. Gallbladder
6. Pylorus
7. Left (splenic) flexure of colon
8. Pancreas
9. Second part of duodenum
10. Right (hepatic) flexure of colon
11. Duodenojejunal flexure
12. Transverse colon
13. Ascending colon
14. Descending colon
15. Terminal ileum
16. Cecum
17. Appendix
18. Sigmoid colon
19. Rectum

four quadrants of the abdomen (upper, lower, right, left) when describing the location of abnormal signs.

Abdominal pain is a common symptom and, in view of the large number of possible causes, it can present difficulty of diagnosis (table 3). A detailed history of the pain is essential. The symptom is often specific to

Table 3 **ACUTE ABDOMINAL PAIN**

ADULTS	ELDERLY	CHILDREN	WOMEN
Appendicitis	Colorectal	Appendicitis	Pelvic
Acute colonic	cancer	Non-specific	inflammatory
diverticulitis	(obstruction	abdominal	disease
Acute	perforation)	pain	Ovarian cysts
cholecystitis	Vascular disease	Mesentric	Ectopic
Dyspepsia	(mesenteric	adenitis	pregnancy
Perforated	infarction,	Intussusception	
peptic ulcer	ruptured aortic	Hernia	
Acute	aneurysm,	Urinary tract	
pancreatitis	embolism)	infection	
Intestinal	Medical causes	Upper	
obstruction		respiratory	
Inflammatory		tract infection	
bowel disease			
Meckel's			
diverticulum			
Ureteric colic			
Rectus sheath			
hematoma			

Table 4 **NON-ABDOMINAL CAUSES OF ABDOMINAL PAIN**

- Myocardial infarction
- Aortic dissection
- Pleuritic pain
- Pulmonary embolism
- Most other intrathoracic lesions
- Herpes zoster
- Disease of the spinal cord
- Diabetes
- Hypercalcemia
- Addison's disease
- Carcinoids
- Hemochromatosis
- Uremia
- Porphyria
- Tabes dorsalis
- Sickle cell crises
- Malaria
- Lead poisoning
- Munchausen syndrome

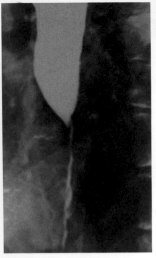

Figure 17 Stricture of upper esophagus.

a diseased organ and specific pathologies, as considered below. No attempt is made to provide a detailed pathway for the investigation of all types of abdominal pain, but the differential diagnosis is considered in each area and selected tables, including extra-abdominal causes of abdominal pain (table 4).

The site of the pain is often helpful in diagnosis. **Epigastric** pain may be related to diseases of the stomach and duodenum, and is often related to meals; weight loss is a particular feature of gastric as well as other intra-abdominal neoplasms. **Gastroenteritis** may produce central abdominal pain and tenderness, and may be accompanied by vomiting and diarrhea. The causes of **dysphagia** are considered in table 5 and figure 17 is an example of one of these disorders.

Biliary pain is commonly in the right hypochondrium and radiates through to the interscapular region. Subphrenic inflammatory irritation, such as an abscess, can present with referred pain to the tip of the shoulder.

Small gut pain is characteristically around the umbilicus and may be colicky in nature, as in intestinal obstruction, and associated with distension, vomiting, and constipation. The commonest cause of intestinal obstruction is **adhesions**, but examine the **hernial orifices** routinely, and specifically whenever obstruction is present.

Table 5 DYSPHAGIA

EXTRINSIC PRESSURE	ABNORMALITIES OF THE ESOPHAGEAL WALL	ABNORMALITIES WITHIN THE LUMEN
Goiter	Strictures:	Foreign bodies
Pharyngeal pouch	Post-traumatic	Webs
Aortic aneurysm	Benign and malignant neoplasms	Schatzki rings
Abnormal aortic arch	Radiotherapy	
Mediastinal tumors	Acute and chronic esophagitis	
Paraesophageal hiatus hernia	Corrosives	
	Crohn's disease	
	Scleroderma	
	Chagas disease	
	Esophageal diverticulum	
	Abnormalities of esophageal contraction:	
	Achalasia	
	Failure of relaxation of the cricopharyngeus	
	Cerebrovascular accidents	
	Diffuse esophageal spasm	

Appendicular pain often starts centrally, at the umbilicus, before moving to the right iliac fossa. Severe central abdominal pain radiating through to the back may be due to acute **pancreatitis**, or ruptured and dissecting abdominal aortic **aneurysms**. In the latter, check for the loss of one or both femoral pulses.

Pain and tenderness in the left iliac fossa may be due to **diverticulitis** or other large bowel pathology. **Alteration in bowel habit** in middle age and later life must be considered as due to cancer until proved otherwise. **Gynecological** problems, such as dysmenorrhea, salpingitis, ruptured ovarian cyst, ectopic pregnancies and the complications of pregnancy, usually present with lower abdominal, often suprapubic, pain.

Renal pain is typically in the lumbar region but may radiate to the inguinal region and scrotum, as can incipient or obstructed hernias. The diagnosis of abdominal pain is further complicated, by radiating pain from the chest or a nerve root, and referred pain from other conditions; **extra-abdominal** causes are considered in table 4.

Vomiting occurs in many abdominal conditions. Examine its contents to detect the smelly and undigested food of pyloric obstruction, or the feculent brown fluid of intestinal obstruction. When associated with

diarrhea the vomiting may be due to gastroenteritis. **Gastrointestinal hemorrhage** may have no abnormal abdominal symptoms or signs, but a full history and examination are essential in its differential diagnosis. A full small gut history and examination is essential in the differential diagnosis of **malabsorption**.

Examination of the Abdomen

As with examination of the thorax, abdominal examination can be considered under inspection, palpation, percussion, and auscultation, inspection and palpation usually providing the most information. In this text, percussion is considered **before** palpation, since it provides useful preliminary information on tenderness and the position of organs, thus modifying the depth of palpation and showing where to palpate for the liver and spleen.

The environment must be warm and the patient relaxed, having emptied their bladder. They should lie supine with one pillow supporting the head, unless this produces dyspnea or discomfort. Hands are placed by the sides, and the legs are extended and uncrossed. The abdomen should be fully exposed. In the male this is up to the nipples, the breasts being covered in the female. The examination must include the genitalia, but these areas are kept covered under a sheet until this part of the examination is reached, in order not to embarrass the patient.

Inspection

Note the size, shape and symmetry of the abdominal wall. These factors may be influenced by fat, a large bladder or uterus (such as in pregnancy or fibroids). Distension may be due to **gas**, fluid (**ascites**) or solid **masses** and viscera (table 6). The wall may be sunken (**scaphoid**) in very thin patients; this is particularly so with starvation and the weight loss of malignancy. The position of the **umbilicus** provides information on symmetry and it may be flattened or everted and contain various amounts of debris related to the age and hygiene of the patient. It may also be the site of a hernia or a congenital discharging sinus (patent urachus). It is occasionally the site of inflammation or a metastatic nodule (**Sister Joseph's nodule**).

The laxity of abdominal skin is related to age and weight gain or loss. Stretch marks of pregnancy are usually laterally placed and are vertical pale scars. They may be slightly bluish, whereas those of Cushing's syndrome have a distinct purplish hue. Excessive hair in the female or absence in the male may be an indication of hormonal abnormalities, requiring examination of other **secondary sexual characteristics**.

The **veins** on the abdominal wall have no valves and may enlarge to provide collateral channels in inferior or superior vena **caval obstruction**

Table 6 ABDOMINAL DISTENTION

Gas
- Gastric dilatation
- Intestinal obstruction
- Megacolon (Chagas, Hirschsprung)
- Toxic dilatation

Fluid - Ascities
Exudative
- Peritonitis acute, chronic (TB, filariasis, schistosomasis, granulomas)
- Pancreatitis acute and chronic
- Trauma to thoracic duct and other abdominal lymphatics
- Benign and malignant (primary and secondary) neoplasm (including Meig syndrome)

Transudative
- Liver failure
- Portal venous hypertension
- Hypoalbuminemia — liver and renal failure, malnutrition
- Hepatic lymphatic obstruction

Abdominal masses
- Abdominal wall tumors: desmoid, endometriosis, mesenteric cysts, neoplasm
- Hepatosplenomegaly
- Aneurysms
- Colonic: inflammatory bowel disease, actinomycosis, TB, amebiasis, helminths (ascariasis, schistosoma), benign and malignant neoplasm
- Pancreatic cyst, neoplasm
- Renal: cysts, hydronephrosis, pyonephrosis, perinephric abscess, benign and malignant neoplasm; full bladder
- Retroperitoneal: sarcoma, hematoma (trauma, anticoagulants, ruptured aneurysm), abscess, pyomyositis
- Uterine pregnancy, neoplasms; ovarian neoplasms

and portal hypertension. They radiate from the umbilicus and, when prominent, produce the pattern termed a **caput medusa** (figure 18). The application of a hot water bottle to the skin produces a characteristic mottled, faint pigmentation (**erythema ab igne**). These markings on the abdomen usually indicate a painful site, indicating that the patient has tried to soothe the pain by the application of heat.

Note recent **wounds**, **dressings**, **fistulae**, **sinuses**, and **stomas**, and the position of old **scars** (figure 19). Ask the patient to explain each one.

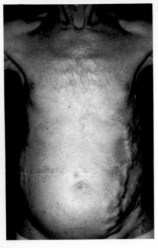

Figure 18 Dilated abdominal veins, secondary to portal obstruction: posthepatic in this case.

The abdominal wall should move freely and symmetrically in quiet (diaphragmatic) respiration. This is not so with diaphragmatic or abdominal wall paralysis. Pain also interferes with these **movements**. The restriction may be limited to one quadrant but is more widespread in **generalized peritonitis**; the maximum is found in **perforated peptic ulcer** and **acute pancreatitis**.

Movements and bulges can be more easily seen if you rest on one knee and bring your eyes down to the level of the anterior abdominal wall (figure 20).

Ask the patient to draw their abdomen in, and then blow it out as far as it will go (figure 21a,b). These maneuvers demonstrate limitation of movement due to tenderness, providing a good deal of information without any manual contact.

Coughing accentuates these differences and also produces pain over tender areas. On coughing, observe the abdominal wall for the presence of **hernias**, particularly over the superficial inguinal rings, old scars for incisional hernias, and the midline for umbilical and paraumbilical hernias, and **divarication of the rectus muscles**. Incisional and midline hernias are often accentuated by asking the patient to raise their head and shoulder off the bed (figure 22).

Movement deep to the abdominal wall may be produced by gut peristalsis or pulsation. **Pulsation** is transmitted from the heart or the aorta, in a thin person, and with abnormalities such as abdominal aortic

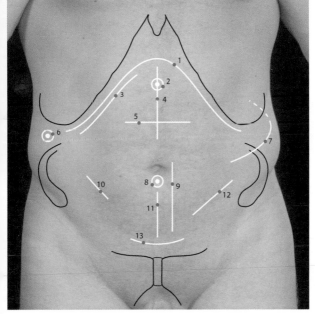

Figure 19 Abdominal incisions.

1. Rooftop
2. Laparoscopy ports for insertion
6. of telescope and operative
8. instruments
3. Right subcostal
4. Upper midline
5. Transverse abdominal

7. Nephrectomy
9. Left lower paramedian
10. Appendix
11. Lower midline
12. Left iliac muscle cutting
13. Suprapubic

aneurysms, a mass in front of the aorta or the pulsatile liver of tricuspid incompetence. Normal gut **peristalsis** is occasionally seen in a very thin individual or in an incisional hernia, when the gut is covered only by skin and fascia. However, visible peristalsis usually represents pathological obstruction, such as **pyloric stenosis**, and upper and lower **intestinal obstruction**, where coils of small gut produce a ladder-like writhing pattern.

The abdominal wall may bulge over normal or abnormal **organs** and **masses**, such as a pregnant uterus, an enlarged liver, spleen, bladder, ovary or gall bladder, segments of gut and mesenteric cysts.

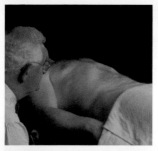

Figure 20 Observing abdominal movements.

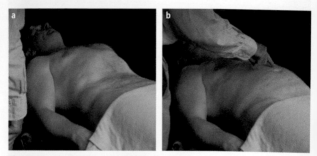

Figure 21 a,b. Drawing in and blowing out abdomen to assess tenderness.

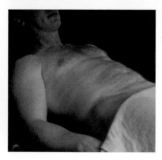

Figure 22 Assessing effect of raising head and shoulders on abdominal symptoms and signs.

Before proceeding to percussion and palpation, ask the patient to point out and personally palpate tender spots. This indicates the extent to which they are willing to have their abdomen indented (figure 23a–c). This is a useful technique in children.

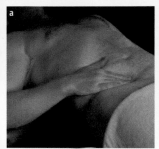

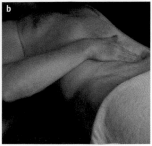

Figure 23 a,b,c. Patient self examination.

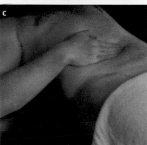

Percussion

Percussion provides a gentle means of localizing abdominal tenderness, and of differentiating between solid and gas-filled structures, thus of defining the borders of solid organ.

Commence with percussion of the four quadrants (figure 24a–d), locate the lower border of the liver (figure 25a) and spleen (figure 25b), the bladder and uterus (figure 25c), and any dullness in the flanks. If the latter is detected it is further assessed for shifting dullness (see below).

To look for tenderness, percuss all four quadrants leaving any known tender area till last. The vibration of gentle percussion is sufficient to produce pain from a sensitive peritoneum (**percussion rebound**). This form of localization is much less painful for the patient than defining tenderness by superficial or deep palpation or by **rebound tenderness** (page 310). The technique is particularly useful in children. Always watch the patient's face while undertaking percussion or any of the palpation techniques described below.

When defining borders of organs and masses, percuss from resonant (gas filled) to dull (solid organ). The **liver edge** is located by percussing

305

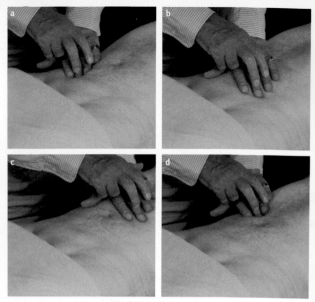

Figure 24 a,b,c,d. Percussion of abdominal quadrants.

sequentially from the right iliac fossa to the costal margin in the right midclavicular line. The dullness is usually located at the costal margin but a very large liver may extend down to the right iliac fossa. Enlargement is expressed in the number of fingers or hand-breadths below the costal margin. The upper edge of the liver usually reaches the fourth right intercostal space, so percuss downwards in the midclavicular line from the second or third interspace. Hyper-resonant lung, such as in emphysema and pneumothorax, and a **pneumoperitoneum** can make it difficult to locate the dullness of the upper margin.

The normal **spleen** is sited posterior to the left midaxillary line and is not easily detected by percussion. It enlarges across the abdomen toward the right iliac fossa. Percussion for splenic dullness therefore starts in the right iliac fossa, passes across the umbilicus to the left costal margin at the anterior axillary line, and then along the tenth rib posteriorly. Percussion from the umbilicus down to the symphysis is usually resonant but dullness may be encountered from the upper border of an enlarged bladder, uterus or ovary, coming out of the pelvis.

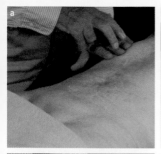

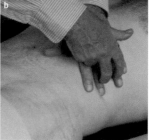

Figure 25 a,b,c. Percussion of liver, spleen and suprapubic region.

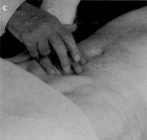

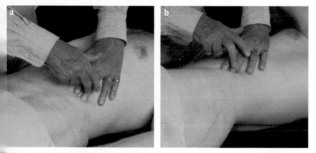

Figure 26 a,b. Examining for shifting dullness.

Abdominal masses are generally dull to percussion and alter normal patterns of resonance.

Ascites produces **dullness to percussion** in the flanks when lying in the supine position (figure 26a). Percuss from resonant to dull, moving the left hand so that the fingers remain parallel to the dull edge being sought. Note the fluid level and then rotate the patient 45 degrees to

307

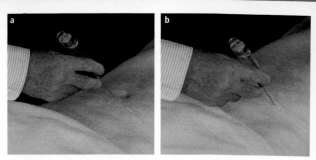

Figure 27 a,b. Paracentesis: subumbilical and left iliac fossa.

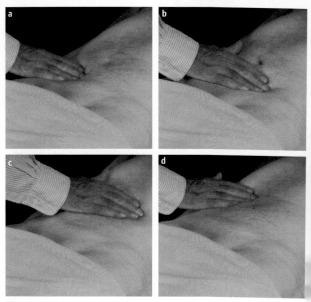

Figure 28 a,b,c,d. Superficial abdominal palpation.

each side in turn (figure 26b). The abdominal wall fluid level changes since the fluid surface remains horizontal, a phenomenon known as **shifting dullness**. Fluid may be drawn off (**paracentesis**), the needle being inserted away from the epigastric vessels; subumbilical or left iliac are common sites (figure 27a,b).

Palpation

The abdomen must not be palpated before thorough inspection or before painful sites have been identified from the history, by the patient pointing them out and by percussion. Throughout percussion and palpation **watch the patient's face** for indications of tenderness and how the examination should proceed. Start with gentle light superficial palpation, proceed to deeper palpation of all regions and then examine specific organs, using **bimanual** techniques as appropriate.

Superficial Palpation

Stand on the right side of the patient and use the flat of your right hand, with fingers together, firm but capable of molding to the contours of the abdominal wall. Feel each quadrant in turn (figure 28a–d). If there is a painful area, leave this till last. Some normal subjects find it difficult to relax the abdominal wall, particularly if the environment or the examiner's hands are cold, or if there is a lack of privacy or any other source of embarrassment. Reassure the patient. Ask them to breathe deeply through an open mouth, and, if necessary, to bend their knees to more than a right angle, and place their feet flat on the couch. Feel specifically for tenderness, guarding, rigidity, and obvious masses.

On palpation, tenderness produces local voluntary tensing (**guarding**) of the abdominal wall. There may also be involuntary reflex contraction (**rigidity**), unrelated to the external pressure or to tenderness, which indicates peritoneal inflammation (**peritonism**). The most extreme form is seen in the **board-like rigidity** often associated with a perforated peptic ulcer. In the latter, it is not possible to depress any part of the abdominal wall and thumping on this board-like abdomen on any quadrant does not necessarily produce any focal tenderness. Guarding and rigidity, however, may be localized, as over an acutely inflamed appendix in the right iliac fossa or diverticulitis in the left iliac fossa.

Deep Palpation

Each region of the abdomen must be systematically examined to identify normal and abnormal viscera and masses. A rigid, flat yet malleable right hand is again used, but placed more steeply than in gentle superficial palpation. Your fingers identify the shape and size of each structure by compressing them through the lax anterior abdominal wall onto the firm posterior abdominal wall, made up of vertebral bodies and muscles. Pressure can be increased by pressing the fingers of the left hand onto the back of the right (figure 29a–d). When examining a mass or a specific organ, note the size, shape, consistency, and any associated tenderness.

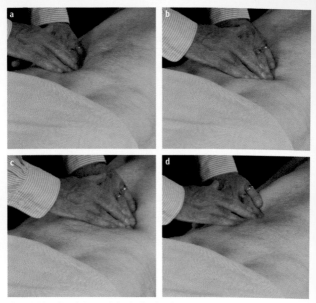

Figure 29 a,b,c,d. Deep abdominal palpation.

Both hands may be used: to measure the approximate sizes of normal and abnormal viscera, to hold mobile structures, and to assess **expansile pulsation**, by pressing on either side of the structure. As with all other aspects of abdominal palpation, watch the patient's face throughout the examination to recognize and minimize discomfort, and ensure that the subject is relaxed and breathing through an open mouth.

Emphasis has already been given to the use of percussion rebound to localize tenderness. The classical method for detecting **rebound tenderness** is to press firmly and deeply with the hand, possibly the left hand pressing down on the back of the right, and suddenly releasing the pressure. The swing of the abdominal wall produces tension on local structures and elicits pain from any sensitive peritoneum. The method is useful in detecting mild and unsuspected tenderness. However, it must **never** be used when obvious tenderness exists, as it can produce severe discomfort.

The **order of palpation** is directed by previous information, based on the site of pain and tenderness, and abnormalities picked up on observation,

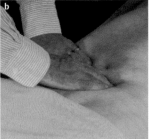

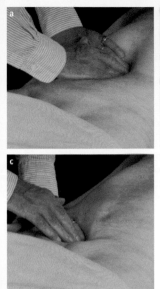

Figure 30 a,b,c. Deep palpation of epigastric, umbilical, and suprapubic regions.

percussion and gentle superficial palpation; particularly the presence of masses and hernias. It is common, after superficial palpation, to start by examining for the liver and spleen in the right and left hypochondria, then the kidneys in each flank, as described for the specific organs below. One danger is to concentrate on the four quadrants and miss midline structures such as an abdominal aortic aneurysm.

A possible order for routine examination is from the right to the left hypochondrium, across the epigastrium, assessing the liver, the pancreas and celiac regions, the spleen and renal masses. Pass downward to the umbilicus to detect the presence of an aortic aneurysm or periaortic masses, and lesions of the transverse colon and stomach. Pass downward into the suprapubic region, considering bladder, ovarian, uterine and small bowel masses, and then into each iliac fossa, with the cecum and appendix to the right and the sigmoid colon on the left (figure 30a–c).

Leave the lumbar regions until last. They are examined bimanually; your left hand is slid behind the region and the hands pressed together to assess structures between, such as kidneys and the ascending and descending colon (see below).

The site gives a strong indication of the underlying anatomy. Define the borders of a structure and whether its surface is smooth, whether it is possible to feel above, below and all around it, and whether it can be moved or moves with respiration. It may be possible to move separate masses, such as omental metastases, or to decide whether a mass is within the omentum, such as a large **omental cyst**, or a **retroperitoneal** structure fixed to the posterior abdominal wall, such as a pancreatic cyst.

Abdominal masses may become more or less prominent when tensing the abdominal wall. Prominence is accentuated when a mass is superficial to the abdominal muscles, either as part of the wall or a protrusion through it, such as a hernia. The abdominal wall is tensed by coughing, or asking the subject to raise their head and shoulders off the bed without using an elbow.

When a lot of **ascites** is present, structures float and it is possible to bounce large structures, such as a liver or spleen, feeling them hit the posterior abdominal wall or the anterior abdominal wall on rebound: this maneuver is known as **balloting**.

Vibration of fluid (**fluid thrill**) may also be produced by tapping one side of the abdomen and feeling the other. The patient or an observer places the side of a hand along the midline to prevent vibration of the anterior abdominal wall and consequent misinterpretation (figure 31).

Individual Organs

Disease of a specific organ may be suspected from the history, directing attention to this viscus on examination. Suspicion may also have been

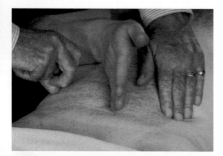

Figure 31 Examining for fluid thrill.

raised during inspection and percussion. In a thin subject, it is not uncommon to palpate a number of normal viscera, including a smooth liver edge, the lower pole of each kidney, the cecum, the ascending, transverse and sigmoid colon, and the abdominal aorta. Other structures which may be misinterpreted as abnormal are: a long **xiphisternum**, which may extend to near the umbilicus, prominent **rectus abdominis muscles**, their intersections and **divarication**, and **calcification** in an old scar.

Liver

The liver is subject to multiple pathologies many of which produce **hepatomegaly**, sometimes associated with **splenomegaly**. A large number of organisms infect the liver sometimes with abscess formation. They include **viruses** (hepatitis A–G, hemorrhagic), **bacteria** (particularly from the gut, possible producing a portal pyemia), **protozoa** (amebiasis, malaria, toxoplasmosis) and **worms** (a large number of tropical diseases, including hydatid, fascioliasis, schistosomiasis). Schistosomiasis, like tuberculosis, syphilis and sarcoid, is also associated with **granuloma** formation.

The liver is a prime site for **secondary malignant disease** and **primary** tumors are found particularly in tropical areas, often associated with schistosomiasis. The liver may not be enlarged with **cirrhosis** (from its various causes) or metabolic disorders such as Wilson disease and hemochromatosis, but many of these diseases progress to **liver failure** and **portal hypertension**. Tables 7 & 8 consider causes of liver enlargement and associated **jaundice**. Biochemical tests are indicators of whether jaundice is due to primary hepatic disease, hemolytic disorders or posthepatic obstruction. MRI and CT provide valuable information and occasionally it may be necessary to biopsy the organ (figure 32); ensure that full information is available on clotting status; preparation includes the administration of vitamin K.

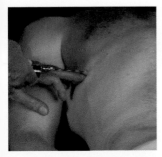

Figure 32 Liver biopsy: use ultrasonic guidance, aseptic technique, through seventh intercostal space, in midaxillary line in sustained expiration.

Table 7 HEPATOMEGALY

INFECTION	CELLULAR PROLIFERATION	METABOLIC	CELLULAR INFILTRATIVE	CONGESTIVE	SPACE-OCCUPYING LESIONS	NEOPLASTIC DISEASE BENIGN	NEOPLASTIC DISEASE MALIGNANT
Viral: Hepatitis A-G Hemorrhagic hepatitis Infectious mononucleosis Bacterial: Abscess Cholangitis Portal pyemia Protozoal: Hydatid disease Amebic abscess Schistosomiasis	Leukemia Lymphoma Polycythemia rubra vera	Hemochromatosis Wilson disease Galactosemia Drugs	Amyloidosis Sarcoidosis Reticuloses	Right-sided heart failure Budd-Chiari syndrome	Abscess Simple cyst Polycystic disease Granuloma Hemangioma	Adenoma	Hepatocarcinoma (hepatoma) Cholangio-carcinoma Metastatic, e.g., colorectal, breast, stomach, melanoma

Table 8 **CAUSES OF JAUNDICE**

Prehepatic (hemolytic disorders)	Hereditary spherocytosis Hypersplenism Sickle cell Thalassemia Acquired hemolytic anemia	
Hepatic (liver dysfunction)	Hepatitis Cirrhosis Metabolic disorders	
Posthepatic (obstruction to biliary flow)	In the lumen	Gallstones
	In the wall	Benign and malignant strictures, including congenital defects
		Sclerosing cholangitis
	Outside the wall	Hepatic tumors
		Tumors of the porta hepatitis
		Periampullary tumors
		Pancreatitis
		Pancreatic cysts
		Pancreatic malignancy

The **livers** move downwards on inspiration and its anterior edge becomes palpable if it extends beyond the costal margin: this occasionally occurs in the normal individual. A large liver extends down toward the right iliac fossa, and the edge is often firm and easily palpable. Use the flat of your outstretched right hand, with the thumb tucked under the palm, placed at right angles to the costal margin. Press the radial border of your index finger into the abdomen during expiration and retain in this position during inspiration, when the descending edge of an enlarged liver is felt against the index finger (figure 33a–d). Preliminary percussion will have indicated the lower edge of liver dullness. If in doubt start to palpate in the right iliac fossa and move upward one or two fingers breadth at a time, until a liver edge is defined or the costal margin is reached.

Repeat the maneuver to the left of the midline to detect an enlarged left lobe of the liver. An alternative technique is to use the fingertips of both hands, placed alongside each other, parallel with the costal margin pressing inwards and upwards during inspiration, along the same pathway, or using the pulps of your fingers superiorly to detect the descending liver edge (figure 34a,b). It is also possible to feel a firm liver edge from above (figure 34c).

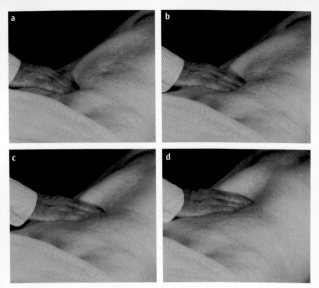

Figure 33 a,b,c,d. Palpation for liver edge.

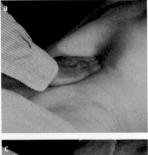

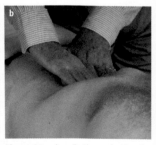

Figure 34 a,b,c. Further palpation for liver edge.

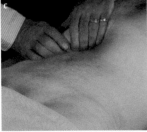

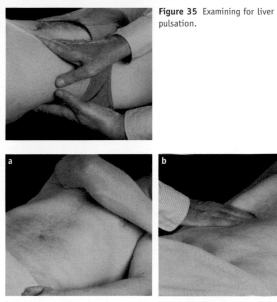

Figure 35 Examining for liver pulsation.

Figure 36 a,b. Observing for a visible distended gallbladder and eliciting Murphy's sign.

The liver edge is measured in finger- or hand-breadths below the costal margin. Note also the shape, consistency, nodularity, and tenderness. A soft, one-finger-breadth liver edge can be normal as may be a palpable Riedel's lobe. An enlarged left lobe may be palpable across the midline. Rectus abdominis intersections can be confused for an edge and well developed abdominal musculature can make a soft liver edge difficult to palpate.

Liver pulsation, as in tricuspid regurgitation, is best felt bimanually. Place your right hand over the right upper quadrant and your left opposite it, in the right loin (figure 35).

Cholecystitis is the commonest gall bladder disease encountered in most countries, and is often associated with **gall stones**. **Carcinoma** of the biliary tree may give rise to an enlarged gall bladder and progressive jaundice.

An enlarged gall bladder extends downward, usually as a smooth enlargement from the liver edge in the midclavicular line. Rolling the patient to 45 degrees on the left side increases its visibility as well as facilitating palpation (figure 36a). A **mucocele** of the gall bladder is often palpable, but enlargement usually indicates malignant obstruction.

An enlarged gall bladder may also be palpable bimanually and may be confused with a palpable right kidney, the latter being further posterior.

Tenderness over the gall bladder is present in acute cholecystitis and, with the hand depressed over the site of the gall bladder, ask the subject to breathe in deeply (figure 36b). Tenderness, producing sudden stopping of inspiration, elicited in this fashion is called a positive **Murphy's sign**.

Spleen

The spleen is subject to **trauma**, particularly from overlying fractured ribs. **Splenomegaly** is often accompanied by **hepatomegaly**, as in **blood disorders** (sickle cell, Mediterranean anemia, leukemia, Hodgkin and non-Hodgkin lymphoma) and **lipid storage** diseases (Gaucher and Niemann-Pick). It is also enlarged with many liver **infections**, such as glandular fever, brucellosis, typhoid, relapsing fever, kala-azar, malaria, toxoplasmosis, trypanosomiasis, schistosomiasis. The spleen becomes rather fragile in some of these conditions, particularly the malarial spleen, and can be ruptured independent of rib fractures. Table 9 considers causes of splenic enlargement.

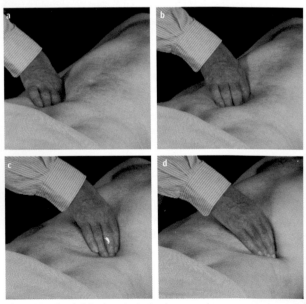

Figure 37 a,b,c,d. Palpation of splenic edge.

Table 9 **SPLENOMEGALY**

INFECTION	CONGESTIVE	CELLULAE INFILTRATION/ METABOLIC	CELLULAR PROLIFERATION/ BLOOD DYSPLASIAS	COLLAGEN DISEASE	SPACE OCCUPYING LESIONS	INFARCTION
Viral: Infectious mononucleosis	Portal hypertension Hepatic vein obstruction Right-sided heart failure	Amyloidosis Gaucher disease Porphyria	Leukemia Myelofibrosis Polycythemia rubra vera Pernicious anemia Hereditary spherocytosis Thalassemia Sickle cell disease Thrombocytopenic purpura Idiopathic	Felty syndrome Still disease	Solitary cyst Polycystic disease Angioma Lymphoma	Embolic Splenic artery/vein thrombosis
Bacterial: Typhoid Typhus TB Syphilis Leptospirosis Septicemia/abscess						
Protozal: Malaria Schistosomiasis Trypanosomiasis Tropical splenomegaly Hydatid cyst Kala-azar						

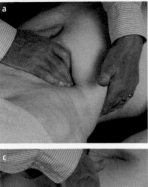

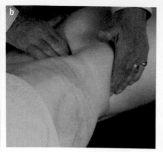

Figure 38 a,b,c. Additional maneuvers to identify splenic edge.

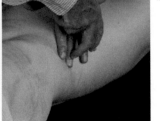

The spleen enlarges from beneath the left costal margin, across the umbilicus, to the right iliac fossa. Like the liver, it descends with inspiration and the same hand movements are used to define and dip under the notched anterior margin.

Start palpation below and to the right of the umbilicus, pass upward across the midline, and end subcostally in the midaxillary line (figure 37a–d).

Palpation is facilitated by bimanual palpation and turning the patient 45 degrees to the right side; the spleen is first "tipped" in the midaxillary line (figure 38a,b). Normal splenic dullness should never extend beyond this point. Check the position again by percussion (figure 38c).

Epigastrium and Umbilical Regions
Stomach and **pancreatic** masses, and aortic **aneurysms** are palpable in the epigastrium and behind the umbilicus (figure 39a,b). In the latter, place your fingertips of each hand on either side of the aneurysm to demonstrate **expansile** pulsation and also to gain some indication of the

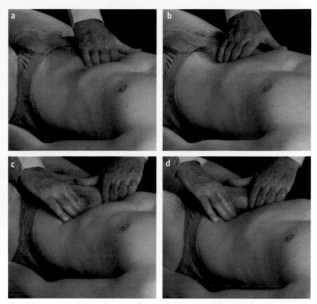

Figure 39 a,b,c,d. Examination of epigastric and umbilical regions for stomach and pancreatic masses, periaortic nodes and aortic aneurysms.

transverse diameter (figure 39c,d). Very few aneurysms are suprarenal in origin, even when the palpating fingers cannot dip over the upper border. Aneurysms occasionally involve the common iliac arteries, in which case the aortic bifurcation may be palpable. Small aneurysms may be difficult to palpate in an obese abdomen. A normal aorta can be palpated against the vertebral bodies in a thin individual: press deeply but gently as this maneuver can produce discomfort.

Para-aortic **nodes** and fixed retroperitoneal or **pancreatic masses** can mimic aneurysms and may transmit aortic pulsation. A **gastric neoplasm** presenting as a mass in the epigastrium or umbilical region may be partly mobile in all directions. In the neonate, the pyloric tumor of **pyloric stenosis** may be palpable, after a meal, on the right side of the epigastrium. **Retroperitoneal** masses, hematomas, and tumors may also extend into the loin and become palpable bimanually. Imaging techniques provide essential additional information for the diagnosis of these lesions (figure 40).

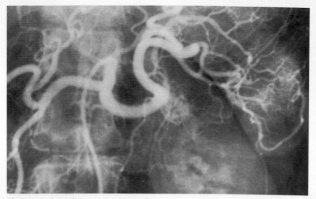

Figure 40 Superior mesenteric arteriogram. Usually reserved for ischemic problems, as MRI is effective for retroperitoneal pathology. However, a blush can be just seen in the center of the pancreas due to an insulinoma.

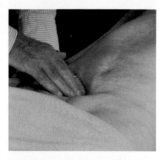

Figure 41 Examination of the suprapubic region for pelvic masses.

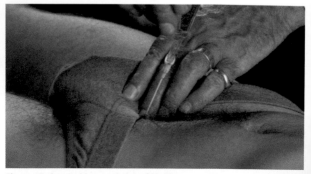

Figure 42 Suprapubic cannulation of bladder.

Subrapubic Region

The suprapubic region is usually resonant and empty to palpation (figure 41). The commonest mass coming out of the pelvis, which you cannot get below and is dull to percussion, is the **pregnant uterus**. A large **bladder** and **ovarian** masses can have similar signs; in the former the patient usually has accompanying urinary symptoms; suprapubic drainage is occationally required (figure 42).

Gynecological problems may present as acute or chronic disorders, including abdominal pain. **Ovarian** disease includes cystic change, and **cysts** may enlarge, twist, bleed, and rupture. Ovarian **cancer** can present with vague and non-specific symptoms, such as weight loss and malaise, before gross enlargement of a pelvic mass, ascites, and the symptoms of invasion and intestinal obstruction. Infection of the uterine tract may produce acute **salpingitis**, presenting with severe lower abdominal and back pain, and vaginal discharge, often with associated urinary symptoms. Sequelae include a **hydro-** or **pyosalpinx**.

Disorders of the body of the uterus include **fibroids**, **endometriosis**, and **sarcomas**. **Menorrhagia** is a common presentation and differential diagnosis. Carcinoma of the cervix is an important lesion to identify and treat in the early stages; this is facilitated by population screening. **Pregnancy** is commonly accompanied by **constipation**, **gastroesophageal reflux** and **urinary tract infection**, and the complications of pregnancy include **antepartum hemorrhage**. Other conditions, such as appendicitis, can occur in pregnancy and present problems of differential diagnoses.

Obstetric injury to the pelvic floor may interfere with its normal functions of pelvic visceral support, maintaining intra-abdominal pressure in straining and coughing, and directing the presenting part in labor. This may interfere with urinary and bowel continence, and present with organ prolapse.

Gynecological examination follows the same principles as described for the alimentary tract, with a general examination of the patient, and in the abdomen paying particular attention to signs in the suprapubic region. Pelvic examination is further considered below; laparoscopy originated in the gynecological field, and is used for many diagnostic and therapeutic procedures.

The Colon

Gaseous colonic enlargement occurs in **obstruction**, **intussusception**, and **volvulus**, and palpable abscess formation may occur with **diverticulitis**, **inflammatory bowel disease**, and **malignancy** of the gut.

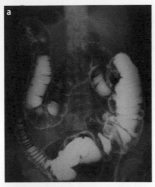

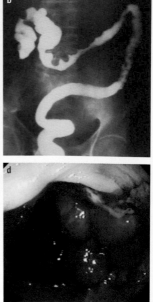

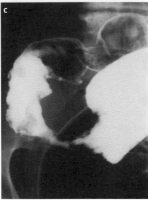

Figure 43 a. Normal barium enema; b. ulcerative colitis, showing colonic narrowing and loss of haustral pattern; c. stenosis due to colonic carcinoma; d. endoscopic view of colonic carcinoma.

The colon may be palpable in most of its course, when loaded with solid or semi-solid fecal material, or if it is distended, as in intestinal obstruction. It is often smooth, ill defined and sausage shaped, with some side-to-side mobility. The contents may be indented. The cecum, in the right iliac fossa, is more rounded.

The **transverse colon** dips across the epigastrium and umbilical regions. The sigmoid colon passes across the left iliac fossa, descending into the pelvis. It is commonly felt in thin individuals and can be identified by its indentible fecal content. The ascending and descending portions of the colon can be felt in the right and left lumbar regions by direct palpation or bimanually. The gut is well visualized with barium studies and each end and stomas provide access for endoscopic examination (figure 43 a–d).

Table 10 **HEMATURIA**

KIDNEY	URETER	BLADDER	PROSTATE	URETHRA	BLEEDING DISORDERS
Cancer of the kidney	Cancer	Cancer	Cancer	Urethritis	
Cancer of the pelvis	Stone	Cystitis	Hyper-plasia	Cancer	
Intrinsic disorders	Retro-peri-toneal fibrosis	Trauma	Prostatitis	Stone	
Trauma		Stone		Trauma	
Stone		Schisto-somiasis		Stricture	
Tuberculosis					
Polycystic					
Arteriovenous malformation					

Lumbar Region

The kidney in **chronic renal failure**, due to **glomerular nephritis** and **nephrotic syndrome**, is not usually palpable, but solitary or **polycystic** disease, **hydronephrosis**, **pyonephrosis** and **neoplasms** may become so, as can a **perinephric abscess**. **Hematuria** must be fully investigated; causes are considered in table 10; figure 44a–d provides examples of the use of imaging in the urogenital system.

The contents of the lumbar region are best felt bimanually. Place your left hand behind the right loin, in line with the right, and press your two hands together when the patient takes a deep breath (figure 45a). Rolling the patient slightly to the opposite side, placing their right arm across their chest, can facilitate palpation of a normal or abnormal kidney (figure 45b).

To examine the left lumbar region, either pass your left hand across behind the subject's back, or lean over the subject to slide your left hand behind the loin (figure 46a,b). Rolling the patient onto the opposite side may again facilitate palpation (figure 46c).

Renal tenderness is usually maximal posteriorly. The kidneys descend on inspiration and may be felt between your two hands. The lower poles may be palpable in normal subjects, particularly that of the lower placed right kidney. A large low-lying or mobile kidney may be caught between your two hands, and felt to recoil when let go. The surface marking of the kidneys is shown in figure 47 and, although renal biopsy is usually undertaken under ultrasonic guidance, anatomical knowledge is essential (figure 48).

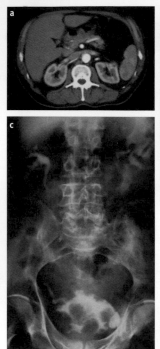

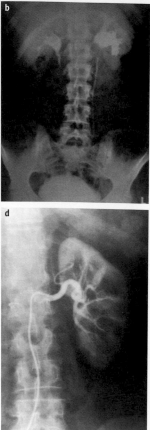

Figure 44 a. MRI: transverse section through both kidneys; b. IVU: carcinoma of left renal pelvis; hilar obstruction is present; c. multiple tumors within bladder; d. normal renal arteriogram.

A **renal mass** may be resonant (rather than dull) to percussion, due to overlying colonic gas. A colonic mass is more anteriorly placed and may be dull to percussion.

Auscultation

Normal gut sounds may be audible even without a stethoscope, particularly after meals and with hunger. At other times sounds may be

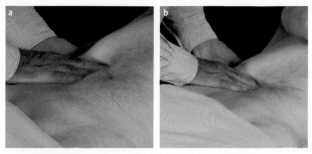

Figure 45 a. Bimanual examination of right kidney; b. with trunk rotation.

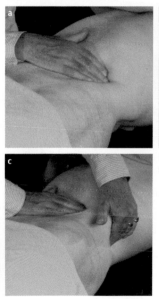

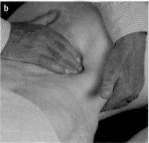

Figure 46 a,b. Examination of left kidney; c. with trunk rotation.

remarkably few, occurring up to every 10 seconds. These **borborygmi** (gurgles) can be best heard by placing the stethoscope on each side of the umbilicus. The sounds are markedly accentuated in **intestinal obstruction**, particularly during the contractions of colic. They are also increased by irritation from blood in the bowel or in any form of diarrhea.

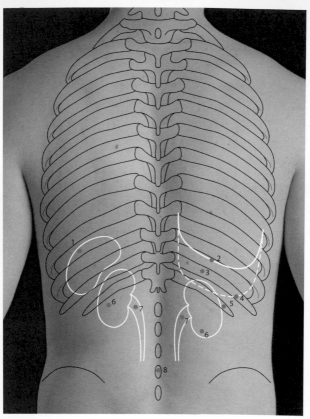

Figure 47 Surface anatomy of kidneys.

1. Spleen
2. Lower border of lung
3. Eleventh rib
4. Lower border of pleura
5. Twelfth rib
6. Kidney
7. Ureter
8. Spine of fourth lumbar vertebra (supracristal plane)

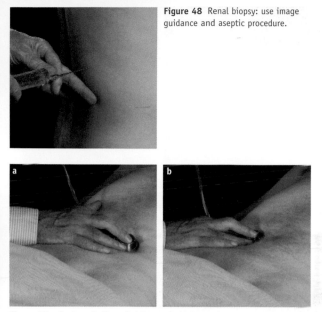

Figure 48 Renal biopsy: use image guidance and aseptic procedure.

Figure 49 a,b. Auscultation of abdomen for gut sounds.

Excess fluid in the gut, as for example in pyloric stenosis, may splash around when the abdomen is gently shaken by holding either side of the pelvis. This **succussion splash** may also be present two to three hours after a meal. It may be audible without a stethoscope. If not, ask the patient to hold the instrument in position, while you use both hands to shake the abdomen from side to side.

Paralyzed gut (**paralytic ileus**), such as postoperatively or in generalized peritonitis, is silent. But listen intently for a few minutes (figure 49a,b). In the late stages of intestinal obstruction, the gut may be markedly dilated and atonic, with few gut sounds, but with marked hyper-resonance (a condition known as **tympanites**) and tinkling sounds of fluid dripping from one distended loop to another. In complete paralysis, breath and heart sounds may be clearly audible over the abdomen. In established obstruction a large amount of fluid accumulates in the gut; this can be shown on a plain radiograph as fluid levels. An occasional level may be seen normally, but many horizontal lines are present in obstruction; the patient can be sitting or standing, or lying on their side (figure 50).

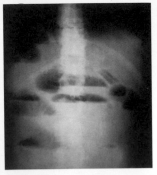

Figure 50 Erect plain radiograph of abdomen, showing fluid levels of intestinal obstruction.

A **peritoneal rub** is produced by friction between roughened peritoneal surfaces, such as in inflammation and neoplasia. It disappears as fluid accumulates, if the surfaces adhere or the condition improves. Rubs over liver abscesses and splenic infarcts may be misinterpreted as arising from a pleural rub from pulmonary disease or pericarditis.

Bruits may be heard in the epigastrium down to the umbilicus and onwards to each mid-inguinal point in aortoiliac arterial stenotic disease (figure 51a–f). Increased portasystemic flow in portal hypertension may produce venous sounds: these are increased on inspiration and during a **Valsalva** maneuver.

Renal artery bruits may be more audible posteriorly (figure 52a); they are an important diagnostic sign in renal artery stenosis. Turn the patient onto their right side. While in this position, percuss for splenic dullness and palpate for the spleen and left kidney. Sacral edema (figure 52b) may also be noted (page 231).

INGUINAL REGION, GROINS, GENITALIA, AND PERINEUM

The abdominal examination is completed by exposure and full examination of the inguinal regions – the scrotum and penis in the male and the vulva in the female. Although the anterior superior iliac spines are palpable, the pubic tubercles and symphysis pubis may be difficult to palpate in obese subjects.

The **inguinal ligament** extends from the **anterior superior iliac spine** to the **pubic tubercle** (figure 53). Direct and indirect inguinal hernias extrude through the superficial inguinal ring, above and medial to the pubic tubercle. Inguinal hernias often reduce spontaneously in the

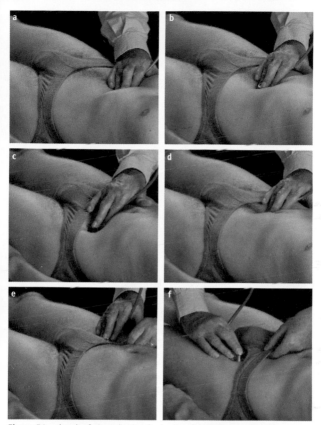

Figure 51 a,b,c,d,e,f. Auscultating for bruits of aortoiliac system.

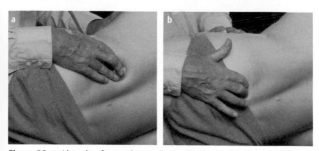

Figure 52 a. Listening for renal artery bruit ; b. checking for sacral edema.

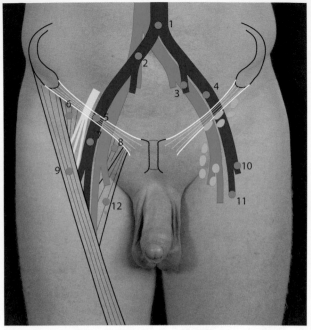

Figure 53 Anatomy of inguinal region.

1. Aortic bifurcation
2. Right common iliac artery
3. Left internal iliac artery
4. Left external iliac artery
5. Midinguinal point
6. Iliopsoas muscle
7. Right common femoral artery
8. Pectineus muscle
9. Sartorius muscle
10, Left profunda femoris artery
11. Left superficial femoral artery
12. Adductor longus muscle

supine position, but usually reappear on asking the patient to cough or stand.

Place your middle and ring fingers over the **superficial inguinal ring** and ask the patient to **cough** (figure 54a–c). If a hernia is present, the gut can be felt to extrude through the ring. This has to be differentiated from tensing of the abdominal wall and the slight bulging of the suprainguinal region just lateral to the tubercle, often present in normal individuals and termed a **Malgaigne's bulge**. Both inguinal regions must be examined, even if a patient is complaining of just a unilateral lump, since the condition is often bilateral.

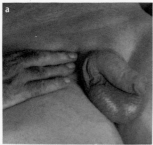

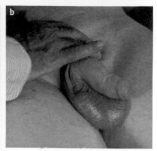

Figure 54 a,b,c. Palpating for cough impulse over superficial inguinal rings.

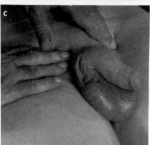

Figure 55 Cough impulse in standing position.

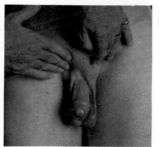

If a hernia is not obvious, ask the patient to stand up and cough again. If there is still doubt, ask the subject to don some clothes, and walk and climb some stairs, but on return to remain standing until examined in this position again (figure 55).

In the male it is possible to **invaginate** the upper part of the scrotum superiorly, subcutaneously into the superficial inguinal ring, even in an obese patient, and for the cough impulse of a hernial sac to be felt (figure 56). This maneuver, however, must be undertaken very gently, as

333

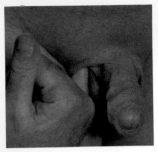

Figure 56 Invagination of scrotum to superficial inguinal ring, to assess cough impulse.

it may cause discomfort, and the invagination of the scrotum must start low enough to follow the line of the spermatic cord, deep to subcutaneous fat.

Once a hernia has been found it is important to be sure that it is **reducible** and, once reduced, to differentiate between a **direct** and an **indirect inguinal hernia**, by seeing if the cough impulse can be controlled by pressure over the deep inguinal ring. Whether you test this in the lying or standing position depends on the ease of reducing and reproducing the hernia by coughing. The deep inguinal ring is situated just above the midpoint of the inguinal ligament. Place your finger over this site after hernia reduction, and ask the subject to cough, either in the standing or lying position, depending on how the hernia is most easily reproduced.

A number of structures produce masses below the inguinal ligament. Common findings are **inguinal lymph nodes** and **femoral hernias**. The latter appear below and lateral to the pubic tubercle; they are usually more difficult to reduce than their inguinal counterparts. A tender, irreducible hernia is difficult to differentiate from a tender lymph node in this region. Other lumps in this region include a **saphenous varix**, a **femoral aneurysm**, **abscesses**, from degenerate lymph nodes or the extension of a psoas abscess, and a psoas bursa.

Penis and Scrotum

The penis is formed of three longitudinal cylinders of erectile tissue, the corpus spongiosum and the two corpora cavernosa. The corpus spongiosum is adherent to the perineal membrane posteriorly, and contains the penile urethra. It is expanded anteriorly as the glans penis, and covered by a fold of skin, the foreskin or prepuce. The scrotum contains, on each side, the testis, epididymis and the contents of the

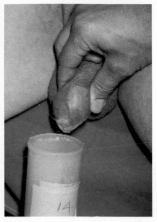

Figure 57 Severe phimosis with pinpoint opening.

spermatic cord. An indirect inguinal hernia may follow the spermatic cord into the scrotum.

Diseases of the penis include the congenital anomalies of **epispadias** (urethra opening on the dorsal aspect of the penis), and **hypospadias** (a proximal ventral opening). Infective **urethritis** is a common venereal disease and this may be accompanied by **epididymo-orchitis** and a late onset **urethral stricture**. The prepuce can be strictured beyond the glans penis (**phimosis** - figure 57) or proximal to it (**paraphimosis**); circumcision may be required in their treatment. **Circumcision** also reduces the incidence of **balanitis** (infection beneath the foreskin), acquired immunodeficiency syndrome (AIDS) and carcinoma of the penis. Prepubertal **epididymal cysts** contain clear fluid but, after puberty, contain sperm (**spermatocele**). Fluid may collect within the tunica vaginalis, the sac surrounding the testis (**hydrocele**). Prominence of the pampiniform venous plexus of the testis (**varicocele**) is more common on the left side.

The testes may be absent bilaterally (**cryptorchidism**), **undescended** (when sited within the inguinal canal or the posterior abdominal wall) or **maldescended** (when the testis has emerged from the superficial inguinal ring but resides outside the scrotum). **Torsion** of the testis is usually of an abnormally developed testis, when it lies horizontal and has an incomplete attachment to the epididymis (producing the clapper bell deformity); the condition is often bilateral.

Tumors of the testis in early life are almost invariably germ cell in origin (**seminomas**, **teratomas**). Early diagnosis is essential, as the excellent

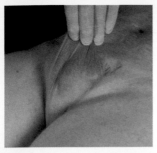

Figure 58 Withdrawing scrotum onto anterior aspect of thighs.

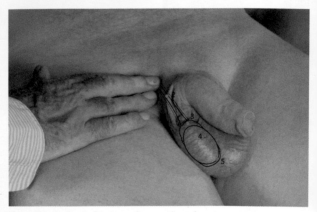

Figure 59 Anatomy of testes and spermatic cord.

1. Middle finger on superficial inguinal ring
2. Spermatic cord
3. Superior pole of epididymis
4. Body of testis
5. Inferior pole of epididymis

results of treatment are reduced when the tumor breaches the testicular capsule, extends beyond regional nodes or presents with extralymphatic spread. Presentation is usually with testicular enlargement and loss of testicular sensation: examine the abdomen and image for enlarged para-aortic nodes.

Examination of the penis and scrotum is usually in the lying position. Ask the patient to spread his legs to allow the scrotum to be raised onto the front of the thighs. This can be done by pulling on the inferior scrotal skin, but do not hold the testes during this movement, as it is painful (figure 58). Examine the skin of the posterior as well as the anterior surface of the scrotum. Note the distribution of hair around the pubis and scrotum and any skin abnormality.

Examine the contents of the scrotum one side a time (figure 59). The testis is sensitive to pressure and during gentle palpation observe the subject's face. Check the oval, vertical orientation of the normal 3-cm adult testis with superior, posterior and inferior epididymis, and the vas deferens passing cranially behind the testis from the inferior pole (figure 60a,b).

The spermatic cord is palpated at the neck of the scrotum, where the contents can be rolled between finger and thumb, and the prominent vas deferens is palpable (figure 61). It is at this site that the vas deferens is manipulated to a subcutaneous position for the operation of vasectomy.

If a scrotal mass is present, first decide whether it is possible to get above it. If not, the **inguinoscrotal** extension is probably an indirect inguinal hernia. If the mass is confined to the scrotum, check whether the testis can be palpated as a discrete entity or whether it is

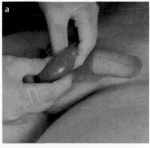
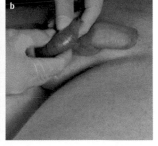

Figure 60 a,b. Examination of testis.

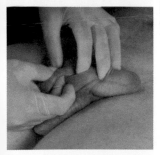

Figure 61 Palpation of spermatic cord.

surrounded by the mass; this is the case in a hydrocele. The latter may be tensely filled with fluid and the testis difficult to palpate. Cysts of the epididymis are usually sited above the testis and can be palpated separate from it, although occasionally they may occur within a hydrocele sac.

The prepubertal testis and epididymis are the same shape as in the adult. Note the absence of secondary sexual hair. Testicular size is assessed by comparison with a standard size set of oval beads. Differentiation of cystic and solid structures is aided by **transillumination**. A varicocele is a collection of varicosities (of the pampiniform plexus), which has been aptly described as a **bag of worms**.

When examining the penis, note whether the subject has been circumcised. If not, retract the foreskin to ensure there is no underlying lesion and check the normality of the urethral orifice (figure 62). Always replace the retracted foreskin to avoid risk of a paraphimosis.

When examining a patient for venereal disease, observe the meatus for discharge and massage the penile urethra from proximal to distal to express a sample (figure 63a,b).

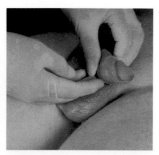

Figure 62 Retracting prepuce to examine glans.

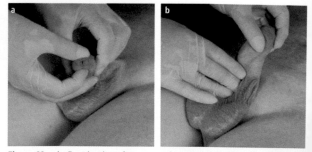

Figure 63 a,b. Examination of meatus and urethral massage.

Rectal and Vaginal Examination

The anal region is subject to a number of specific diseases. Hemo... (**piles**) are mucosal prolapse, initially occurring on straining, but... advanced cases remaining as external lumps. They present with ble... perianal lumps, and the complications of thrombosis and strangulatio... **Rectal prolapse** is extrusion of the full thickness of the rectal wall and... is usually only seen in patients incapable of controlling their bowel habit. An **anal fissure** is a longitudinal linear ulcer across the anal margin that causes pain and spasm; it may bleed. Sepsis may present as a **perianal** abscess: an **anal fistula** is an inflammatory tract where an abscess, initially in communication with the anal canal, discharges onto the surface, producing a tract between anal mucosa and the perianal skin, usually bypassing muscular control.

A **perianal hematoma** (external pile) is a thrombosed subcutaneous vein that is an extremely tender lump; it fortunately soon resolves. Other perianal lesions include **Crohn's disease** and **malignancy** of the anal canal. All these perianal lesions can produce discharge, local irritation, inflammation, and **pruritus** (table 11). **Anal warts** are of venereal origin and also occur around the vulva and glans penis. **AIDS** sufferers are subject to additional infections, including herpes simplex virus, cytomegalovirus, *Mycobacterium avian-intercellulare* and *Candida*.

Pilonidal disease and **hidradenitis suppurativa** are two other infective conditions occurring in the perineum but not of anorectal origin. The former commences in a congenital midline pit over the sacrum, between the buttocks, and infection may progress to abscess formation. Hidradenitis is a chronic suppurative disease of apocrine glands, affecting the groins and extending into the perineum; it may also occur in the axillae.

Table 11 PRURITUS ANI

ANAL DISORDERS	SOILING	INFECTION	GENERAL
Piles	Fecal	STD including	Skin disorders
Fissures	incontinence	warts	including eczema
Fistulae	Urinary	Candidiasis	and allergies
Rectal prolapse	incontinence	Trichomoniasis	Obstructive jaundice
Crohn's/TB	Vaginal	Scabies	Diabetes
Malignancy	discharge	Lice	Hyperparathyroidism
	Diarrhea	Threadworms	Myeloproliferative
	Sweating		disorders
	Poor hygiene		Lymphoma
			Psychological

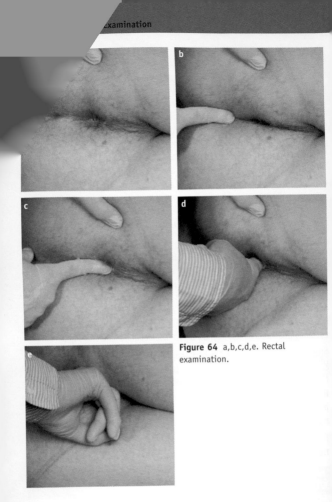

Figure 64 a,b,c,d,e. Rectal examination.

Examination of the alimentary tract is completed by examination of the perineum, including rectum, and sometimes vagina, these examinations are usually undertaken with the subject in the left lateral position.

Rectal examination provides valuable information on pelvic organs.

Explain the importance of the procedure to the patient, who should turn onto their left side, so the pelvis is a true vertical, bringing the buttocks to the edge of the couch and drawing their knees up to their chest: ensure adequate lighting to **observe** the perineum. Put on a pair of disposable gloves and first lift up the right buttock to expose the anus, the back of the scrotum or the vaginal margins. Note any abnormality of the skin, protrusions from the anal canal or other lesions. Ask the patient to strain down and note any extrusion of skin or mucosa through the anus (figure 64a).

Dip your gloved right index finger into a lubricant and lubricate the anal margin. Tell the subject that you are intending to insert the finger. Rest the pulp of the finger on the anal margin and gently curl the tip into the anus (figure 64b,c). Proceed slowly and note any tenderness or spasm as the finger passes through the anal sphincter. Extreme tenderness and spasm may indicate a fissure and may prevent further examination unless carried out very slowly and very gently. Usually your finger passes easily through the sphincter into the **anal canal** and the **lower rectum**. Note any surrounding lumps or nodularity within the anal canal.

Systematically **palpate** the contents of the pelvis (figure 64d). First feel the hollow of the **sacrum** and the **coccyx**; this may be examined between your index finger inside and thumb outside.

Turn your hand anticlockwise round the left side of the pelvis to examine anteriorly (figure 64e). In a normal **prostate**, the groove between the two lateral lobes is palpable. The **seminal vesicles** lie above this but are not usually palpable. The tip of your finger, however, is touching the peritoneum of the **pouch of Douglas**, through the wall of the rectum, and detects abnormalities within the pouch, including the tenderness of pelvic peritonitis.

Rotate your finger to examine the right side of the pelvis and ask the patient to strain down as your finger negotiates the lower rectum to note any abnormality of the wall.

Further information may be obtained by **bimanual** examination, your left hand palpating the lower abdomen (figure 65).

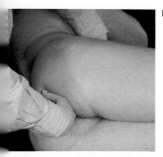

Figure 65 Bimanual examination.

The vagina lies anterior to the rectum. The rounded firm **cervix** with a central canal can be felt through the rectal wall. Lean over the patient and rest your left hand over the suprapubic region to examine the pelvis bimanually, when it may be possible to assess the shape and size of the **uterus**, and any associated abnormalities.

Note any tenderness in the **fornices**, suggesting pelvic inflammatory disease. The ovaries lie on the lateral wall and are not usually palpable but may become so in the presence of an ovarian cyst or other pathology.

Note the presence of fecal material in the rectum and, on removal of your finger, note the consistency of this material and the presence of any blood or mucus on the glove, before disposing of it. Clean the anus with toilet paper then ask the patient to return to the supine position.

Abnormal findings may lead to further examination by proctoscopy, sigmoidoscopy or colonoscopy.

Vaginal disorders include venereal and non-venereal infection and the late sequelae of child-birth – **cystoceles**, **rectoceles**, and **procidentia**.

Vaginal examination should only be undertaken with prior consent, with a chaperone and with full privacy; it is usually in an obstetric or gynecological clinic; it does not form part of a routine abdominal examination.

The examination may be carried out in the left lateral position, but is usually in the supine position, with bent knees and abducted hips. The patient should empty her bladder before the examination.

Initial examination is of the vulva and introitus (figure 66); a good light is essential. Examine the anatomy, hair distribution, skin condition, swellings, discharge, bleeding, and organ prolapse, at rest and on straining.

Figure 66 Vulval anatomy.

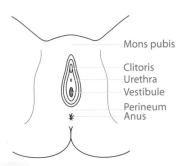

Mons pubis

Clitoris
Urethra
Vestibule
Perineum
Anus

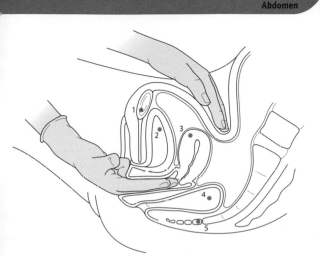

Figure 67 Bimanual examination of female pelvis.

1. Symphysis pubis
2. Emptied bladder
3. Anteverted uterus
4. Rectum
5. First coccygeal vertebra

Gloved right ring and middle fingers palpating and fixing cervix; for uterus to be palpated by the abdominal hand.

Digital examination must be unhurried and gentle, and wearing surgical gloves; explain to the patient what you are going to do at each stage, and develop a set and reliable routine. Initially insert a single digit and a second only if accommodated.

A bivalved speculum is usually introduced, having excluded any obstruction and determined the size of instrument required. Observe the shape and color of the cervix, and any discharge. Note any cervical abnormality and take a swab and smear. In the latter, know the details of the package you are going to use, read and follow the full instructions, have all the apparatus you need laid out ahead of time, and ensure the required patient details are on the specimen.

Bimanual examination provides information on the cervix, uterus, and adnexia (the fallopian tubes and ovaries). The normal cervix is firm to palpation (the consistency of the cartilage of your nose), but it softens in pregnancy to the consistency of your lip. Determine whether the uterus is ante- or retroverted (figure 67); it may be difficult to palpate if

343

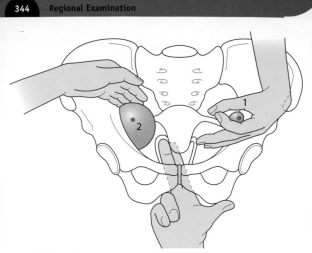

Figure 68 Bimanual examination of enlarged ovary.

1. Normal ovary: not palpable, but the subject's left hand (with its side resting on the anterior superior iliac spine) indicates the normal ovarian position
2. Abnormal ovary may be palpable bimanually: gloved fingers placed in the fornix of vagina, the other hand palpating the abdomen

the latter. Note the size, shape, consistency, and other abnormalities, including associated discomfort.

The adnexia are normally impalpable, except in very thin individuals (figure 68). If palpable, determine the shape and size and features of any mass, and tenderness. The final part of the examination is palpation of the pouch of Douglas, to identify any intraperitoneal abnormality, as with a rectal examination.

Pain and tenderness must be kept to a minimum in the examination, but they are an important physical sign of pelvic inflammatory disease and some disorders of pregnancy. Your technique must be gentle enough to differentiate between discomfort from the examination and existing pathology.

On completion of the examination, provide the patient with appropriate tissues and privacy to rearrange her clothing.

Neurological

The collection and grouping of symptoms facilitate anatomical localization of lesions within the central and peripheral nervous systems. Cerebration can be altered in psychiatric as well as organic disease and its various components, such as **behavior**, **attitude**, **emotion**, **thought process**, **intelligence**, and **insight.**

Of particular note in the neurological history are disturbances of **consciousness** (table 1), **orientation in time and space**, **memory**, **speech**, **vision**, and **motor and sensory** function. **Headache** is a common symptom, particularly in raised intracranial pressure, but it lacks specificity since it occurs in many other complaints. The **Glasgow Coma Scale** (table 2) provides a grading system of coma in relation to head injuries that is used for the initial assessment and monitoring progress.

Note the frequency, timing, duration and progress of symptoms, and what the patient was doing at the time of onset of faints, falls or fits. **Epileptic fits** may be accompanied by tongue biting and urinary incontinence. Associated chest pain, palpitations or dyspnea may indicate a cardiac or respiratory etiology for these symptoms.

Speech disturbances are primarily due to abnormalities of articulation (**dysarthria** and **anarthria**) or of the organization of language (**dysphasia**, **aphasia**). The muscles of the palate, tongue, larynx, and pharynx have bilateral cortical innervation. Thus disturbances of articulation require damage to a lower motor neuron (cranial nerve), the nucleus (**bulbar palsy**) or bilateral upper motor neuron damage (**pseudobulbar palsy**). Basal ganglia disease produces slow and monotonous speech, whereas cerebellar disorders characteristically produce staccato or scanning speech.

Damage to Broca's area (precentral cortex of the dominant hemisphere) produces an **expressive dysphasia**, the patient knowing what to say but unable to produce words. Mild degrees present as failure to name common objects and names (nominal aphasia). These conditions are commonly accompanied by inability to write (**agraphia**).

Dysphasia may also be produced by lesions of the parietal region due to failure of understanding of the spoken or written word (**receptive aphasia**, **word deafness**, and **word blindness**). If Broca's area is not affected the subject may produce a stream of disconnected words (**jargon aphasia**). More commonly, extensive lesions affect the expression as well as the understanding of speech (**global aphasia**).

Table 1 COMA

Drugs/chemicals	Anesthetics Overdose Reaction (e.g., Reye syndrome) Addictive/recreational Alcohol Poisons (e.g., weedkiller, carbon monoxide)
Infection: encephalitis, meningitis	Prion disease Viral: hemorrhagic, non-hemorrhagic Bacterial: brucellosis, meningococcal, syphilitic, tuberculous Protozoa and worms: amebic, cysticercosis, malaria, dracunculiasis, toxoplasmosis, trichinosis, visceral larva migrans, trypanosomiasis (sleeping sickness), schistosomiasis
Trauma	Cerebral damage, hemorrhage, edema
Endocrine	Hypo/hyperglycemia Hypo/hypercalcemia Myxedema Pituitary and adrenal disorders
Metabolic	Metabolic acidosis. Hypo/hypernatremia
Organ failure	Hepatic, renal, respiratory
Benign and malignant, primary and secondary tumors	Space-occupying lesions
Vascular	Infarction Hypertensive encephalopathy Thrombosis Embolism Hemorrhage (intracerebral, brainstem, subarachnoid)
Miscellaneous	Postepileptic seizure, hypothermia, hyperpyrexia, Wernick's encephalopathy

Table 2 **GLASGOW COMA SCORE**

RESPONSE	DETAILS	SCORE
Best eye response (E)	Eyes open spontaneously	4
	Eye opening to verbal command	3
	Eye opening to pain	2
	No eye opening	1
Best verbal response (V)	Orientated	5
	Confused	4
	Inappropriate words	3
	Incomprehensible sounds	2
	No verbal response	1
Best motor response (M)	Obeys commands	6
	Localizing pain	5
	Withdrawal from pain	4
	Flexion to pain	3
	Extension to pain	2
	No motor response	1

Coma Score = E + V + M (minimum = 3; maximum = 15)
Coma Score of 13 or higher correlates with a mild brain injury, 9–12 is a moderate injury and 8 or less a severe brain injury: but the components should be presented with the score

Disturbances of **memory** may be short or long term; the former is frequently due to organic disease and may be reversible. **Visual** symptoms are considered with the cranial nerves (page 29).

Motor symptoms include **paralysis**, **spasticity**, **incoordination**, and **abnormal movements**. Mild paresis may present with fatigue and weakness, such as diminution of grip, dropping things and toe catching when walking. Spasticity may be due to pyramidal or extrapyramidal disease. In milder forms it presents with stiffness.

Cerebellar dysfunction interferes with everyday activities, such as writing and eating, or may produce a mild **intention tremor** and loss of balance. Abnormal movements include the tremor of **Parkinson** disease, **tics** and **choreiform movements**.

The distribution of the **sensory** disturbances of **anesthesia**, **paresthesia** (pins and needles), numbness, increased sensation (**hyperesthesia**), and **pain** provide important information on the localization of lesions; visceral pain may be referred to somatic **dermatomes**.

NEUROLOGICAL EXAMINATION

Neurological examination may be a detailed assessment of the nervous system, following up a specific symptom or suspected disease, or a survey of the system, as part of a routine general examination. A detailed neurological examination can be time consuming and exhausting for a patient, and information obtained from a tired, fatigued, uncooperative or ill patient can be misleading. Initial examination should therefore be targeted on the suspected abnormality, such as a peripheral nerve injury, returning one or more times to complete the observations. Follow-up of neurological findings is critical when abnormalities have been found or are suspected.

Diseases may affect single cortical areas, spinal tracts or peripheral nerves, but lesions often involve more than one pathway. Localization of the disease is helped by a precise history. However, it is important to keep an open mind, as it is easy to follow a wrong lead as to the level of a lesion, and be blinkered about the possibility of disease at other levels or at multiple sites.

One gains an overall impression of neurological function from the patient's **gait**, **posture**, and **speech**. Examination of the current mental state includes psychiatric assessment, but a few simple tests should be applied. These include **orientation** in time and place (what are the day and date, where are you?), short and long term **memory** (repeat three to five words or numbers and request again after a short interval; birthday, place of birth, anniversaries); **general knowledge** (names of presidents, ministers, capitals); **mathematical skills** (take 7's from 100); **interpretation of proverbs**.

Detailed examination of the peripheral nervous system includes assessment of the cranial nerves, followed by examination of motor and sensory function of the rest of the body. In this text, the cranial nerves are linked to their special sensory organs, and are considered with the head and neck (page 27); this section considers the assessment of somatic function.

MOTOR FUNCTION

Examination of the motor system can be divided into assessment of **power**, **tone**, **coordination**, **reflexes**, and **abnormal movements**. During this examination, also look for wasting and other muscular abnormalities. Muscle abnormalities may be indicative of **musculoskeletal** as well as neurological disease and are also considered on page 71.

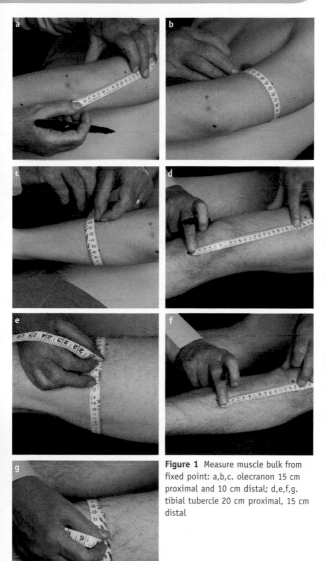

Figure 1 Measure muscle bulk from fixed point: a,b,c. olecranon 15 cm proximal and 10 cm distal; d,e,f,g. tibial tubercle 20 cm proximal, 15 cm distal

Muscle

Observe the symmetry and shape of muscles for evidence of
hypertrophy, **wasting**, **abnormal shape** (e.g., torn tendons and
contractures), and **abnormal movement**. **Palpation** of muscles allows
the assessment of **tone** and also localization of symptomatic and
unsuspected **tenderness**. **Hypotonia** may be present in muscle wasting
disease (myotonia or peripheral nerve injuries) and **hypertonia** in
established upper motor neuron disease.

Muscle bulk is related to age, sex, physical activity, and to nutritional
status. **Atrophy** may indicate primary muscle disease or peripheral nerve
damage. Measurement of the amount of **wasting** can be obtained with a
tape measure, comparing two limbs or by repeated measurements after a
timed interval. Measure the circumference at set distances from a bony
landmark such as the tip of the shoulder in the upper arm, the olecranon
for the forearm, and the tibial tubercle for the thigh and calf (figure
1a–g).

The small muscles of the hand provide an early indication of **general**
muscular wasting, as well as peripheral nerve injury. This is seen
particularly on the dorsum of the **hand**, with loss of substance of the
interossei of the thumb and index finger, and loss of muscle bulk deep
to the long extensor tendon (figure 2a,b).

Local causes of muscular wasting in the hand include carpal tunnel
syndrome, lesions of the median and ulnar nerves and their roots, **motor
neuron disease**, **poliomyelitis**, **syringomyelia**, **peripheral neuropathy**,
and **rheumatoid arthritis**. If the hands are placed with their palms
together, and then back-to-back, the thenar and hypothenar muscles can
be compared on the two sides (figure 3a,b). The adductor pollicis
facilitates downward pressure in a thumb grip; ulnar nerve damage can
be highlighted by deficiency of this movement (**Froment's sign** – figure
4), flexor pollicis is used to compensate for the deficit.

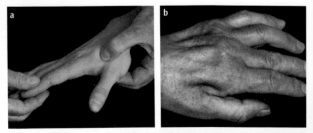

Figure 2 a,b. Assess wasting in first dorsal interosseous.

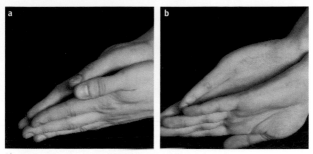

Figure 3 Compare: a. thenar and b. hypothenar eminences.

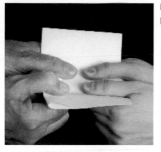

Figure 4 Right ulnar palsy with positive Froment's sign.

At some sites, peripheral nerves can be **palpated** for thickening and associated tenderness (e.g., the ulnar nerve behind the medial epicondyle of the humerus and the common peroneal nerve over the neck of the fibula); this is a diagnostic feature of leprosy. Tapping along the course of a nerve may give an indication of the site of damage (over the median nerve at the wrist in carpal tunnel compression) or the level to which regeneration has taken place after nerve transection (**Tinel's** sign).

Power

Power is assessed by **active** movement of each joint, in each direction, comparing right with left, and then adding **resistance** to these movements. Individual joints are considered with the musculoskeletal system.

Power can be graded from 0 to 5. Zero indicates no contraction; 1, a flicker of movement; 2, active movement with gravity excluded; 3, active

351

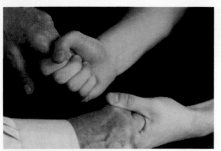

Figure 5 Comparing grips.

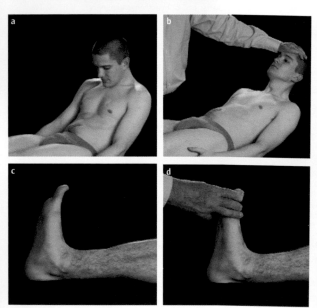

Figure 6 Active and resisted: a,b. spinal flexion and c,d. dorsiflexion of right ankle.

against gravity; 4, active against gravity and resistance (plus and minus signs are used to divide this group); 5, normal.

Assessment of the power of active movement begins with observation of **posture** and **gait**. It is then determined in each joint and individual muscle groups; testing specific movements, while eliminating the action of accessory muscles, and tricks that overcome and mask any individual muscle weakness. When assessing this power, an indication is also obtained of the control of antagonistic muscles, the smoothness and coordination of movements, and whether they are limited by pain, contractures or joint abnormalities.

Initially gross movements are used to compare the limbs, such as a handshake, and flexion and extension of joints. Compare the grip on the two sides (figure 5), and active and resisted, spinal flexion and dosiflexion of the ankle (figure 6a–d).

Tone

Passive movement assesses tone, **spasticity** of upper motor neuron lesions and the **clasp-like cog-wheel rigidity** of diseases of the basal ganglia; it also locates joint **pain** and **stiffness**, and identifies **contractures**, as considered in the musculoskeletal section. Passive movement must always be preceded by active movement; the degree of pain and disability can then direct the extent of your subsequent examination (watch a patient's face for signs of discomfort during all movements).

Tone in the upper and lower limbs is assessed by passive movement of the major joints, and by palpation of the bulk of large muscles and muscle groups, such as gluteus maximus and the erector spinae muscle mass (figure 7a–f).

Coordination

Coordination of upper limb movements is assessed by the subject alternately touching your finger and their own nose. Move your finger from side to side, and then leave it in position and ask the patient to repeat the movement with their eyes closed (figure 8a–c). Ask the patient to draw imaginary circles in space or screw up imaginary jam jars (figure 8d).

Fine movement can be assessed by tapping the dorsum of one hand with the other, and then alternately with the front and back of this hand (figure 8e,f). A more practical approach is to ask the patient to undo a button and write with a pen; various types of grip are further considered in the musculoskeletal system (page 131).

In the lower limb, ask the patient to place each heel in turn on the shin of the contralateral limb, and move it from the knee to the ankle and back. Ask the patient to touch your strategically placed finger with the great toe of each foot, then with their eyes closed; to describe circles

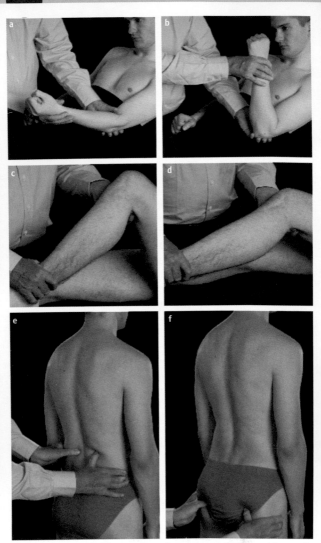

Figure 7 Assessment of tone: a–d. passive movement of elbow and knee; e,f. palpation of erector spinae and gluteus maximus.

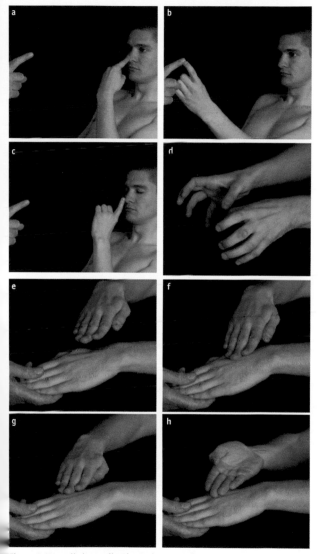

Figure 8 Upper limb coordination: a,b,c. nose-finger, moving target and eyes closed; d. closing imaginary jam jar; e–h. tapping on back of hand; front and back hand placement.

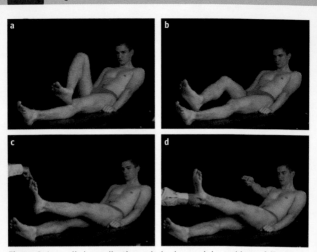

Figure 9 Lower limb coordination: a,b. heel up and down shin; c. following movements with tip of toe and d. "shooting" moved toe with closed eyes.

with their great toe, or with their eyes closed, to "shoot" the great toe with two fingers, after you have passively moved the foot (figure 9a–d).

Observe the patient walking (figure 10a); disturbances of gait can be accentuated by asking the subject to walk a straight line and repeat this heel-toe fashion (figure 10b). **Ataxia** (incoordination of gait) may be due to an altered state of consciousness (e.g., excess alcohol, head injury, upper motor neuron spasticity), altered tone of cerebellar or basal ganglia disease and abnormalities of sensory input, when the patient is unaware of their position in space. **Apraxia** is failure to organize movements that are otherwise intact, and is associated with frontal lobe lesions.

Standing on toes and heels, and walking backwards on the heels are further tests of coordination (figure 10c-e), but also depend on position sense, muscle power, and normal joints. The altered coordination in cerebellar disease is characteristically slow, awkward, and incomplete. It requires a few tries to complete a movement and it is often broken down into its component parts (**disdiadochokinesis**). Abnormalities of posture may be accentuated by asking the patient to stand still, with their feet together and their eyes closed (**Romberg's sign** – figure 11).

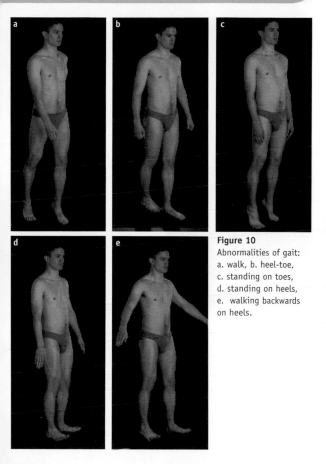

Figure 10
Abnormalities of gait:
a. walk, b. heel-toe,
c. standing on toes,
d. standing on heels,
e. walking backwards
on heels.

Reflexes

Assessment of deep and superficial reflexes provides information on the integrity of reflex arcs at different levels in the central nervous system. They may be abolished by disease of the lower motor neuron or sensory neurons in the reflex arc, and may be modified by central damage, such as in hyper-reflexic upper motor neuron lesions.

A number of reflexes are assessed with the cranial nerves (page 27); these include those of the special senses, as well as somatic motor and sensory function.

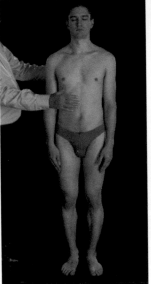

Figure 11 Posture: Romberg's sign.

When testing limb reflexes, the position of the limb is such as to put slight tension on the stimulated muscle, but supporting the weight to avoid any active tension. Appropriate tendons are struck precisely and gently with a patellar hammer from a few centimeters' swing. Asking the patient to clench their teeth, or pull opposing clasped fingers can reinforce sluggish reflexes.

In hyper-reflexia, stimulation of one muscle may produce movements elsewhere, e.g., antagonists or more distal muscles. In marked hyper-reflexia, tension in the muscle alone may produce reflex contraction, and sustained tension can produce repeated jerking movement (clonus), as seen in patellar or ankle clonus (figure 12a,b).

If the stimulated muscle is weak, the stimulus may produce movement in powerful antagonist muscles (**paradoxical** or **inverted reflexes**). **Hyporeflexia** may persist after motor recovery in a peripheral nerve injury; it is not a good indicator of the severity of the lesion. Reflexes may persist until late in the course of muscular disease.

Reflexes are graded by the degree of contraction: 0, not elicited; 1, elicited with reinforcement; 2, normal; 3, brisk; 4 and 5, unsustained and sustained clonus.

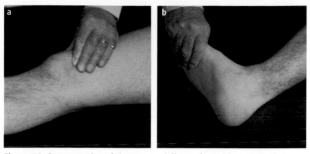

Figure 12 Demonstration of clonus: a. patellar push; and b. sustained dorsiflexion.

Specific reflex nerve root levels are: biceps, C5,6; supinator and triceps, C6,7; knee, L3,4; ankle, S1,2. Specific reflexes are shown in the figures 13a–l.

Of the superficial reflexes, the **Babinski** response is routinely examined (figure 14a). It is elicited by scratching the outer edge of the sole, from the heel forwards with a key or other implement. A normal response is curling downwards of the toes. A positive (abnormal) response is extension and fanning of the toes. This is present at birth, but after this it is indicative of an upper motor neuron lesion.

Abdominal reflexes are elicited by scratching diagonally across the four quadrants; each normally produces contraction of the underlying muscles (figure 14b).

The cremasteric reflex is contraction of the cremaster muscle of one side, by scratching the adjacent thigh (figure 14c). It is easily elicited in children but less so in later life.

A number of reflexes are only prominent at birth. Examples are the grasp reflex, produced by stroking the palm (figure 14d), and the placing response, elicited by stroking the outer border of the foot.

At the end of the examination of the motor system look for spinal tension signs. Neck rigidity (**Kernig's sign**) occurs in meningitis (figure 15).

Pain from a nerve root lesion is accentuated by stretch tests. The tension of straight leg raising on the lower spinal roots is increased by dorsiflexion of the foot and raising the head off the pillow (figure 16a–c).

The femoral nerve stretch test is carried out prone: knee flexion increases tension and associated pain (figure 17).

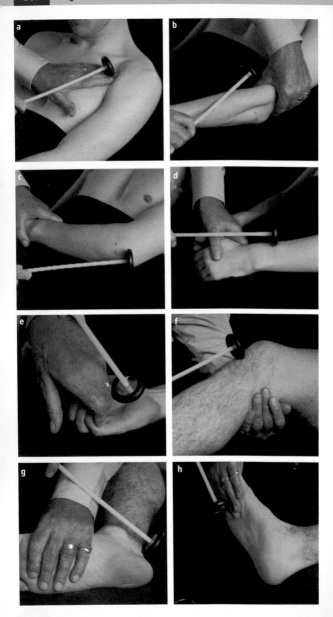

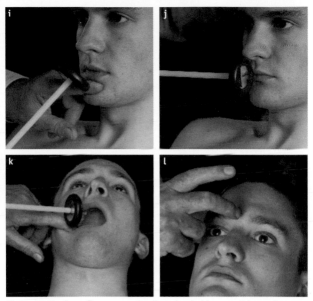

Figure 13 Tendon reflexes: a. pectoralis major; b. biceps; c. triceps; d. supinator; e. finger flexion; f. knee; g,h. ankle jerk; i. jaw jerk; j. pouting reflex; k. oroangular reflex; and l. glabellar tap.

Abnormal Movements

Abnormal movements include epilepsy, **tremor** (figure 18; e.g., Parkinson disease), **spasm**, the **clonus** of upper motor neuron disease, and the **athetoid** and **choreiform** movements of birth injuries and chorea. **Fascicular** movements (flickering) of muscles occur in motor neuron disease and may indicate a hyperexcitable muscle; the movements are precipitated by gentle tapping.

In summary, upper motor neuron lesions initially produce paralysis and hypotonia but subsequently develop in to weakness, spasticity, hyper-reflexia, and an extensor plantar response. Extrapyramidal lesions interfere with the balance of muscle activity, affecting tone, coordination, and involuntary movement, without marked loss of power. Cerebellar lesions produce hyptonia and ataxia; lower motor neuron lesions produce weakness, wasting, hypotonia, and areflexia.

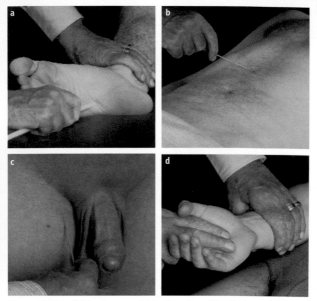

Figure 14 Superficial reflexes: a. Babinski response (dorsiflexion and fanning of toes in newborn and upper motor neuron lesions); b,c,d. abdominal and cremasteric reflexes in childhood, and grasping in new born, but indicative of upper motor neuron damage in later life.

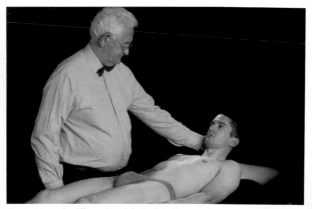

Figure 15 Neck stiffness (Kernig's sign) indicative of meningeal irritation.

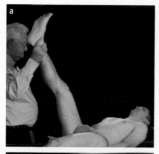

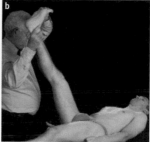

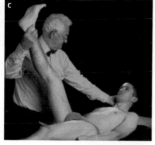

Figure 16 a. Straight leg raising produces posterior thigh pain with lumbosacral nerve compression; accentuated by b. foot dorsiflexion and c. neck flexion.

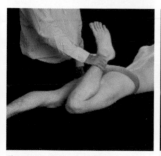

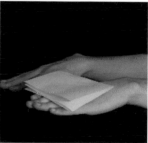

Figure 17 Femoral nerve stretch test. **Figure 18** Tremor accentuated by paper.

SENSORY FUNCTION

Altered sensation varies from total loss (anesthesia) to excess (hyperesthesia). Be sure the patient is not using the term "numbness" to describe limb weakness. Ask the patient to outline any abnormal area of sensation. Another point of possible misinterpretation is to label sensory

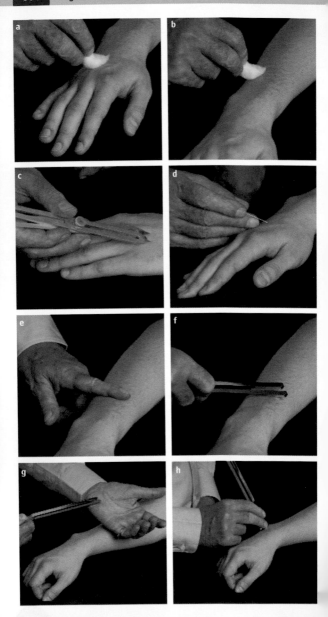

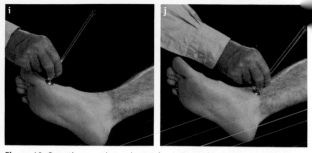

Figure 19 Somatic sensation: a,b. touch, most notable across axial line; c. two-point discrimination; d. altered sensation to blunt sterile needle; e,f. hot and cold, warm finger, cold tuning fork; and g–j. vibration in upper and lower limbs.

inattention as sensory loss. In the former, patients may require a good deal of verbal encouragement to pay attention during the examination.

In examination of an asymptomatic patient, examine the limb extremities first: if these are normal, detailed proximal examination is not usually necessary. During sensory examination, expose the area of interest, together with the equivalent part of the opposite side of the body.

Observation of the skin provides information on sensory innervation before examining each sensory modality. Insensitive skin is susceptible to damage from unnoticed minor trauma. An extreme example of these **trophic changes** is in leprosy, where the long-term sequela is loss of digits.

Examination

When examining an abnormal area, ask the patient to close their eyes and say "yes" every time contact is made. When looking for changes in sensation, ask whether each stimulus is normal or abnormal. Move from insensitive to normal areas or from normal to hyperesthetic, varying the rate and the rhythm of the stimuli. Gently mark the boundaries of change with a biro or skin pencil. This enables you to check consistency of response and also to reproduce these markings in diagrammatic form.

Start with the wrist and ankle on each side; progress proximally to the olecranon and acromion, and to the patella and anterior superior iliac spine, if there is a distal sensory abnormality.

 touch and light **pressure** are transmitted in the dorsal column to the postcentral cortex. Initially test them by finger contact over the affected area, and then detailed mapping with a wisp of cotton wool or an artist's paintbrush (figure 19a,b). Initially let the patient watch while you apply the stimulus, to ensure a positive response is appreciated: compare it with the contralateral side.

Two blunt **points** are distinguished as separate contacts at varying distances in different parts of the body (figure 19c): lips and tongue 2–3 mm; fingertips 3–5 mm; dorsum of the fingers 4–6 mm; palms 8–15 mm; dorsum of the hands 20–30 mm; dorsum of the feet 30–40 mm; and the back 40–50 mm.

Pain and temperature are carried to the level of sensory awareness in the spinothalamic tract. Test the former with a sterile pin or a partially blunted needle (figure 19d). Ask the patient to respond to each contact, stating whether it feels dull or sharp.

Gross **temperature** difference is detected by comparing the warmth of the side of your finger with the cold of the side of a tuning fork (figure 19e,f). More precise mapping is with test tubes of warm and cold water. Temperature changes may be more consistent than those with a pinprick. Mapping follows the same routine as that described for touch.

Vibration sensation is assessed by applying the base of a clinical tuning fork to a bony prominence (figure g–j). The stimulus is generated by lightly tapping the fork on your hypothenar eminence. Strike the tuning fork before each application and ask the patient, with their eyes closed, whether vibration is present and when it stops. Occasionally deliberately stop the vibration of the tuning fork to assess the accuracy of response. The feet are particularly important to assess for distal neuropathy in a diabetic patient.

Graphesthesia is assessed by writing numbers or letters on each palm, forearm or the anterior compartment of each shin (figure 20). Use a blunt object, such as the blunt end of a pen or pencil. With the patient's eyes closed, give examples for orientation and then assess; the numbers 3 and 8 are useful stimuli.

Assessment of size, shape, and weight (**stereognosis**) is with common objects placed in the palm of the hand, with the patient's eyes closed. Useful stimuli are pens, pencils, and keys (figure 21).

Sensory inattention is typical of parietal lobe lesions. It is elicited by the simultaneous application of stimuli on the two halves of the body (figure 22). The patient has their eyes closed and occasionally only one side is touched.

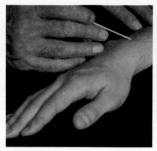

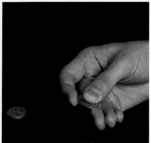

Figure 20 Graphesthesia, write 3's and 8's.

Figure 21 Stereognosis.

Figure 22 Sensory inattention.

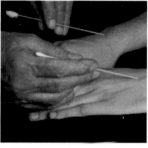

Examine joint **position** sense in the upper and lower limbs, starting distally and moving proximally if a defect is elicited. Hold the hand or foot with your left hand and with the right index finger and thumb gently grasp each side of the terminal phalanx of the index finger or great toe. Indicate to the patient up and down movements and then, with their eyes closed, ask them to identify a series of movements, inserting ups and downs in a random fashion. The normal subject can perceive minimal change of angulation (figure 23a–d).

Check for **deep** pain sensation by squeezing the tendo Achilles from side to side or pressing the base of the thumb or great toenail.

A useful initial test of neurological function of the upper limbs including position sense, power, and coordination is to ask the patient to extend both arms with the palms outwards, and upwards or downwards with their eyes closed and observe any unconscious drift (figure 24a,b).

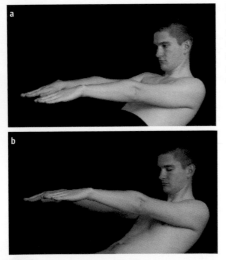

Figure 23 a,b,c,d. Position sense: hold sides of digit, demonstrate up and down movement before patient closes eyes.

Figure 24 a,b. Maintaining position with eyes closed; downward drift occurs in neurological disorders.

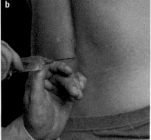

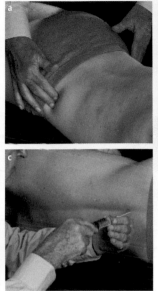

Figure 25 Lumbar puncture: a. above or below fourth lumbar spine (supracristal plane); b. sitting or c. lying (using aseptic technique).

The Romberg sign (see above) is associated with asking the patient to stand upright with their feet together and eyes closed. Make sure you guard against any fall. An initial gentle sway of the body is normal but in abnormalities of dorsal column function, the patient is unable to stand unaided.

Lumbar puncture provides access to the epidural and subarachnoid spaces: both of these sites are used in various anesthetic techniques. In examination of the nervous system, the technique is used primarily to sample cerebrospinal fluid, it must **never be undertaken in cases of known or suspected raised intracranial pressure** and, as with all invasive procedures described, full aseptic precautions must be in place.

The entry site is above or below the fourth lumbar spine (sited in the supracristal plane (figure 25a). The procedure may be undertaken in the sitting or lying position (figure 25b,c). In the former, have the patient leaning forward over the back of a chair, or over the side of a bed. In the latter, their head and knees should be tucked into the body, with their back near, and parallel to, the edge of the bed.

Autonomic Nervous System

Denervation of the sympathetic supply of the limb produces vasodilatation and loss of sweating. Initially there is rosy coloring of the digits, due to capillary dilatation, but this may progress to mottling, edema, and lowering of the temperature. Degenerative (trophic) changes may develop, giving smooth skin and some spindling, due to pulp atrophy. Hyperkeratinization may develop on traumatized areas, together with loss of hair, trauma lines across the nails, and clubbing.

Abnormalities of the sacral parasympathetic innervation include altered tone in the anal and urinary sphincters, and impotence. Changes associated with cranial nerve lesions are considered on page 60.

PERIPHERAL NERVE INJURIES

Peripheral nerve injuries are diagnosed by mapping cutaneous sensory loss, and detecting weakness in specific muscles or groups of muscles. The cutaneous nerves and dermatomes are shown in figures 26a,b.

The **skin** of the **upper limb** is supplied by the **brachial plexus** (anterior roots of C5–T1), with contributions from C4, over the tip of the shoulder and the clavicle, and T2 and 3, along the inside of the upper arm and axilla. T6 supplies the skin over the thumb and C8 the little finger; C7 has a variable supply over the central fingers. As there is marked overlap between dermatomes, sensory loss is most easily defined across **axial**

Figure 26
a. Cutaneous nerves and dermatomes, anterior.

1. Supraclavicular
2. Upper lateral cutaneous of arm
3. Anterior cutaneous (branch of 5.)
4. Intercostobrachial
5. Medial cutaneous of arm
6. Lateral cutaneous of forearm
7. Medial cutaneous of forearm
8. Palmer cutaneous of ulnar
9. Palmer cutaneous of median
10. Radial digital
11. Median digital
12. Ulnar digital
13. Subcostal
14. Lateral cutaneous of thigh
15. Genitofemoral
16. Ilioinguinal
17/19. Medial/intermediate cutaneous of thigh
18. Obturator
20. Saphenous
21/22. Lateral cutaneous of calf
23. Superficial peroneal
24. Sural
25. Deep peroneal

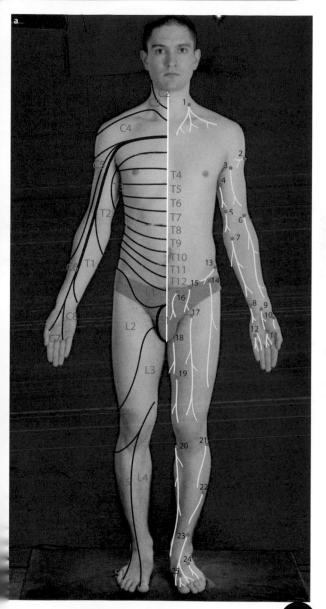

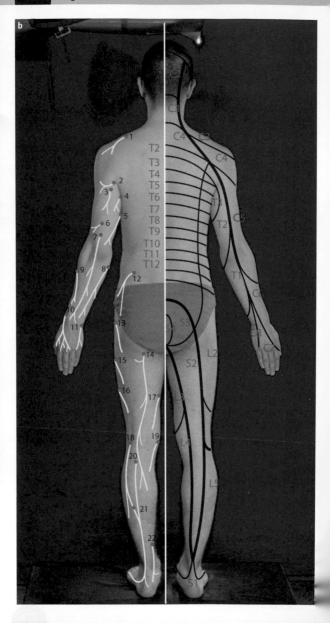

lines, where separated dermatomes lie adjacent to each other. The **muscle** innervation of the limb differs from that of sensation, in that the proximal muscles are supplied by the upper nerve roots, and T1 supplies the small muscles of the hand. The biceps reflex is supplied by C5/6; supinator, C6; and triceps, 6/7.

The **brachial plexus** may be damaged by penetrating injuries and by severe traction injuries at birth, pulling either downwards, avulsing the upper roots (**Erb's palsy**), or upwards, pulling on the C8 and T1 roots (**Klumpke's palsy**). Motorcycle accidents are also notorious for dragging the shoulder downwards, while the helmet sustains an upward pull. Pressure around the thoracic inlet, such as from a cervical rib, damages T1. **C5/6** injuries produce weakness of deltoid, supraspinatus, infraspinatus, teres minor, biceps, and brachialis. The limb hangs limp by the side, medially rotated and fully pronated in the "waiter's tip" position. Sensory loss is over the outer aspect of the arm and forearm. **T1** injuries produce weakness of the hand and sensory loss over the inside of the arm.

The **long thoracic** nerve, to serratus anterior, may be damaged during axillary dissection; paralysis of this muscle produces a winged scapular. The **thorocodorsal** nerve may also be damaged in radical axillary dissection; weakness of latissimus dorsi may produce remarkably few symptoms. The **axillary** nerve passes around the surgical neck of the humerus, and is easily damaged in fractures at this site and in shoulder dislocation. In these conditions, the resultant paralysis of deltoid and teres minor is painful to demonstrate, therefore look for the associated sensory loss, over a small area of skin, near the humeral attachment of the deltoid.

Figure 26

b. Cutaneous nerves and dermatomes, posterior.

1. Supraclavicular
2. Upper lateral cutaneous of arm
3. Posterior cutaneous of arm
4. Intercostobrachial
5. Medial cutaneous of arm
6. Lower lateral cutaneous of arm
7. Posterior cutaneous of forearm
8. Medial cutaneous of forearm
9. Lateral cutaneous of forearm
10. Superficial radial
11. Dorsal branch of ulnar
12. Iliohypogastric
13. 15. 16. Lateral cutaneous of thigh
14. Posterior cutaneous of thigh
17. Obturator
18. Lateral cutaneous of calf
19. Medial cutaneous of thigh
20. Sural
21. Sural communicating
22. Saphenous

The **radial** nerve may be damaged in fractures of the shaft of the humerus, as it passes along the radial groove. This produces a disabling paralysis of wrist extension (wrist drop) but minimal sensory loss, over the first dorsal interossei.

Median nerve injuries are usually associated with carpal tunnel compression, producing weakness of the thenar muscles, and sensory loss over the palmer aspect of the lateral three and a half fingers. Night pain is a disturbing symptom, and wasting gradually becomes obvious. Injury at the level of the elbow may accompany elbow dislocation, fractures, and misplaced injections. There is loss of flexion of the thumb, and index and middle fingers. Retained adductor pollicis (ulnar) and extensor pollicis muscles (radial) turn the thumb into the plane of the palm (simian palm). This, together with the outstretched (extended) index finger, produces the "benediction sign," when the hand is raised and facing forward.

Ulnar nerve damage is classically at the elbow, where the nerve is superficial, as it passes behind the medial epicondyle; it may also be trapped as it passes through the cubital tunnel, between the heads of flexor digitorum profundus. There is weakness of this muscle, all the interossei, the medial two lumbricals, and the adductor pollicis: Froment's sign is diagnostic for the latter (page 141). Interossei weakness may be demonstrated by failure to grip paper between the fingers, and weakness of the pinch grip between the fingers and the thumb. With more distal ulnar nerve lesions the loss of wrist and finger flexion is less marked.

In long-standing median and ulnar nerve lesions, due to ischemia and other chronic conditions such as leprosy, there is also marked muscle contracture, and this may produce a claw hand (**main-en-griffe**). The claw appearance is accentuated by interosseous muscle wasting. Clawing of the little and ring fingers is most marked with ulnar nerve injuries at the wrist. In lesions of the ulnar nerve at the elbow joint, additional paralysis of the medial finger tendons of the flexor digitorum profundus prevents flexion deformity of the interphalangeal joints; this produces the **ulnar nerve paradox**: the higher the lesion the less the deformity.

The **lower limb** is supplied by the **sacral plexus** (L4–S3), the distribution of the sensory dermatomes corresponds to those of the arm – along the outer surface to the periphery, and then proximally along the medial aspect of the limb (figure 26a,b). The groin and anterior thigh gain additional sensation from L1–3; thus you kneel on L3/4, walk on S1, and sit on S3. The knee jerk is supplied by L3/4, the ankle by S1 and the plantar reflex by S1/2; L5 is not represented in these reflexes, but can be specifically tested in dorsiflexion of the great toe.

The roots of the sacral plexus are well protected within the pelvis. T. **sciatic** nerve may be damaged as it passes outwards through the grea sciatic notch over the ischium, posterior to the head of the femur. In posterior dislocation of the hip, there is usually an associated fracture of the acetabular rim. The injury typically occurs in motorcycle accidents, when force applied to the bent knee is transmitted along the femur to the flexed hip. Sciatic palsy produces a flail limb.

Nerve injuries around the knee joint spare the hamstring muscles, but damage to the **tibial** nerve produces loss of plantar flexion and sensory denervation of the sole and lateral aspect of the foot (**sural** branch). Injury below this level produces paralysis of the small muscles of the sole; the unopposed action of the long flexor and extensor muscles produces a high arched sole. If the sural nerve is spared, there is still sensory loss over the sole, but sensation over the lateral aspect of the foot is preserved.

Injuries to the **common peroneal** nerve usually occur as it passes over the lateral aspect of the neck of the fibula, through direct trauma and fractures at this site (bumper fracture). The paralysis of the peroneal and anterior muscles produces a characteristic foot drop, with flopping of the foot during the gait. Sensory loss is over the anterolateral aspect of the lower leg and foot. The foot becomes inverted by the unopposed action of the tibialis posterior muscle. Sensory loss from damage to the **deep peroneal** nerve is limited to the dorsal skin of the first web.

The **femoral** nerve (L2,3,4) can be damaged by surgery around the psoas muscle and its sheath. A dramatic temporary paralysis may be produced by a spontaneous retroperitoneal bleed in patients on anticoagulants; there is usually a mass in the loin. The resultant disability is marked, with sensory loss over the anterior and medial thigh, and along the course of the saphenous nerve, on the medial aspect of the leg and foot. There may be paralysis of iliopsoas (L1,2) and pectineus, with loss of hip flexion, as well as paralysis of quadriceps, with loss of knee extension and instability of the knee joint. The patient is unable to extend the knee when sitting on the edge of an examination couch. The femoral nerve can also be the site of diabetic neuropathy.

Damage to the **obturator** nerve (L2,3,4) may occur in femoral hernia repair, particularly if the nerve takes an aberrant course, over the posterior aspect of the body of the pubic bone. Paralysis of the adductors is not total, since the adductor magnus receives part of its nerve supply from the sciatic nerve, together with the remainder of the hamstring muscles.

lateral **cutaneous** nerve of the thigh (L2,3) may be compressed
in the lateral fibers of the inguinal ligament, producing pain,
peresthesia and sensory loss over the lateral aspect of the upper thigh
(meralgia paresthetica).

LOCAL ANESTHESIA

Local anesthesia is produced by local anesthetic agents reversibly
blocking sodium transport across neural membranes. The anesthetic may
be absorbed through a **mucous membrane**, **infiltrated** into an operative
area, injected in close proximity to a **peripheral nerve**, or placed in the
extradural (**epidural** and **caudal anesthesia**) or subarachnoid (**spinal
anesthesia**) space. Subcutaneous infiltration is useful for minor surgical
procedures, such as excising lumps and suturing wounds. Wound edges
may also be infiltrated with a long-acting anesthetic to aid
postoperative pain relief. Infiltration should not be undertaken through
infected tissues and it is difficult to obtain adequate anesthesia of
inflamed areas.

This section considers common sites for neural blockade. The **choice** of
anesthetic depends on the length of anesthesia required (**short-acting**,
e.g., lidocaine, acts within a few minutes and lasts 30–60 minutes,
whereas **long-acting**, e.g., bupivacaine takes 15–30 minutes to act and
lasts for a few hours). The **dosage** varies with the preparation used, the
effect required, the vascularity of the region, and the age, weight,
physique, and clinical condition of the patient: 1% and 2% solutions are
usually available, but for larger areas and epidural use, solutions of
0.25% and 0.5% are appropriate. A large number of proprietary
preparations exist, and you must **read the manufacturer's instructions
and seek expert advice** for the agent you intend to use; particularly
note recommended doses for **children**. The **maximum dose** is usually
200 mg for an adult for short-acting and 400 mg in 24 hours for long-
acting preparations. This maximum dosage may be doubled when
preparations include **adrenalin**; this produces local vasoconstriction and
reduces the usual dilatory effect of the local anesthetic. Adrenalin
preparations also prolong the anesthetic effect. The usual concentration
of adrenalin is 1:200 000 (up to 1:80 000 in dental practice). **NB**
Adrenalin preparations must **NEVER** be used in digital anesthesia, as
they may produce severe vasoconstriction of the digital vessels with the
potential for ischemic damage.

An aseptic technique is essential when injecting a local anesthetic. It
often precedes an operative procedure, and full skin preparation and
toweling of the region may be required. Adequate time must be allowed

for the anesthetic to work before commencing any operative proce
You must be aware of the potential **complications** of local anesthet
These are dose related, and more likely to occur with inadvertent
intravascular injection. You must therefore always withdraw the plunge
of the syringe before injecting the anesthetic, and the injection must be
given slowly, to detect any immediate untoward effects before the full
dose is administered.

Read the manufacturer's instructions concerning drug interactions, these
include beta-blockers, vasoconstrictor, and some antiviral preparations.
The effects of toxicity and the occasionally encountered hypersensitivity
include myocardial depression and arrhythmias, and cerebral excitation;
you should therefore monitor the effects of an injection for at least 30
minutes. Management may include cardiopulmonary resuscitation and
the maintenance of fluid and electrolyte balance. Other complications
relate to the damage of adjacent structures and anatomical knowledge is
essential when undertaking regional blockade.

The **scalp** commonly requires suturing after head injuries. The first
priority is to establish the severity of the injury and to ensure that you
are not dealing with a skull fracture or an underlying intracerebral
hemorrhage. During this time, digital pressure can be applied to the
wound edge and then firm bandaging to reduce the heavy blood loss
that may occur from this vascular structure. Anesthesia is usually by
local infiltration, allowing debridement, removing just enough hair to
determine the extent of the laceration. The mobility of the scalp over
the periosteum and the rapid healing, due to its vascularity, allow you
to close most defects.

The whole scalp can be anesthetized by injecting anesthetic around the
nerves supplying it. The supraorbital nerve emerges from the orbit
through the supraorbital notch or foramen (figure 27a), and the
supratrochlear lies medial to it. The contribution from the maxillary
nerve is through the lacrimal, emerging from the lateral aspect of the
orbit, and the zygomatic branches emerging from the zygomatic bone
(figure 27b). The auriculotemporal nerve passes a centimeter anterior to
the upper part of the ear (figure 27c). The lesser occipital (figure 27d)
passes cranially near the posterior margin of the ear and the greater
occipital (figure 27e) lies 3–4 cm from the midline.

The infraorbital and mental nerves are in line with the supraorbital,
1.5 cm from the midline. The infraorbital (figure 28a) leaves the maxilla
a centimeter below the infraorbital margin, and supplies the **lower
eyelid**, **cheek**, **upper lip**, and **anterior nares**. The mental (figure 28b)
emerges from the mental foramen, directed laterally, about 1.5 cm above
the lower mandibular margin, and supplies the **lower lip** and **chin**.

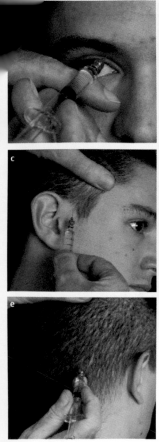

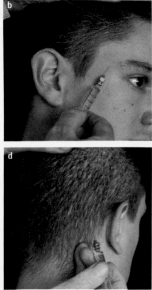

Figure 27 Scalp: a. supraorbital notch (supratrochlear injection placed medially to this point); b. zygomatic branches of maxillary; c. auriculotemporal; d. lesser occipital; e. greater occipital.

Ocular surgery may be undertaken under local anesthesia. As well as infiltrating the nerves already described, supplying the skin around the orbit, peribulbar injection (figure 29a–c) is through the lid or, by retracting it, through the underlying conjunctival sac. The needle passes backwards below the eyeball along the orbital floor for 3–4 cm.

The **mandibular nerve** (figure 30) emerges through the foramen ovale. This site, in the pterygoid fossa, is about 4 cm deep to the mandibular

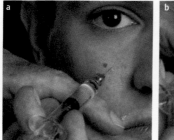
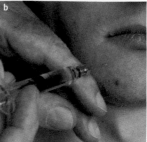

Figure 28 Face: a. infraorbital; b. mental.

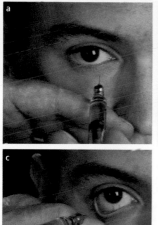
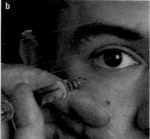

Figure 29 a,b,c. Periorbital and orbital: infraorbital through lower eyelid, medial, lateral, subconjunctival.

notch. The surface markings of the notch can be found by asking the subject to open their mouth. Place your finger on the condyle of the mandible and, on closing the mouth, your finger rests over the mandibular notch. Pass the needle horizontally and medially for 4 cm in the coronal plane, from this point.

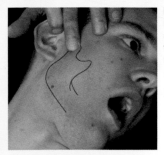

Figure 30 On closing the mouth, the needle is advanced at the point marked with the index finger, through the mandibular notch, to the mandibular nerve: about 4 cm.

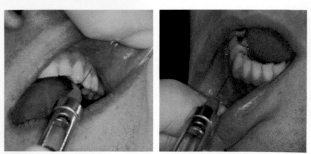

Figure 31 a,b. Local infiltration of upper and lower teeth.

Teeth

The **upper teeth and gums** are supplied by the superior and posterior alveolar branches of the maxillary nerves. The labial surface of the gums receives additional supply through the infraorbital nerve, and the lingual surface from the nasopalatine and greater palatine nerves. The **inferior teeth and gums** are supplied by the inferior alveolar branch of the mandibular nerve, as it passes through the mandibular canal. The labial surface receives additional supply from the buccal and mental nerves, and the lingual surface from the lingual nerve. The incisors receive bilateral innervation.

The upper teeth and lower front teeth (figure 31a,b) are anesthetized by local infiltration of the adjacent gums; the anesthetic diffuses to the alveolar branches of the maxillary and mandibular nerves. The **inferior alveolar (dental) nerve** is anesthetized as it enters the mandibular canal. Place your thumb over the retromolar fossa and direct the needle above it, passing posteriorly and laterally for 1.5 cm along the medial

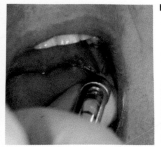

Figure 32 Inferior dental

side of the ramus of the mandible (figure 32). The **lingual nerve** passes just medial to this site and crosses the root of the third molar tooth; an inferior dental block thus also produces anesthesia of the anterior two-thirds of the tongue.

Cervical and Brachial Plexuses

The roots of the **cervical plexus** emerge from the transverse processes between the scalene muscles, and pass laterally. They are approached from behind the posterior border of the sternomastoid muscle to avoid the carotid sheath (figure 33a–d).

The **interscalene block** is a useful approach to the brachial plexus: the anesthetic is placed deep to the prevertebral fascia between the scalenus anterior and scalenus medius. In thin subjects, the lateral border of the scalenus anterior can be seen and palpated (figure 34a,b). The needle is aimed at the transverse process of the sixth cervical vertebra; this is at the level of the cricoid cartilage. The entry point is usually just behind the external jugular vein.

A **brachial plexus block** is lower and more laterally placed than the scalene block (figure 35), and passes close to the dome of the pleura and lung; these structures may be damaged. The entry point is 2 cm above the middle of the clavicle, passing posteromedially and downward at 45 degrees, toward the C7 transverse process. The anesthetic is again placed deep to the prevertebral fascia.

The prevertebral fascia follows the cords of the brachial plexus around the axillary artery as the **axillary sheath**, passing through the cervico-axillary canal into the upper arm. The cords are closely applied to the artery, and identification of the artery is the key to an **axillary block**. The anesthetic is placed within the axillary sheath but outside the artery (figure 36a,b). The needle is directed at the artery; entry into the sheath

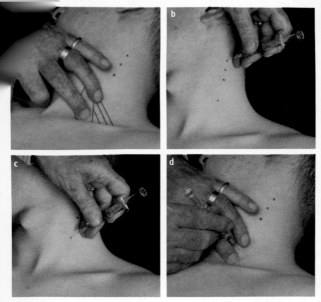

Figure 33 a,b,c,d. Ventral branches of cervical plexus accessed behind sternomastoid: needle passed behind carotid sheath through prevertebral fascia.

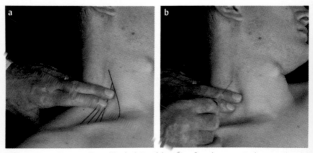

Figure 34 a. Interscalene block: lateral border of scalenus anterior may be both visible and palpable; b. needle advanced at level of cricoid cartilage.

is felt by a slight loss of resistance. Great care is taken to ensure that no blood is withdrawn through the syringe, as this indicates that the needle is within the axillary artery or vein. Once an intravascular

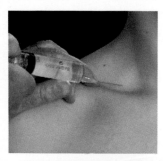

Figure 35 Brachial plexus block: entry point 2 cm above middle of clavicle (i.e., above dome of pleura).

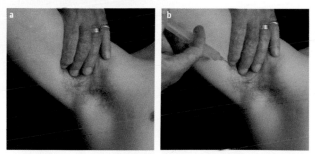

Figure 36 a,b. Axillary artery palpated by lateral pressure onto upper humerus; the needle directed at the artery, but stopping after entering the axillary sheath.

insertion has been excluded, the anesthetic is injected; this diffuses along and outside the artery to the nerves within the axillary sheath.

Anesthesia at the Elbow

The ulnar, medial, and radial nerves can be anesthetized at the level of the epicondyles. The **ulnar nerve** (figure 37a) is palpated and anesthetized behind the medial epicondyle. The **radial nerve** (figure 37b) pierces the lateral intermuscular septum through the origin of the brachialis muscle; it then lies under the medial border of brachioradialis, and gives off its **posterior interosseous** branch. Both nerves are anesthetized by passing the needle deep to the medial border of the brachioradialis at the epicondylar level, and backward toward the capitulum of the humerus. The musculocutaneous nerve also passes superficially at this site. The **median nerve** lies medial to the palpable brachial artery. Anesthetic placed superficial to the artery also

383

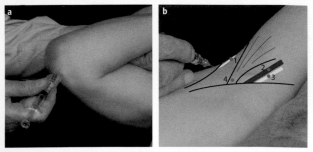

Figure 37 a. Elbow: ulnar nerve behind medial epicondyle; b. radial divides in lateral extreme of cubital fossa – cutaneous branch passes beneath brachioradialis; posterior interosseus, between two heads of supinator; injection also affects musculocutaneous; median is medial to brachial artery.

1. Radial nerve   3. Median nerve
2. Brachial artery   4. Biceps

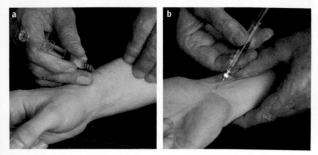

Figure 38 Wrist: a. radial nerve, b. median nerve proximal to flexor retinaculum.

anesthetizes the anterior branch of the medial cutaneous nerve of the forearm and terminal branches of the medial nerve of the arm.

Anesthesia of the Hand

Anesthesia of the **radial nerve** at the wrist is over the lateral aspect of the radius, 2 cm proximal to the wrist joint (figure 38a). Here the nerve can be palpated, as it passes posteriorly over the tendon of brachioradialis, underneath the cephalic vein. The **median nerve** lies behind palmaris longus at the proximal edge of the flexor retinaculum (figure 38b). The **ulnar nerve** passes over the retinaculum medial to the pisiform bone.

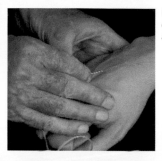

Figure 39 Beir's block: cannulation of dorsal vein, exanguinating bandage and proximal arterial tourniquet.

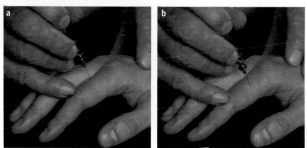

Figure 40 a. Medial and b. lateral palmer digital nerves through dorsal approach.

The hand, including the wrist, can be anesthetized by a **Bier's block** (figure 39). This is an injection of local anesthetic into an empty venous system, using a proximal arterial tourniquet to avoid release of anesthetic into the systemic circulation. A **short-acting** agent is used; this becomes inactive within an hour and reduces the risk of any toxic effects on release of the tourniquet. A cannula is placed within a dorsal hand vein and held with a plaster. An Esmarch bandage is used to exanguinate the hand, over the cannula, before placing a tourniquet around the mid-forearm. The tourniquet is maintained at 30 mmHg above systolic pressure. On completion of the procedure, release the pressure for 15 seconds and reinflate on two or three occasions, over 4–5 minutes, to dilute the effect of any residual anesthetic into the systemic circulation.

Digital blocks are placed from the dorsal aspect of the hand. The palm of the hand is placed on a flat surface and the needle inserted vertically onto the proximal phalanx, either centrally and advanced posteriorly on each side in turn, or as separate medial and lateral injections (figure 40a,b).

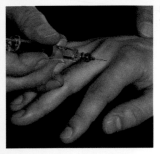

Figure 41 Digital nerves through web.

The injection is made, after initial aspiration, at the level of the anterior border of the phalanx. Alternatively the needle can be directed proximal to the level of the web (figure 41). **NB** Check that the agent used contains **no adrenalin** – this must never be injected at this level.

Intercostal Block

Anesthetizing part of the chest wall usually requires placement of local anesthetic around more than one intercostal nerve. The usual site to begin is in line with the inferior angle of the scapula over the posterolateral aspect of the chest; the inferior angle lies over the seventh rib and this can be palpated on either side of it. The neurovascular bundle runs along the subcostal groove and the proximity of the vessels again emphasizes the need to withdraw the plunger of syringe before any injection. Palpate the rib and insert the needle onto its lower part, then "walk" it down over the lower border (figure 42). The depth of the rib is established in this maneuver and once the lower border is passed, the needle is not advanced to any greater depth for the injection.

Anesthetizing the **lumbar sympathetic chains** is usually undertaken under image guidance. The surface marking is just below the tip of the twelfth rib, at the lateral border of the erector spinae muscle mass on each side. The needle is passed horizontally forwards at 45 degrees toward the vertebral column. It is then advanced to the anterior border of the vertebra, by "walking" the needle along the vertebra until it is felt to disappear. Aspiration is again essential before injection of local anesthetic, as the lumbar vessels and the aorta or inferior vena cava may be entered (figure 43).

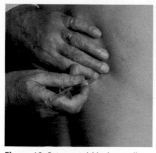

Figure 42 Intercostal block: needle "walked over" lower border of rib.

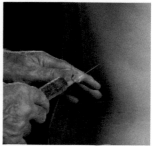

Figure 43 Sympathetic chain: use longer needle and ultrasonic guidance.

Lower Limb

The **femoral nerve** lies outside the femoral sheath, **lateral** to the femoral artery. The surface marking is by palpation of the femoral artery at the midinguinal point (halfway between the anterior superior iliac spine and the midline), just below the inguinal ligament. The needle is passed posteriorly, deep to the fascia lata, reaching the nerve as it enters the thigh on iliopsoas, from under the inguinal ligament (figure 44).

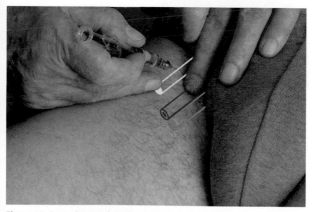

Figure 44 Femoral nerve: lateral to mid-inguinal point (left middle finger on palpable femoral artery).

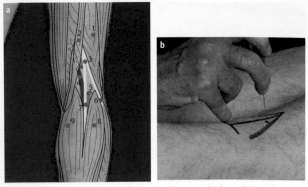

Figure 45 a,b. Popliteal fossa: single injection anesthetizes tibial and common peroneal nerves.

1. Semimembranosus
2. Biceps
3. Low division of sciatic nerve
4. Popliteal artery
5. Popliteal vein

6. Common peroneal nerve
7. Tibial nerve
8. Lateral head of gastrocnemius
9. Medial head of gastrocnemius

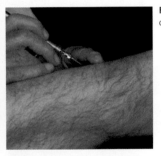

Figure 46 Common peroneal at neck of fibula.

The sciatic nerve usually divides in the upper thigh, but may be closer to the popliteal fossa. The **tibial** and **common peroneal** are closely related at the apex of the popliteal fossa, and lie in a plane between the deeply placed artery and the superficial veins. The two nerves are anesthetized with a single injection placed 5 cm above the popliteal crease and 1 cm laterally; the needle passes backward toward the back of the femur for 3 cm (figure 45a,b). The common peroneal nerve can also be palpated and anesthetized as it crosses the **neck of the fibula** laterally (figure 46). The **saphenous nerve** may be anesthetized at a knee or ankle level

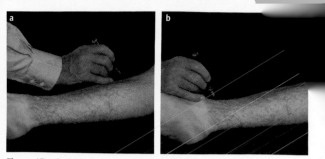

Figure 47 a,b. Saphenous nerve at knee and ankle.

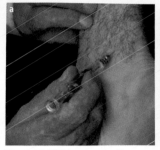

Figure 48 Tibial nerve at ankle.

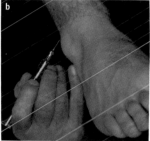

Figure 49 Sural nerve behind lateral malleolus.

(figure 47a,b); the former is over the anteromedial aspect of the tibial plateau. At the ankle, the nerve lies alongside, usually medial to the palpable great saphenous vein on the anterior aspect of the medial malleolus.

At the ankle, the **tibial nerve** (figure 48) passes with the posterior tibial vessels in the groove behind the medial malleolus. Palpation of the artery at this site allows placement of the injection just lateral to the vessel; again check for extravascular delivery of the anesthetic. The **superficial peroneal** and the **sural nerves** (figure 49) pass just behind the lateral malleolus; the **deep peroneal nerve** crosses the ankle joint just lateral to the tibialis anterior tendon; it may be in close relationship to the anterior tibial artery (figure 50).

Digital anesthetic can be delivered from the dorsal aspects of the proximal phalanx. The needle is passed from the posterior aspect of the

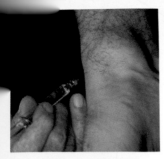

Figure 50 Deep peroneal nerve lateral to tibialis anterior.

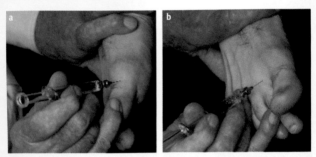

Figure 51 Digital nerves; needle passed vertically alongside proximal phalanx: a. medial; b. lateral.

phalanx and then "walked over" its edge, and advanced to its anterior border. The great toe usually requires separate medial and lateral injections (figure 51a,b). Anesthetic may initially be placed centrally, over the dorsum of the toe, to reduce the discomfort of subsequent injections. It is again emphasized the need to check that the anesthetic preparation does **not contain any adrenalin**.

A **Bier's block** (figure 52) is also applicable to the foot; first place a venous needle or cannula, exanguinate the foot over it and apply a proximal calf tourniquet. A dorsal foot vein or the great saphenous vein at the ankle is used for the intravenous injection. The needle is placed before exanguination and the tourniquet pressure is 30 mmHg above systolic, to prevent blood flow during the procedure. The short-acting anesthetic wears off in about an hour; release within half an hour should be controlled by briefly letting down and then re-inflating the tourniquet a number of times over 4–5 minutes, to prevent sudden release and potential systemic toxicity.

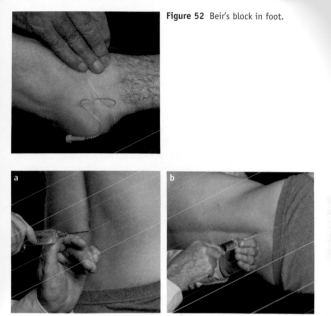

Figure 52 Beir's block in foot.

Figure 53 Lumbar puncture: a. in sitting or; b. left lateral position, above or below fourth lumbar spine; needle advanced in mid-line, with slightly cranial angulation.

Lumbar Puncture

Lumbar puncture may be undertaken with the subject sitting or lying in the left lateral position (figure 53a,b). In the latter, ask the patient to draw their legs up to their chest, to keep their back vertical and near the edge of the bed, to ensure that the needle is advanced horizontally in the midline. The entry point is above or below the spine of the fourth lumbar vertebra, which is identified in the supracristal plane (passing between the upper borders of the iliac crests). A lumbar puncture needle approximately 5 cm long is advanced through the supraspinous and interspinous ligaments into the extradural space. Various techniques are used to show the sudden release of pressure on a syringe as it enters the space, but still lies outside the spinal meninges.

An **epidural anesthetic** is delivered into the extradural space; a catheter is left *in situ* to provide long-term pain relief postoperatively. Further anterior advancement of the needle is felt to hit the dura and then, on

... it, cerebrospinal fluid (CSF) can be withdrawn (page 369). ...ion of anesthetic at this level produces a **spinal anesthetic**. The ...ent's shoulders are slightly raised, to retain the anesthetic around ...e nerves of the cauda equina. **NB** the dosage of anesthetic required is ...ess for spinal anesthesia, and therefore differentiation of the site for extradural and spinal anesthesia is essential to avoid an overdose.

In a **caudal block,** anesthetic is placed in the sacral canal, through the sacral hiatus. It is undertaken in the left lateral position. The surface marking of the hiatus is the apex of an equilateral triangle, based on the two posterior superior iliac spines (the dimples of Venus). The hiatus is also palpable and is covered by the sacrococcygeal membrane. The needle is passed through the skin and the membrane, the latter being felt as a slight click. The needle (or cannula) is then advanced for a centimeter cranially. The dural sac ends at S2, but aspirate to exclude both CSF and blood before injection. There should be minimal resistance; observe and palpate to exclude a subcutaneous delivery.

Appendices

Appendices

Appendix 1

ANATOMICAL ORIENTATION

To find a location one needs directions from a known point on a map. In the body, specific anatomical terms are used for directions. Bony prominences are usually used as reference points and the body's map is the **anatomical position** (figure 1). In the latter, the subject stands upright, with their arms down by their sides, and head, trunk, palms, and toes facing forward.

The **sagittal plane** passes vertically from front to back, the **midsagittal (median) plane** is in the midline, and **parasagittal** planes are to either side of it. The **coronal (frontal) plane** passes vertically from side to side at right angles to the sagittal plane and the **transverse (horizontal) plane** passes horizontally at right angles to the other two (producing a cross-sectional/axial/transaxial radiological image). Outer structures are **superficial** to inner, **deep**, structures. The **median line** passes vertically downward at the junction of the midsagittal and midcoronal planes. In the anatomical position, the body's **center of gravity** is in the midline, just anterior to the second piece of the sacrum.

When relating two points in the coronal plane, the point nearest the midsagittal plane is **medial** to the second, and the second point is **lateral** to the first (in figure 1, **A** is medial to **B** and **B** is lateral to **A**). When comparing two points along a limb, the point nearer to the trunk is **proximal** and the one furthest away is **distal**. Ipsilateral refers to structures on the same side of the body; **contralateral**, the opposite.

The front of the body in the anatomical position is termed **anterior** and the back **posterior**. **Ventral** is usually synonymous with anterior and **dorsal** with posterior (in figure 1, **E** is anterior to **F** and **F** posterior to **E**). An exception is the foot where, due to inward twisting during development, the dorsal aspect of the foot comes to lie in front and the ventral aspect behind. Later, when taking up the upright position, the ventral part becomes the sole. When relating two points in the horizontal plane, the one above is **superior** (**cranial**, **rostral**) to the second, and the second point is **inferior** (**caudal**) to the first (in figure 1, **G** is superior to **H** and **H** is inferior to **G**).

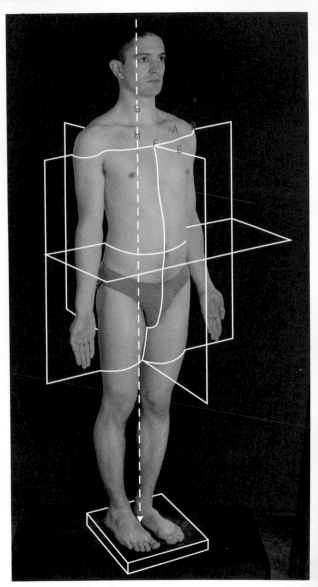

Figure 1 Anatomical position.

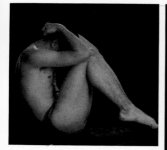

Figure 2 Subject in flexed position.

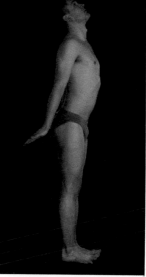

Figure 3 Subject in extended position.

The direction of joint movements is also described in relation to the anatomical position. The posture of the subject in figure 2 is in the flexed position and figure 3 extended.

Forward movement of the distal part of the limb from the anatomical position is termed **flexion** (of the wrist in figure 4a) and backward movement **extension** (of the wrist and hip in figure 4b,c): note that the description relates to the anatomical position not to the position of the joint in space.

Movement of the head and the trunk to one side is termed **lateral flexion** (figure 5a,b), movement of a limb away from the midline is termed **abduction** (figure 6a) and towards the midline **adduction** (figure 6b). In digital movement, the midline is taken as the middle finger and the second toe: figure 7a,b show finger abduction and adduction respectively. In development, the thumb rotates inwards through approximately 90 degrees, and its movements are described in relation to this acquired position, i.e., to the plane of the thumbnail (figure 8 shows thumb extension). In addition, movement of the thumb toward the fingers is termed **opposition**.

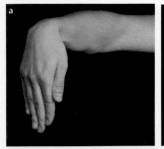

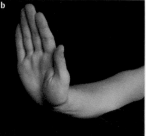

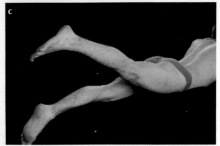

Figure 4 a. Wrist flexion and b. extension, and c. hip extension.

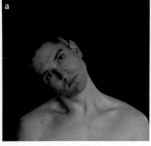

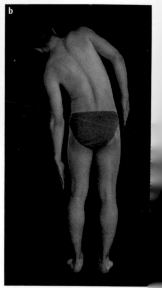

Figure 5 a,b. Lateral flexion of head and trunk.

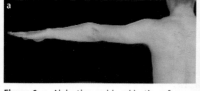

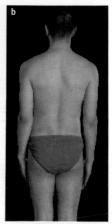

Figure 6 a. Abduction and b. adduction of shoulder.

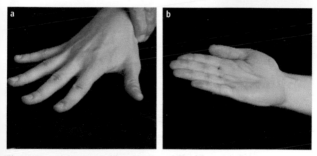

Figure 7 a. Abduction and b. adduction of fingers.

Figure 8 Extension of thumb.

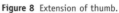

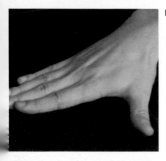

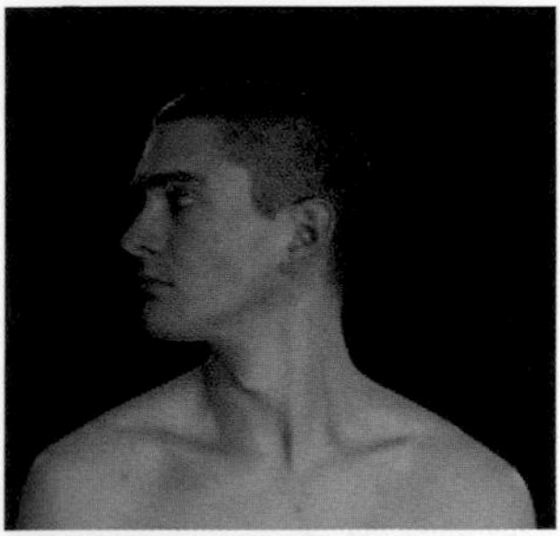

Figure 9 Rotation of head to right.

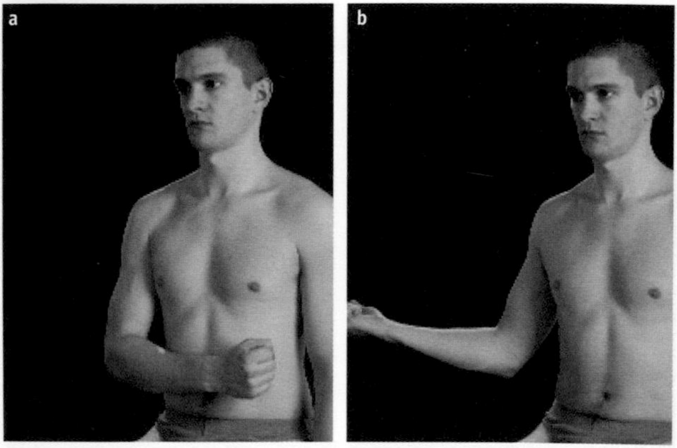

Figure 10 a. Medial and b. lateral rotation of shoulder.

Rotation of the head and trunk is to the right or the left (figure 9 shows rotation of the head to the right). In the joints of the limbs, rotation that moves the thumb or the big toe from the anatomical position toward the midline is termed **medial (internal) rotation** (figure 10a), and away from the midline, **lateral (external) rotation** (figure 10b). Rotation of the lower limb occurs mainly at the hip joint, but is also demonstrable in the bent knee: figure 11a shows medial rotation from the anatomical position (figure 11b); figure 11c, lateral rotation.

Medial (internal) rotation of the forearm at the elbow is termed **pronation** (figure 12a) and lateral (external) rotation, **supination** (figure 12b). Circular movement of the distal part of a limb, e.g. the hand at the wrist, is termed **circumduction**.

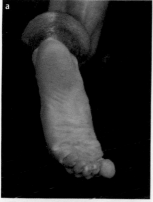

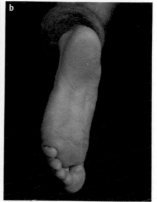

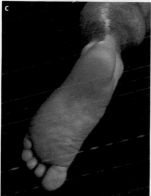

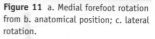

Figure 11 a. Medial forefoot rotation from b. anatomical position; c. lateral rotation.

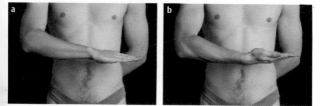

Figure 12 a. Pronation and b. supination of forearm.

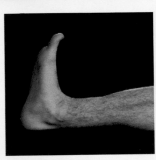

Figure 13 Dorsiflexion.

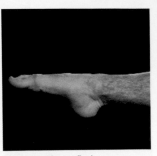

Figure 14 Plantar flexion.

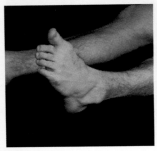

Figure 15 Inversion.

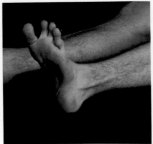

Figure 16 Eversion.

The rotation of the lower limb during development also affects the description of movements of the knee, ankle, and foot joints. Backward movement of the distal part of these joints is flexion and forward movement, extension. In the ankle, specific terms are used: upward movement of the foot is **dorsiflexion** (figure 13) and downward movement, **plantar flexion** (figure 14); turning the sole inwards is **inversion** (figure 15) and outwards, **eversion** (figure 16).

Appendix 2

SYSTEMIC HISTORY AND EXAMINATION

General

Mental state, personal care, features, clinical syndromes, posture

Pulse, blood pressure, respiratory rate, temperature

Hands: *skin* (palm and dorsum) color, temperature, moisture, palmar erythema, cyanosis, staining (nicotine, bruising, rashes), pigmentation, tone, thickness, laxity, senile changes Osler's nodes, rheumatoid changes, Dupuytren's contracture

Nails: bitten, pallor, spooned, clubbing, splinter hemorrhages

Muscles: wasting, abnormal movements, flap

Lymphadenopathy

Head and Neck

Cranial Nerves
I: smell

II: visual acuity, color vision, visual fields, fundoscopy

III,IV,VI: pupillary responses to light and accommodation, extraocular movements, ptosis, lid lag, nystagmus, enophthalmos, exophthalmos

V: sensation over the three divisions; corneal reflex, muscles of mastication, jaw jerk

VII: facial expression, whistle, blowing out cheeks against resistance, taste anterior two-thirds of tongue

VIII: hearing: watch, whisper, Rinne's and Weber's tests

IX: gag reflex, taste posterior third of tongue

X: voice, cough, uvular deviation, swallow

XI: shoulder shrugging, neck rotation, head nodding

XII: tongue movements

Nose
Deformity, airway, bleeding

...es

...nflammation, chemosis, pallor, subconjunctival hemorrhage

..., yellow, blue, brown

...ens/iris: scars, abrasions, ulcer, cataract, arcus senilis, ...imbic calcification, coloboma

...phthalmos, enophthalmos, glaucoma

Movements: extraocular movements, conjugate in all directions, nystagmus, fatigability of pursuit movements

Visual fields: to confrontation with finger, and white and red pin heads

Visual acuity: Snellen's chart, reading chart, light and accommodation reflexes, Horner syndrome

Fundi: optic disc, vessels, macula

Ear
Pinna: malformation, gouty tophi

External acoustic meatus: wax, infection

Tympanic membrane: scarring, redness, perforation, bulging (and Valsalva)

Hearing: watch, whisper, Rinne's and Weber's tests

Temporomandibular Joint
Movements

Mouth
Lips: telangiectasia, swelling, ulceration, pigmentation, Koplik's spots, cleft

Gums: gingivitis, hypertrophy, retraction

Teeth: discoloration, caries, periodontal disease

Tongue: glossitis, atrophy, macroglossia, geographic tongue, ulceration, leukoplakia, neoplasia

Tonsil: redness, purulent discharge, gag reflex

Oropharynx: redness, coated, purulent discharge, fetor

Salivary glands: tenderness, swelling, abscess, cysts, tumors, duct calculi

Face
Congenital features, Cushing's, acromegaly

Facial palsy: upper/lower motor neuron

Cachexia, weight loss, edema

Neck

Trachea: deviation, tug

Thyroid: palpable, enlarged, symmetrical, focal lump, cyst, benign, malignant tumours, tracheal deviation, retrosternal extension, bruit, movement on swallowing

Carotid arteries: enlargement, bruits, jugular venous pressure, hepatojugular reflex

Lymph nodes: submental, submandibular, preauricular, postauricular, occipital, deep and superficial cervical lymph chains

Neck movements

Musculoskeletal System

History: localize symptomatic muscles, joints, bones

Pain, stiffness, limited movement, creaking, cracking, locking, giving way, swelling, wasting, contractures, deformities, loss of function

Manual dexterity: dressing, toiletry, eating, writing

Mobility: ability to sit and stand, walking distance, independence, need for assistance or mechanical aids, work and recreational activity

Symptoms of inflammatory disorders: fever, malaise, ocular problems, urethritis, diarrhea

Examination: pain at rest, on movement, Cushingoid, Paget's deformity, weight, fever, malaise, inflammatory eye conditions, blue sclera, gouty tophi, digital trophic changes

Nails: color, discoloration, pitting, ridging, hyperkeratosis

Compare bones, joints and muscles of the two sides of the body. Ensure appropriate exposure and record any abnormalities of asymptomatic joints

Look: skin: creases, scars, color, erythema, atrophy, rashes, sinuses

Shape: swelling of bone, bursae, synovium, effusions, bony alignment (valgus, varus), subluxation, dislocation, shortening, deformity, wasting

Position: at rest and during activity

...ities: swan neck, boutonnière's, z thumb, finger drop, mallet
...puytren's contracture, Heberden/Bouchard nodes, ulnar
...

...e: kyphoscoliosis, neurological and myopathic abnormalities,
...delenburg test

Feel: skin, soft tissue and bones, warmth, tenderness, thickening, nodules, overgrowth, deformity

Abnormal bursae/synovial thickening

Effusions: reducible, fluctuant, ballottable, transillumination

Fractures: tenderness, deformity

Move: active, passive and resisted movements in each joint plane

Pain, power, tone, range, creaking, crepitus, clicking, triggering, locking, hypermobility, telescoping, contractures, stability

Fracture: abnormal mobility, crepitus

Deformity: mobile or fixed

Hand: ability to grip, pinch and do up shirt buttons

Gait: spastic, ataxic, waddling, limp, use of mechanical aids

Measure: range of joint movements (goniometer)

Limb circumference at equivalent levels from fixed bony points on the limbs on each side

True and apparent leg shortening, Bryant's triangle

Proceed to X-ray and image symptomatic areas, to identify abnormal bone and soft tissues

Female Breast

History: Pain: cyclical/persistent

Lump: generalized/discrete, duration, change, previous history

Discharge: milk, pus, blood, serous (color)

Menstrual history: pregnancy, breast feeding, pill and hormone replacement

Family history

Examination: secluded, warm area with subject undressed to waist

Sitting, reaching up, leaning forward, lying

For each breast: pillow behind shoulder and hand behind head

Look for: symmetry, mobility, flattening, swelling, skin dimpling, redness, peau d'orange, ulceration, submammary edema, lumps

Palpate: each quadrant, the retroareolar area and the nipple, for nodularity (general/focal), lumps, mobility

Express from the nipple

Axillary nodes: anterior, medial, posterior, lateral, apical, infraclavicular, supraclavicular

Liver enlargement, spinal tenderness

Cardiovascular System

History: Pain: angina, central chest (radiation), back

Palpitations, edema, cyanosis, fatigue, syncope

Cough, sputum, hemoptysis; dyspnea, orthopnea, paroxysmal nocturnal dyspnea

Hypertension, diabetes, hypercholesterolemia, smoking, family history of vascular disease

Symptoms of stroke: visual, speech, motor, sensory, cranial and peripheral nerves, memory

Claudication, pain in feet at rest, foot ulceration, gangrene

Examination: Marfan, Down, Turner syndromes, cachexia

Hands, fingers and nails: clubbing, peripheral cyanosis, nicotine staining, splinter hemorrhages, Osler's nodes

Head and neck: jugular venous pressure (cannon waves, CV systolic waves), hepatojugular reflex, xanthelasma, pallor, jaundice, central cyanosis, malar flush, fundi

Arterial pulse: rate, rhythm, volume, character, thickening of vessel wall

Tachycardia, bradycardia, sinus arrhythmia, premature beats, atrial fibrillation, hyperdynamic, collapsing (Corrigan), bisferiens alternans, pulsus paradoxus

Radio-femoral delay, radial asymmetry, cardio-peripheral deficit

Peripheral pulses: presence, symmetry, volume, bruits

Blood pressure: standing/lying

Respiratory rate, temperature

Heart: lying at 45 degrees, repeated in supine, rotated and sitting positions, on to Valsalva and squatting maneuvers

Position, force and character of apex beat, abnormal pulsation, thrills, cardiac outline, scars

Auscultation with bell and diaphragm over mitral, aortic, pulmonary, and tricuspid areas, repeat during inspiration and expiration, and appropriate positions

Sounds: first and second, splitting, third and fourth, summation gallop, opening snap, ejection click, mid/late systolic click, pericardial knock/rub

Timing of onset and offset of *murmurs* in relation to systole, diastole and valve closure, point of maximum intensity, grade, radiation, effect of positional and respiratory maneuvers

Systolic: aortic stenosis, HOCM, mitral regurgitation, mitral valve prolapse, ventricular septal defect

Diastolic: aortic regurgitation, mitral stenosis

Continuous: patent ductus arteriosus, venous hum, pulmonary arteriovenous malformation, ruptured coronary sinus

Lungs for basal crepitations, pulmonary effusion

Hepatomegaly, liver pulsation, ascites, peripheral edema

Feet: pulses, trophic changes, pressure sores, ulceration, gangrene, inflammation, abscess formation, neuropathy, postural changes, venous filling time

Respiratory System

History: upper respiratory tract infection, nasal discharge, nasal obstruction, pain over sinus or in ears, cervical lymphadenopathy

Chest pain: related to respiration, angina

Cough: day/night time, dry, productive, sputum (appearance and volume), hemoptysis

Breathlessness: at rest, on exercise, orthopnea, paroxysmal nocturnal dyspnea, wheezing

Pyrexia, rigors, cyanosis, edema, myalgia

Examination: cough, sputum (examine sputum pot: color, consistency, volume)

Pulse, blood pressure, respiratory rate, temperature

Hands, fingers and nails: clubbing; peripheral cyanosis, nicotine staining, wasting of small muscles, wrist tenderness, carbon dioxide retention flap

Head and neck: conjunctival pallor, jugular venous pressure, Horner syndrome, hoarseness of voice

Cervical and axillary nodes

Chest: pattern of respiration, rate, depth, tachypnea, dyspnea, irregularity, stridor, use of accessory muscles, Cheyne-Stokes

Anterior chest wall configuration: pectus excavatum, pectus carinatum

Scars, prominent veins

Vertebral column abnormalities: buffalo hump, barrel chest, lordosis, kyphoscoliosis

Palpate tracheal deviation, tracheal tug

Chest expansion: manual assessment and tape measure

Tactile vocal fremitus, subcutaneous emphysema, rib tenderness

Percussion: resonant, hyper-resonant, dull, stony dull

Coarse percussion

Auscultation: use bell and diaphragm

Breath sounds: normal, vesicular, bronchial, bronchovesicular

Adventitious sounds: crackles (râles), wheezes (rhonchi)

Vocal resonance: egophony, whispering pectoriloquy

Pleural friction rub

Alimentary and Genitourinary Systems

History: weight (current, changes), fatigue, pigmentation

Pain: site, radiation, relation to food

Flatulence, nausea, vomiting, hematemesis

Dysphagia: site, solids/fluids

Stool: frequency, quantity, consistency, mucus, blood (fresh, altered, melena), tenesmus

Perianal pain: lump, discharge, pruritus

Micturition: frequency, nocturia, polyuria, oliguria, hematuria, obstruction, hesitancy, poor stream, dribbling, urgency, dysuria

Urethral discharge/pain

Urine: amount, discoloration, clarity, color, blood, debris

Menstruation: menarche, menopause, dysmenorrhea, menorrhagia, amenorrhea

Dyspareunia: superficial/deep, vaginal discharge, contraception

Pregnancy: past obstetric history, last smear, last menstrual period, expected date of delivery, abdominal pain, vaginal bleeding, venous thrombosis

Examination: presence and features of any vomitus

Weight loss, cachexia, dehydration, obesity, hypo/hyper-pigmentation, encephalopathy

Hands: palmar erythema, telangiectasia, Dupuytren's contracture, skin laxity, muscle wasting, arthropathy, liver flap

Nails: pallor, clubbing, spooning, leukonychia, onycholysis

Head and neck: conjunctival pallor, jaundice, xanthelasma, halitosis (hepatic, uremic, faecal, ketotic), tongue (dry, furred, glossitis, leukoplakia), gingivitis, dentition

Salivary glands: tenderness, swelling

Cervical lymphadenopathy (NB: scalene node)

Abdomen: lying supine with a single pillow, fully exposed, but breasts and genitalia covered until these areas are examined

On inspection: skin: laxity, pigmentation, bruising, scratch marks, striae, hair distribution, scars, sinuses, fistulas, stomas, dilated veins, herniae, divarication of the recti

Umbilicus: position, hygiene, nodules, discharge, hernia

Distension: scaphoid abdomen, respiratory movements, visible peristalsis

Enlarged organs: liver, gall bladder, spleen, bladder, uterus, masses

Discomfort on blowing out/drawing in abdominal wall and coughing

On percussion of the four quadrants: rebound tenderness, hyper-resonance, position of organs (liver, spleen, bladder, uterus), masses, ascites, shifting dullness

On palpation: NB watch patient's face throughout. In children and with sensitive abdomens, start with self-examination to identify tender areas

Superficial/deep four quadrant, tenderness, guarding, rigidity

Organs: liver, gall bladder, spleen, kidneys, bladder, uterus, colon/feces

Masses: stomach, pancreas, uterus, ovarian, large/small bowel, retroperitoneal

Aorto-iliac aneurysms

Ballottable organs/masses, fluid thrill, sacral edema

On auscultation: gut sounds: normal, absent, tinkling, increased

Friction rub

Renal, aorto-iliac bruits/hums

Succussion splash

Inguinal/Femoral Hernia

If not obvious ask the patient to stand

Observe site, overlying skin, cough impulse, reduction by patient

Palpate for tenderness, cough impulse, reducibility, anatomical position of neck, controllability

Inguinal/axillary nodes

External Genitalia

Draw scrotum forward onto the front of the thighs

Observe symmetry, skin, scars, rashes

Swellings: inguino-scrotal, scrotal (testis, epididymis)

Palpate: testis, epididymis, spermatic cord

Relation of cyst/masses to testis/epididymis

Penis: circumcised, retractable foreskin, position and shape of meatus, balanitis, discharge

Rectal/vaginal examination

Nervous System

History: current mental state: level of consciousness, orientation, memory (recent, long term), intellect, understanding, insight, thought content, behavior, mood, hallucinations, delusions

Prior injury, stroke, transient ischemic attack

Headache, fits, faints, falls, dizziness

Disturbances of vision/speech, diplopia, visual loss, dysarthria, dysphasia, aphasia

Disturbances of motor or sensory function of limbs/face, dysesthesia, clumsiness, weakness

Examination: NB compare the two sides of the body

Handedness

Speech: dysphasia (expressive, receptive, global), jargon, scanning, stuttering, dysarthria

Motor function: tone: spasticity, flaccidity, rigidity, clonus

Power: hand grips, wrists, elbows, shoulder, ankles, knees, hips

Coordination finger–nose, heel–shin, dysdiadochokinesis, pyramidal drift

Reflexes: tendon, superficial

Abnormal movements: tremor (static, intention), choreiform, athetoid, convulsions, associated movements, tics

Muscle: wasting, hypertrophy, fasciculation

Abnormalities of posture: upper/lower motor neuron, extrapyramidal, cerebellar, sensory, myopathic, Romberg's sign, standing on toes, walking backwards on heels, heel-toe

Gait: spastic, ataxic, waddling, limp

Sensory function: nerve root, spinal cord level, hemianesthesia

Light touch: cotton wool

Pain: pinprick

Temperature: finger/tuning fork

Vibration: start distally on wrist and ankle

Position sense: hold sides of digit

Graphesthesia: use 3s and 8s

Two-point discrimination. blunt compass, start on hand

Stereognosis: coins, keys

Spinal deformity/tenderness, neck rigidity

Palpate and percuss abnormal superficial nerves

Map out areas of altered sensation

Contractures, neuropathic joints, ulceration

Carotid bruits

Autonomic: sweating, postural hypotension, heart rate response to a Valsalva maneuver

Appendix 3

TOOLS OF EXAMINATION AND DIAGNOSIS

Surprisingly few tools are required for most clinical examinations. You should carry a **watch** to count the pulse and respiratory rate, and carry a **stethoscope**, a **torch** and a **tape measure**. On the wards and outpatient

Table 1 CHECK LIST FOR LUMPS AND ULCERS (bold = both)

	LUMPS	ULCERS
Site	**Tissue of origin** **Relations**	
Exterior	**Size** **Shape** **Surface** **Color** **Tenderness** **Temperature** **Mobility**	Edge flat sloping punched out undermined raised everted
Interior	Consistency Indentation Fluctuation Fluid thrill Transillumination Expansion Compressibility Reducibility Cough impulse Pulsation Bruit Discharge	Floor depth covering discharge Base penetration fistulation
Surroundings	**Induration** **Tethering/fixation** **Invasion:** **nerves** **vessels** **other tissue** **Nodes** **Related disease**	

departments you can expect (but check) disposable **gloves**, wooden **spatulas**, and a **sphygmomanometer**, an **ophthalmoscope** and an **auroscope**. Additional tools are required for ENT (**nasal speculum, mirror and endoscope**), neurological (**odorants**, Snellen and colour vision charts, **cotton wool, sterile pin, tuning fork**, 2 point **retractor, patellar hammer**), musculoskeletal (**goniometer**) and pelvic examination (**proctoscope** and **vaginal speculum**).

Ask the patient to demonstrate an abnormality, to direct your own examination: disease represents loss or modification of form and function, but be aware that the full house of classical signs of a specific disease is not present in every patient.

Diagnostic Sieve

- The **history** and **examination** are usually sufficient to provide a provisional diagnosis and a management plan; **investigations** provide further evidence on the diagnosis and help monitor progress
- The **systems review** (table 2) is an effective means of surveying the activity of the whole body, identifying problems not volunteered or noticed by the patient, and helping the diagnosis of the presenting and subsidiary problems
- When there is still difficulty in making a diagnosis, consider the **anatomy** of the region involved, and systematically go through the potential causes of disease (the diagnostic sieve)
- When considering the anatomical structures (table 2), also think of the nerve supply to the symptomatic area, as the pain could be due to radiation from proximal nerve damage or referred from a deeper structure supplied by the same dermatome
- The **diagnostic sieve** originated from the five pathologies of the **surgical sieve** – congenital, infection, trauma, neoplasia, and degenerative disease. The other pathologies in table 2 are less common surgical problems and infection has been expanded to inflammation
- **Inflammation** is the "body's response to injury," where the injury may be infective (viruses, bacteria, fungi, protozoa, parasites), but also due to trauma, neoplasia and to "foreign" protein, giving rise to an antigen/antibody response, as in autoimmune disease
- In **neoplasia**, consider benign and malignant, and in the latter, primary and secondary disease
- **Degenerative** disease includes arterial, arthritic, dementia and other diseases of the old, and sometimes not so old

Table 2 **CONSIDERATIONS IN DIAGNOSIS**

SYSTEM	ANATOMY	PATHOLOGY	
Cardiovascular	Skin	Congenital	Metabolic
Respiratory	Subcutaneous tissues	Inflammatory	Hormonal
Gastrointestinal	Vessels and nerves	Traumatic	Hematological
Genitourinary	Muscles	Neoplastic	Poisons
Musculoskeletal	Bones	Degenerative	Chemicals
Neurogenic	Joints		Iatrogenic
Endocrine	Viscera		Idiopathic
Hematopoietic			Psychiatric

Glossary

*The descriptions are of commonly encountered terms and condition.
include text entries but not all items from the tables. Infective disea
not included.*

Abscess – localized collection of pus. The site is added (sometimes with a prefix): subphrenic, subungual, subcutaneous (under the diaphragm, nail, skin); intrahepatic (in the liver), para/perinephric (around the kidney); retrocecal, retroperitoneal (behind the cecum, peritoneum)

Acanthocytosis – crenated red cells on a blood film

Acanthosis nigricans – skin pigmentation, often associated with malignancy

Accommodation – the process of focusing an image onto the retina, through ciliary muscle contraction

Accommodation reflex – changes in the pupil size that occur on changing between distant and near vision

Achalasia – failure of muscle relaxation, usually with reference to the esophagogastric junction

Achondroplasia – hereditary disorder of epiphyseal ossification, resulting in dwarfism

Acidosis – reduction of normal tissue pH (usually measured in the serum)

Acquired immunodeficiency syndrome (AIDS) – viral infection producing a defect in cell-mediated immunity

Acromegaly – clinical syndrome due to increased growth hormone

Acute – sudden onset; also used to define severe and to differentiate an acute inflammatory response to certain bacteria from the chronic inflammatory granuloma produced by others

Addison disease – clinical syndrome due to adrenal cortical insufficiency

Adenoids – enlargement of the lymphatic tissue in the roof of the nasopharynx

Adhesions – sticking together of two normally separate parts, e.g., loops of gut, visceral and parietal, pleura and pericardium

Agenesis – failure of development

**– loss of taste

a – inability to interpret a sensation, e.g., visual

phia – inability to write

exia – inability to read aloud

Allen's test – test of hand blood flow

Allergy – body's reaction to foreign material (the substance may not be identified)

Alveolitis – inflammation of the alveoli

Amnesia – loss of memory

Amniocentesis – withdrawal of amniotic fluid

Anacrotic – abnormal pulse wave, with an additional notch on the ascending limb

Anaphylaxis – acute hypersensitivity to a foreign substance, such as a protein, drug or mismatched transfusion, giving rise to a state of shock

Anarthria – inability to articulate

Anatomy – study of body form

Anemia – reduction of circulating red cells, hemoglobin or packed red cell volume

Anencephaly – congenital absence of the brain

Anesthesia – loss of sensation, local or general

Aneurysm – localized dilatation of a blood vessel, usually an artery

Angina – chest pain from myocardial ischemia

Angioma – benign tumor of blood or lymphatic vessels

Ankylosis – fusion of parts, usually a joint

Anosmia – loss of smell

Aortic incompetence – *see* incompetence

Apgar score – scoring system of physical activity in the newly born

Aphasia – inability to speak; may be partial, as in nominal (loss of names), jargon (senseless speech)

Aphthous – small idiopathic mouth ulcer

Apnea – cessation of breathing

Apraxia – impaired voluntary control of an otherwise intact motor function

Arteriovenous malformation/fistula – abnormal communication between arteries and veins, may be congenital/acquired (including surgically produced)

Arthritis – inflammation of a joint, usually qualified by the type, e.g., **osteoarthritis** – wear and tear of cartilage covering the articular surface; **rheumatoid arthritis** – a chronic inflammation involving cartilage and soft tissues

Ascites – collection of intraperitoneal serous fluid (table 6; page 301)

Asystole – cardiac rest

Ataxia – loss of control of voluntary movement

Atelectasis – collapsed, non-aerated lung, usually due to a blocked bronchus, but may be congenital

Atheroma/atheromatous/arteriosclerosis – arterial occlusive disease

Athetosis/athetoid – abnormal involuntary movement

Atresia – congenital failure to open, or pathological closure, of a lumen, e.g., gut or vessel

Atrial septal defect (ASD) – abnormal opening between the two atrial cavities of the heart

Atrophy – wasting of a tissue, as in malnutrition or muscle denervation

Audiometry – test of hearing

Auscultation – listening to sounds produced by the body, usually through a stethoscope

Autopsy – postmortem examination of a body to determine or confirm the cause of death

Babinski response – extensor plantar response; occurs in pyramidal tract disease, on stroking the lateral aspect of the sole of the foot there is spontaneous dorsiflexion of the great toe, with "fanning" of the toes

Bacteriology – study of bacteria

Balanitis – inflammation of the glans penis and prepuce

Balloting – feeling an object bouncing within a fluid collection, e.g., on tapping of fetal head or an abdominal mass within ascites

Basal cell carcinoma (BCC) – malignant skin lesion

Beau's lines – transverse ridges in a nail, indicating periods of defective growth

Benign – non-malignant tumor; a disease with mild characteristics or with a good prognosis

Biopsy – tissue sample taken from known or suspected disease for classification

Bjerrum screen – black screen with a central white target, used for mapping the visual fields

Blood dyscrasia – disorder of the blood

Borborygmi – rumbling or gurgling sounds made by passage of flatus through the intestines

Bovine cough – cattle-like cough due to vocal cord paralysis, secondary to recurrent laryngeal nerve damage

Bradycardia – slowing of the heart

Bronchiectasis – bronchial dilatation with infection

Bronchitis – inflammation of bronchial mucosa

Bronchoscopy – examination of the bronchial tree with a bronchoscope

Bruising – bleeding into tissues

Bruit – abnormal sound heard with a stethoscope over a large (usually narrowed) artery

Bryant's triangle – anatomical marking made in the supine position, by dropping a vertical line from the anterior superior iliac spine to a horizontal line through the greater trochanter; used to detect shortening of the femoral neck

Bulbar palsy – paralysis from damage to the cranial nerve nuclei in the brainstem

Bursa – cushioning synovial-lined cavity over or between pressure points

Cachexia – extreme general state of ill-health, with malnutrition, wasting, anemia, and muscle weakness

Calcemia – calcium level in the body: hyper- (excess) or hypo- (reduced)

Calculus – an abnormal concretion, usually of inorganic matter; occurring in reservoir organs and ducts

Campbell de Morgan spots – small red hemangiomas, usually on the trunk, having no pathological significance

Cannula – hollow tube placed within or introduced into a cavity or vessel, for withdrawal or delivery of fluid

Caput medusa – periumbilical network of veins, secondary to hepatic venous obstruction (portal hypertension)

Carcinoma – malignant epithelial tumors, characterized by invasion and metastasis

Caries – tooth decay

Cataract – opacity of the lens and/or its capsule

Celiac – malabsorption disease of gut

Cesarean section – delivery of the fetus through a uterine incision

Chalazion – *see* meibomian cyst

Cheyne-Stokes respiration – rythmical alternation of rapid and absent periods of breathing, due to damage to the respiratory center: usually a preterminal state

Cholecystitis – inflammation of the gall bladder

Chorea – neurological disorder, characterized by irregular involuntary (**choreiform**) movements of the limbs and face

Chronic – persistent, e.g., pain, discharge or infection. In the latter, the term has a specific pathological meaning, with production of a granuloma

Circumcision – surgical removal of the prepuce of the glans penis

Cirrhosis – chronic perilobular fibrosis of the connective tissue of the liver

Cleft lip – congenital malformation of the upper lip, due to failure of fusion of the maxillary and frontonasal processes; frequently associated with **cleft palate**

Clonus – increased reflex activity, characterized by repetitive muscular contraction induced by stretch: usually occurring with upper motor neuron lesions

Clubbing – digital disorder, usually of the fingers, characterized by longitudinal and lateral curving of the nails, and bulbous endings: occurring in a number of conditions, including congenital cardiac, chronic pulmonary and inflammatory bowel disease

Coarctation of the aorta – congenital narrowing of the aorta

Colic – painful powerful contractions of a muscular tube, usually due to obstruction of the intestine, ureter or biliary tree

Colonoscopy – examination of the colon with a colonoscope

Coma – unrousable state of consciousness

Congenital defect – developmental abnormality, present at birth

Coning – compression of the brain through the tentorium cerebelli or the foramen magnum, secondary to raised intracranial pressure – usually a terminal event. NB it can be precipitated by lumbar puncture

...unctivitis – inflammation of the conjunctiva

...sensual – reflex excitement of a part, in response to stimulation of ...other, as with a contralateral pupil response to light

Consolidation – conversion into a firm mass, as occurs in the lung in pneumonia

Contracture – deformity, usually due to muscle shortening. This may be permanent, when fibrosis is present, or temporary if in respose to a stimulus such as anesthesia or cold

Contralateral – occurring on the opposite side of the body

CPR – cardiopulmonary resuscitation

Craniotomy – operation on the skull

Crepitus – irregular noise or palpable feeling on moving abnormal tissues, as with a fractured bone, osteoarthritic joints, inflamed tendons or gas in tissues

Cricothyroidotomy – opening into the trachea through the cricothyroid membrane, usually undertaken as an emergency for an obstructed airway

Crohn's disease – inflammatory bowel disease

Cryptorchid – bilateral absence of testes within the scrotum, due to non-descent or congenital absence

Cushing's disease – clinical syndrome due to hypersecretion of adrenal cortical hormones, in response to a local abnormality, an extrinsic stimulus, or from an ectopic site

CVP – central venous pressure

Cyanosis – blue discoloration of the skin and mucous membranes due to an abnormal amount of reduced hemoglobin, usually due to pulmonary or cardiac disease

Cyst – retained collection of fluid, from a variety of sources, e.g., exocrine and endocrine glands, congenital rests (dermoid, thyroglossal), degenerative, e.g., pancreatitis and parasitic (hydatid)

Cystocele – bladder bulging into the vagina, usually a complication of vaginal childbirth

Dacrocystitis – inflammation of the lacrimal apparatus

Decussation – crossing, usually referring to a neural pathway

Dehydration – reduced body fluid due to low intake or loss

Demyelination – removal or destruction of the myelin of nerve tissue

De Quervain's synovitis – inflammation of the te...
side of the wrist

Diabetes insipidus – clinical syndrome due to the lack...
hormone

Diabetes mellitus – clinical syndrome due to the lack of, or c...
abnormal response to, insulin

Diarrhea – increased frequency and/or quantity, and looseness of st...
(but document precisely the patient's description)

Diastole – period of the cardiac cycle from the closure of the aortic and pulmonary valves to the beginning of the next ventricular contraction

Diplopia – double vision

Discharge – leaking of fluid from the body through a normal (e.g., nose or anus) or an abnormal opening (e.g., an ulcer or fistula)

Dislocation – loss of the normal proximity of structures, usually the bones of a joint

Divarication – separating or stretching, as between the rectus abdominis muscles

Diverticulum – pouch or cul-de-sac from a hollow organ or duct

Douglas (pouch of) – rectouterine/rectovesical peritoneal pouch, palpable on rectal examination

Down syndrome – clinical syndrome of genetic origin

Dupuytren's contracture – thickening and contraction of the palmar fascia, causing a digital flexion deformity, usually of the ring and little finger

DVT – deep vein thrombosis

Dysarthria – difficulty in articulation

Dysdiadochokinesis – impared voluntary movement of cerebellar origin

Dysfunction – general term for impaired activity of an organ or part

Dyskinesia – impairment of voluntary movement

Dysmenorrhea – pain occurring at or about the time of menstruation

Dyspareunia – difficulty or pain on intercourse

Dyspepsia – general term covering symptoms from the upper alimentary tract

Dysphagia – difficulty or pain on swallowing

. speaking

or discomfort in breathing; **paroxysmal nocturnal** a occurring when supine, usually secondary to left

ain or difficulty in passing urine

– inappropriately sited tissues or organs, as with an ectopic ancy

tropion – eversion of the edge of an eyelid

Eczema – non-contagious inflammatory disease of the skin

Edema – excess of tissue fluid

Effusion – fluid collection, such as in a joint or pleural cavity

Egophony – sound of speech through a pleural effusion: like the bleat of a goat

Ehlers-Danlos syndrome – inherited disorder of elastic tissue, producing laxity of tissues

Electrocardiogram (ECG) – a record of the electrical activity of heart muscle

Embolism – sudden blocking of a blood vessel, usually an artery, by blood clot, clumps of bacteria or other foreign material transported in the circulation

Emphysema – dilatation of pulmonary alveoli

Empyema – pus in the pleural cavity

Encephalitis – inflammation of the brain

Endocarditis – inflammation of the endocardium, usually involving the valve cusps

Endometriosis – ectopic endometrium, usually within the pelvis or abdominal wall

Enophthalmos – recession of the eyeball into the orbit

Entropion – inversion of the edge of an eyelid

Epididymo-orchitis – inflammation of the epididymis and the testis

Epilepsy – cerebral disorder producing excessive and disordered discharge of cerebral neurons, resulting in paroxysmal recurrent movements, often with tongue biting and incontinence, and usually accompanied by unconsciousness – the **epileptic fit**

Epispadias – congenital malformation of the urethra, opening on the dorsal aspect of the penis

Epistaxis – bleeding from the nose

Erythema – redness of the skin due to hyperemia

Erythema ab igne – pigmented reticular cutaneous discoloration, due to exposure to heat; often on the shins from sitting in front of a fire, or on the abdomen, from a hot water bottle, applied for pain relief

Esophagoscopy – examination of the esophagus through an esophagoscope

Exophthalmos – prominence or protrusion of the eyeball

Expansile – expanding, usually an aneurysm or pulsatile vascular mass

Failure – end-stage loss of function of an organ, e.g., cardiac, pulmonary, hepatic or renal failure

Fallot's tetralogy – congenital cardiac anomaly, the classical four abnormalities are pulmonary artery stenosis; ventricular septal defect; an overriding aorta; and an enlarged right ventricle

Fasciculation – involuntary ripple-like twitching of voluntary muscles

Fatigue – tiredness and lethargy that usually accompany cardiac failure

Feculent – like feces

Fibrillation – spontaneous independent contraction of the auricular or ventricular cardiac muscle; spontaneous contraction of recently denervated skeletal muscle

Fibroid – resembling fibrous tissue; smooth muscle tumor (fibroma) commonly of the uterus

Fibrosis – abnormal production of fibrous (scar) tissue, often interfering with function

Fissure – deep groove, may be normal, e.g., in the brain, but may be a breach of a normal lining, e.g., the longitudinal ulcer of an **anal fissure**

Fistula – an abnormal connection between epithelial/endothelial surfaces, e.g., anal (from anal canal to external skin), between two loops of gut or arteriovenous

Fit - *see* epilepsy

Forceps – gripping instrument used in surgery; **obstetric forceps** applied to the fetal head to facilitate delivery

Fracture – discontinuity of a structure, usually a broken bone

Froment's sign – use of flexion of the interphalangeal joint of the thumb to grip, when the adductor pollicis is paralyzed

Galactorrhea – excessive lactation or milk discharge outside the normal period of lactation

Gallstone – concretion within the biliary tree

Gangrene – death and anerobic putrefaction of ischemic tissue

Gas gangrene – infection with gas-producing organisms, notably *Clostridium perfringens*, but also anaerobic staphylococci and streptococci; a potentially lethal condition

Gastroduodenoscopy – endoscopic inspection of the stomach and duodenum

Gastroenteritis – inflammation of the stomach and intestine

Gibbus – prominent hump/lump on the back

Glands of Montgomery – prominent sebaceous glands of the areola of the breast; they enlarge in pregnancy

Glasgow Coma Scale (GCS) – system of assessing cerebral damage

Glaucoma – increased intraocular pressure

Glossitis – inflammation of the tongue

Goiter – enlargement of the thyroid gland

Granuloma – small tumor produced by the chronic cellular response to certain infections and other agents, such as tuberculosis and foreign bodies

Graphesthesia – the ability to recognize letters or figures traced on the skin by blunt pressure

Guarding – voluntary contraction of abdominal wall muscles in response to painful palpation

Halitosis – fetid or offensive breath

Hashimoto disease – chronic thyroiditis associated with autoimmune antibodies to thyroxin

Heart block – condition in which the transmission of impulses from the sinoatrial node through the atria, atrioventricular node and bundle of His to the ventricles is delayed or interrupted

Heberden's nodes – bony phalangeal nodules of osteoarthritis

Hemangioma – benign tumor of blood vessels

Hemarthrosis – bloody joint effusion

Hematoma – discrete collection of blood in the body following a bleed

Hematuria – blood in the urine

Hemianopia – loss of half of the visual field, of one or bo[...]
homonymous hemianopia – to one side (nasal of one eye a[...]
of the other), seen in unilateral cortical lesions; **bitemporal he[...]**
– due to lesions of the optic chiasm

Hemiplegia – paralysis of one side of the body

Hemochromatosis – deposition of iron throughout the body, due to metabolic defect or excess transfusion

Hemodialysis – removal of waste products from the body by an external device, in patients with renal failure

Hemoglobinopathy – abnormal hemoglobin

Hemolysis – release of hemoglobin from damaged red cells

Hemoptysis – coughing of bright red blood from the lungs, bronchi or trachea

Hemorrhage – bleeding; the escape of blood from any part of the vascular system; **splinter hemorrhage** – linear hemorrhage under the nails, seen in bacterial endocarditis

Hemorrhoid (pile) – swelling at the anal margin

Hemothorax – collection of blood in the pleural cavity

Hepatitis – inflammation of the liver

Hepatocellular dysfunction – abnormal liver function

Hepatoma – tumor originating in the hepatic parenchyma

Hepatosplenomegaly – enlarged condition of the liver and spleen

Hernia – protrusion of the contents of a cavity through its wall

Hickman line – external catheter device for long-term venous access, often passed into the subclavian or internal jugular veins

Hidradenitis – inflammation of the sweat glands

Hodgkin disease – tumor of lymphatic tissue

Horner syndrome – damage of the cervical sympathetic chain producing: enophthalmos, miosis, ptosis, with narrowing of the palpebral fissure, facial flushing, loss of sweating and stuffiness of the nose, on the side of the lesion

Howell-Jolly bodies – spherical, eccentrically placed granules or nuclear remnants in red blood corpuscles, usually in hemolytic or toxic anemia, and after splenectomy

Hydrocele – circumscribed collection of fluid, usually in the tunica vaginalis of the testis

– abnormal increase of cerebrospinal fluid within the

...rosis – obstructed dilated renal pelvis filled with urine

...alpinx – obstructed dilated uterine tube filled with clear fluid

...er/hypo – abnormal increase/low level (e.g., cholesterol, sodium, ...cium, glucose)

Hyperdynamic – abnormally great muscular or nervous activity; extreme functional energy

Hyperemia – excess of blood in any part of the body; **reactive hyperemia** – increased blood flow after temporary ischemia

Hyperesthesia – excessive sensitivity of the skin, due to local causes or to peripheral nerve damage

Hyperhidrosis – excess sweating

Hyperkalemia – high body potassium level

Hyperkeratinization – horny thickening of epithelium, particularly of the palms and soles; characteristic of chronic arsenical poisoning and vitamin A deficiency

Hyperkinesia – abnormally powerful movement, as in muscular spasm

Hyperparathyroidism – abnormally increased activity of the parathyroid glands due to a neoplasm or to hyperplasia

Hyperpnea – increased rate/depth of breathing

Hypertension – high arterial blood pressure usually in the systemic circulation. It may also be in the pulmonary arteries, secondary to lung disease, and in the portal venous system, due to liver disease

Hypertonia – excessive tension, as in arteries, muscle or intraocular

Hypertrophic obstructive cardiomyopathy (HOCM) – congenital overgrowth of cardiac muscle, particularly affecting the left ventricle and interventricular septum

Hypertrophic pulmonary osteoarthropathy – proliferative periostitis at the distal end of long bones, particularly of the wrist and ankle, always associated with gross clubbing, and usually indicative of carcinoma of the bronchus

Hypertrophy – an increase in the size of the cells of a tissue; **ventricular hypertrophy** – enlargement of heart muscle

Hypocarbia – low carbon dioxide on blood gas analysis

Hypoglycemia – low blood sugar concentration

Hypokalemia – low body potassium

Hyporeflexia – reduced reflex action

Hypospadias – congenital malformation of the urethra, opening onto the ventral aspect of the penis

Hypothyroidism – clinical syndrome, due to thyroid hormone insufficiency

Hypotonia – reduced tension in a body structure, such as in arteries, muscles and the eye

Hypoxemia/hypoxia – insufficient oxygen to maintain normal tissue respiration

Iatrogenic – disorder produced by therapy

Idiopathic – disease of unknown cause

Ileus (paralytic) – obstructed gut (non-motile)

Impaction – forceful driving of one structure into another, such as broken bones, a misdirected tooth or feces into a poorly evacuating rectum

Imperforate anus – congenital defect of anal canal development

Impotence – inability to perform the sexual act

Incompetence – regurgitation through a defective valve, e.g., related to the heart or varicose veins

Infarct – area of dead tissue, with or without hemorrhage, produced by obstruction of an end-artery

Infection – invasion of the body by pathogenic organisms, and their subsequent multiplication

Inflammation – body's response to cellular damage, whether this be physical or chemical injury, bacterial invasion or other disease

Innervation – nerve supply

Intermittent claudication – skeletal muscle pain on exercise, due to inadequate blood supply

Intracranial pressure – pressure within the skull: if there is free circulation of the cerebrospinal fluid and the patient is recumbent, this is the same as the pressure measured by lumbar puncture

Intubation – passage of a therapeutic tube; this is usually through an existing anatomical pathway, such as the trachea or urethra

Intussusception – invagination of a loop of proximal into distal bowel

...l – occurring on the same side of the body

...ia – insufficient blood supply to a part to sustain its normal
...on

...hara chart – multi-colored dotted charts, designed to identify color-
...and subjects

Jaundice – clinical syndrome of excessive circulating bile pigments,
giving rise to yellow discoloration of the sclera, skin, and mucous
membranes

Kernig sign – reflex contraction of neck muscles in meningitis

Ketosis – excessive ketones within the body

Klinefelter syndrome – congenital chromosomal defect of gonadal
hormone production

Koilonychia – spoon-shaped nails related to certain forms of anemia

Koplik spots – whitish-blue specks on the oral mucous membrane in
measles

Korotkoff – sounds heard on release of a cuff when measuring blood
pressure

Kussmaul breathing – rapid breathing of diabetic coma

Kyphosis – spinal curvature in which the concavity of the curve is in a
forward direction, generally seen in the thoracic region

Laparoscopy – inspection of the contents of the peritoneal cavity by
means of a laparoscope

Laparotomy – inspection of the peritoneal contents through an
exploratory abdominal incision

Left bundle branch block – *see* heart block

Lesion – non-specific term for a pathological abnormality

Leukemia – disease of the white blood cells

Leukonychia – white spots on a nail

Leukoplakia – thickened white patches on mucous membranes, the
lesions are chronic inflammatory but have malignant potential

Lichen planus – disorder of skin and mucous membranes, producing
patchy discoloration

Lordosis – spinal curvature in which the convexity of the curve is in a
forward direction, generally found in the lumbar region

Lymphadenitis – inflammation of lymph nodes

Lymphadenopathy – enlargement of lymph nodes

Lymphedema – excess tissue fluid, due to failure of lymphatic dr

Lymphoma – tumor of lymphatic tissue

Macrognathia – abnormal enlargement of the jaw

Malabsorption – defective absorption of fluids and other nutrients from the gut

Malgaigne's bulge – muscular bulge along the line of the inguinal canal, due to tissue laxity rather than an underlying hernia

Malignant – life-threatening pathological process, usually characterized by invasion and metastasis

Malnutrition – insufficient nutriment, due to inadequate intake or failed absorption

Mammography – soft tissue radiographic technique for examining the breasts

Marfan syndrome – congenital hereditary disorder of mesodermal tissue, its features include tall stature, increased span, long thin digits, subluxation of the lens, and arterial dissection

Mass – non-specific term of a collection of cells or tissues, usually implies a palpable or visible abnormality

McMurray test – test to demonstrate damage to the knee menisci

Meconium – gut content of the newly born

Meconium ileus – bowel obstruction of the newborn, due to inspissated meconium

Mediastinoscopy – examination of the mediastinum by means of an endoscope inserted suprasternally

Mediterranean disease (thalassemia) – a congenital hemoglobin abnormality

Meibomian cyst – infection of sebaceous gland on eyelid margin

Meiosis – process of cell division with reduction of diploid status

Menarche – onset of the menses

Menopause – cessation of the menses

Menorrhagia – excessive and/or prolonged menstrual bleeding

Mesothelioma – malignancy of pleura, pericardium and peritoneum, due to exposure to asbestos

Metastasis – spread of malignant disease from its primary site to distant parts of the body, by way of natural passages, blood vessels, lymphatics or by direct continuity.

...obin – congenital hemoglobin abnormality, when part of the ...cule is in the oxidized ferric form and unavailable for oxygen ...t

...yocardial infarction) – death of a segment of heart muscle due to ...emia

Microcephalus – small sized head

Microcytosis – small red blood cells

Micrognathia – undersized jaw, usually applied to the mandible

Mikulicz syndrome – symmetrical enlargement of the lacrimal and salivary glands

Mitral incompetence – *see* incompetence

Mole/nevus – congenital benign pigmented skin lesion; **hydatidiform mole** – abnormal intrauterine fetal development, producing a polycystic mass of chorionic villi

Motor neuron disease – progressive degeneration of motor neurons

Mucocele – mucus-filled cyst, e.g., in the mouth or the gall bladder

Mucoid – of the nature of mucus

Mucopurulent – containing mucus and pus

Mucus – viscous secretion of mucus membranes

Multiple myeloma – tumor arising from the bone marrow

Multiple sclerosis – demyelinating disease of the brain and spinal cord

Murmur – sound related to blood flow and heard on auscultation, usually indicating an abnormality of heart valve origin. A machinery (continuous) murmur may be heard over arteriovenous malformations. Other blood vessel sounds are usually referred to as bruits

Murphy's sign – subcostal tenderness elicited on inspiration, in patients with cholecystitis

Myasthenia gravis – disorder of the motor end-plate, giving rise to abnormal muscle fatigability

Myelocele – *see* spina bifida

Myelodysplasia – imperfect development of any part of the spinal cord

Myelopathy – impaired function of striated muscle

Myocardial infarction (MI) – death of a segment of heart muscle due to ischemia

Myotonia – abnormality of muscle relaxation after effort

Myxedema – a clinical syndrome, due to reduced thyroid hormone production

Nausea – feeling of sickness with the desire to vomit

Nelaton's line – line joining the anterior superior iliac spine and the ischial tuberosity on radiograph

Neoplasia – generic term for a new growth, whether benign or malignant

Nephritis – inflammation of the kidney; may be congenital or acquired

Nephrotic syndrome – degenerative renal disease

Neuritis – inflammation of a nerve

Neuroma – non-specific term for a benign neural tumor, or a painful post-traumatic mass of disorganized regenerating nerve endings

Neuron – functional unit of the nervous system: upper motor neuron – passing from the cortex to the spinal cord; lower motor neuron – from the spinal cord to the muscle

Neuropathy – altered neuronal function

Nevi (spider) – acquired cutaneous capillary dilatation, with central spot and radiating capillaries, often seen in hepatic failure

Nevus (strawberry) – congenital benign pigmented cutaneous lesion of vascular origin

Niemann-Pick disease – abnormality of reticuloendothelium

Nocturia – getting up at night to pass urine

Nodule – a small aggregation of cells

Nystagmus – congenital or acquired involuntary eye movement, particularly in horizontal plane, usually related to labyrinthine or cerebellar disease

Orthopnea – breathlessness on lying flat

Osler's nodes – painful digital nodules of infective endocarditis

Osteitis fibrosa cystica – generalized rarefaction of bone, with cyst formation and fibrous replacement, due to excess parathormone production

Osteoarthritis – degenerative joint disease associated with wear, tear, and aging

Osteochondroma – benign tumor of bone and cartilage

Osteomalacia – decalcification of the bones

...omyelitis – bone infection

...eoporosis – rarefaction of bone

...titis – inflammation of the external (externa) or middle (media) ear

Paget disease – of the nipple: periareolar, eczematous skin changes related to an underlying carcinoma; of bone (osteitis deformans): inflammatory disorder producing bowing of long bones and skull thickening

Palpitations – awareness of the heartbeat, often because of increased force, rate or irregularity

Pancoast syndrome – apical lung tumor, producing a Horner syndrome and damage to the T1 root of the brachial plexus

Pancreatitis – inflammation of the pancreas

Papilledema – edema of the optic disc, observed on ophthalmoscopy

Paracentesis – sampling or removing abnormal peritoneal fluid, usually through a wide-bore needle

Paralysis – weakness of neural or neuromuscular origin

Paralytic ileus – *see* ileus

Paraphimosis – constriction ring of the prepuce, proximal to the glans penis

Paresthesia – abnormal somatic sensation, usually numbness or tingling

Parkinson disease – chronic neurological disease producing muscle weakness, rigidity and tremor (**parkinsonism**)

Paronychia – infection around the nail

Patent ductus arteriosus – persistence of fetal communication between the aorta and the left pulmonary artery

Pathological – disease state

Pathology – study of disease

Peau d'orange – obstructive edema, producing dimpling of the skin, typically in infiltrating carcinoma of the breast

Pectus carinatum – pigeon chest

Pectus excavatum – depressed anterior chest wall

Percussion – process of striking the surface of the body to hear and feel the underlying resonant effects

Perforation – hole through the full thickness of a tissue, such as the gut wall

Pericardial rub – noise produced by movement of inflamed layers of pericardium

Pericardial tamponade – compression of the heart by fluid within the pericardial cavity

Pericarditis – inflammation of the pericardium

Perimetry – use of a perimeter to measure visual fields

Peristalsis – wave-like contraction of a hollow organ

Peritoneal rub – noise produced by movement of inflamed layers of peritoneum

Peritonism – abdominal tenderness associated with peritonitis. Guarding is usually present, as may be **percussion rebound** (pain on percussing the abdomen)

Peritonitis – inflammation of the peritoneum

Perseveration – a repetitive activity without an appropriate exciting stimulus

Perthe's – **disease** of the neck of the femur; **test** of lower limb deep vein patency

Pheochromocytoma – tumor of the adrenal medulla

Philadelphia chromosome – usually found in bone marrow cells of patients with chronic myeloid leukemia

Phimosis – narrowing of the preputial orifice, preventing retraction of the foreskin and, in its extreme, the passage of urine

Pile – *see* hemorrhoid

Pleurisy – inflammation of the pleura

Pneumonia – inflammation of the lung

Pneumoperitoneum – gas within the peritoneal cavity

Pneumothorax – gas within the pleural cavity

Polycystic – multiple cysts, may be congenital or acquired, e.g., kidney, ovary, pancreas

Polycythemia – increase in the number of circulating red blood cells usually associated with an increase in hemoglobin, packed red cell volume and blood viscosity

Polyhydramnios – excessive amniotic fluid

Polyp – pedunculated epithelial tumor

Polypectomy – removal of a polyp

Polyuria – increased urine excretion

Priapism – persistent penile erection

Primary biliary cirrhosis – imflammation of the bile ducts, producing fibrosis and destruction, with associated jaundice

Procidentia – complete prolapse, e.g., uterus or rectum

Proctoscopy – examination of the anal canal and lower rectum by means of a proctoscope

Prolapse – bulging of a lax wall, e.g., vagina into the rectum, or of cardiac valves, e.g., mitral valve

Proptosis – bulging of eyeball

Pruritus – itching (*see also* table 11, page 339)

Pseudobulbar palsy – upper motor neuron paralysis of the cranial nerve nuclei, in the brainstem. This indicates bilateral cerebral lesions, as the lower cranial nerve nuclei are bilaterally innervated

Pseudocyst – fluid collection lined by diseased tissue of varied origin

Ptosis – prolapse or drooping of an organ, such as the upper eyelid

Pulsatile – beating with the pulse (*see also* expansile)

Pulsus paradoxus – pulse becoming less pronounced with inspiration rather than expiration

Purulent – containing pus

Pyemia – pus-forming organism in the bloodstream

Pyo- – purulent infection of an organ

Pyonephrosis – obstructed dilated renal pelvis filled with pus

Pyosalpinx – obstructed dilated uterine tube filled with pus

Pyrexia – raised temperature

Râles – fine pulmonary added sounds

Ramsay Hunt syndrome – herpes zoster infection of the geniculate ganglion

Rash – cutaneous eruption

Rebound – reflex response to withdrawal of a stimulus, e.g., sudden pain on withdrawal of the hand in deep palpation of a painful abdomen

Rectocele – prolapse of the rectum into the vagina

Reflex – involuntary response to a stimulus, e.g., knee extension to a patellar tap

Reflux – back flow, e.g., through an incompetent gastroesophageal junction, or through valve-less lower limb veins

Regurgitation – reversal of flow, as with swallowed food into the mouth or of blood through incompetent cardiac valves

Resuscitation – restoration of life or consciousness, in the apparently dead or collapsed patient

Retention – retaining substances in the body that are normally excreted

Retinopathy – disorder of the retina

Rhabdomyoma – tumor of striated muscle; **rhabdomyosarcoma**, malignant form

Rheumatic fever – infection accompanied by abnormalities of cardiac valves

Rheumatism – non-specific term applied to pain of musculoskeletal origin

Rheumatoid nodules – aggregations of cells and tissues, situated in various soft tissues of the body, often over bony prominences

Riedel's lobe – a congenital anomalous lobe of the liver, projecting downward from the right side anteriorly

Right bundle branch block – *see* heart block

Rigidity – state of stiffness and inflexibility

Rinne's test – auditory test

Romberg's sign – with the feet together the patient closes their eyes: swaying or falling is indicative of sensory ataxia, due to loss of position sense in the lower limbs; **rombergism** – exhibiting a positive Romberg's sign

Ronchi – coarse pulmonary added sounds

Rub – audible movement of inflamed surfaces, e.g., pericardium, pleura

Salpingitis – inflammation of the uterine tubes

Sarcoid – systematic inflammatory disease, characterized by non-caseating granulomas

Sarcoma – malignancy of non-epithelial tissue

Scar – connective-tissue replacement of mesodermal or ectodermal tissue that has been destroyed by injury or other disease

Scoliosis – lateral curvature of the spine

Scotoma – loss of part of the visual field

Secondary – *see* metastasis

Seminoma – malignancy of the testis

Septal defect – hole in the interatrial or interventricular septum, or both

Septicemia – severe infective state, in which the bloodstream is invaded by large numbers of bacteria

Sickle cell – hereditary abnormality of hemoglobin

Sigmoidoscopy – inspection of the rectum and pelvic colon with a sigmoidoscope

Sinus – infected tract communicating with the skin, or the lumen of a hollow viscus

Sinus arrhythmia – irregularity of heart rhythm, caused by changes in vagal stimulation of the sinoatrial node during respiration

Sinus rhythm – normal heart rhythm, due to conduction of impulses from the sinoatrial node to the atrioventricular node, through the atrial muscle, and thence the conducting system

Sister Joseph's nodule – umbilical metastasis

Sjögren syndrome – syndrome characterized by deficient secretion of the lacrimal, salivary or other glands, giving rise to keratoconjunctivitis sicca, dry tongue, and hoarse voice

Snellen chart – test of visual acuity

Spasm – sudden, powerful, involuntary contraction of muscle

Spastic hemiplegia – hemiplegia with increased muscle tone

Spasticity – persistent muscle contraction, producing stiffness and rigidity, or loss of controlled movement, usually following an upper motor neuron lesion

Speculum – instrument for the inspection of a tube or passage

Spherocytosis – abnormal thick, almost spherical, red blood cells (spherocytes)

Sphincterotomy – incision of a sphincter

Spider nevus – small red, cutaneous vascular dilatation from which capillaries radiate, and resemble a spider

Spina bifida – imperfect development of the spinal cord and vertebral covering

Splenomegaly – enlarged spleen

Splinter hemorrhages – longitudinal hemorrhagic subungual streaks, usually due to bacterial endocarditis

Splitting – of the heart sounds: due to asynchronous closure of the mitral and tricuspid, and the pulmonary and aortic valves

Spondylolisthesis – subluxation of the lower lumbar vertebrae on the sacrum

Sputum – material expelled from the respiratory passages by coughing or clearing the throat

Squint – condition in which one eye deviates from the point of fixation

Status epilepticus – recurrent epileptic fits without any periods of recovery or regain of consciousness

Steatorrhea – excessive fat in the stool, as in celiac disease

Stenosis – narrowing of an orifice or a lumen, as with a cardiac valve, an atheromatous artery, or benign and malignant lesions of the gut

Stereognosis – ability to recognize the shape and character of an object by means of touch

Stoma – opening, such as a colostomy on the abdominal wall

Strangulated hernia – gut ischemia due to constriction of the lumen and blood vessels at the neck of a hernial sac

Stricture (stenosis) – narrowing of a lumen, e.g., gut or duct, may be congenital or acquired

Stridor – harsh respiratory sounds due to an obstructed airway

Stroke – sudden paralysis, due to cerebral damage; **stroke volume** – blood ejected by a contraction of the left ventricle

Stye – inflamed eyelid sebaceous cyst

Subluxation – partial dislocation

Subungual – beneath a nail

Sulfhemoglobin – abnormal hemoglobin produced by hydrogen sulfide

Suppuration – production or exudation of pus

Syncope – transient loss of consciousness, as with a faint, but may also accompany cardiac disease

Synovitis – inflammation of the synovial membrane, of a joint or tendon sheath

Systolic – relating to cardiac systole

Tachycardia – rapid beating of the heart

Tachypnea – rapid breathing

Talipes – congenital deformity of the foot

Tamponade – pathological compression of an organ, e.g., the heart from a pericardial effusion

Target cell – abnormal red blood cell, with a ringed appearance on staining, assocated with certain types of anemia and postsplenectomy

Telangiectasia – dilated capillaries, often multiple forming an angiomatous mass: **hereditary telangiectasia** (Rendu-Osler-Weber disease) there is often a secondary anemia, due to recurrent mucosal bleeding in the gut

Tenesmus – painful, often unsuccessful attempts at defecation or urination

Tenosynovitis – inflammation of a tendon sheath

Teratoma – congenital embryonic cell malignancy of the testis or ovary

Thalassemia – hereditary anemia, due to a hemoglobin abnormality

Thomas test – test for fixed hip flexion

Thoracotomy – surgical exposure of the thorax

Thrill – palpable vibration of abnormal blood flow, such as through a diseased heart valve or arteriovenous malformation

Thromboembolic disease – passage of blood clot through the circulation

Thrombosis – intravascular coagulation

Thyrotoxicosis – clinical syndrome, due to an overactive thyroid gland

Tic – uncontrolled local repetetive movement, commonly affecting the face

Tinel's sign – tingling sensation on percussion of a regenerating nerve ending

Tinnitus – subjective noise in the ear

Tone – tension in normal muscle; altered by neuromuscular disorders

Tophi – sodium biurate deposits in gout, often subcutaneous on the ear

Torsion – twisting, usually of the stalk of a structure, e.g., of a cyst, ovary or testis

Tracheostomy – opening in the trachea, usually to relieve an obstructed airway

Traction – act of pulling

Tremor – rhythmic, involuntary, purposeless, oscillating movement, resulting from the alternate contraction and relaxation of opposing muscle groups

Trendelenburg sign – dipping of the contralateral side of the pelvis when standing on an abnormal hip; **Trendelenburg gait** – spastic gait

Trendelenburg test – a tourniquet test for determining the competency of superficial veins of the lower leg

Tricuspid incompetence – *see* incompetence

Trigger finger – nodule in a long flexor tendon in the palm, clicking through a concomitant stricture of its sheath

Trophic changes – wasting of tissues, due to ischemia or denervation

Tumor – swelling

Turgor – increased tissue tension, usually due to edema

Turner syndrome – congenital genetic abnormality affecting gonadal development

Tympanitic – hyper-resonant

Ulcer/ulceration – discontinuity of epithelial surface

Ulcerative colitis – inflammatory bowel disease, characterized by ulceration with passage of blood and mucus, and variable systemic effects

Uremia – terminal stage of renal failure, with retention of waste products

Urethritis – inflammation of the urethra

Urinalysis – analysis of urine

Valgus – displacement away from the midline, the distal portion projecting laterally, as with hallux valgus

Valsalva maneuver – forcible exhalation against a closed airway, used to produce vagal stimulation

Valvotomy – operation of splitting a stenosis, as with a diseased heart valve

Varicocele – abnormal plexus of varicose veins of the pampiniform plexus around the spermatic cord

Varicose veins – dilated thin tortuous superficial veins, usually of the lower limb

Varix (saphena) – tortuous dilated vein segment (at the saphenous opening)

Varus – displacement toward the midline, the proximal portion projecting laterally, as with bow legs (genu varus)

Venepuncture – puncture of a vein to withdraw blood, or introduce fluids or drugs

Venereal – sexually transmitted

Ventricular septal defect – abnormal opening between the ventricular cavities of the heart

Vertigo – giddiness, a sense of instability, often with a sense of rotation

Virology – study of viruses

Viscus – internal organ

Vocal fremitus – palpable chest wall vibration produced by speech

Vocal resonance – sounds heard over the chest while a patient is talking, when markedly increased it is termed **bronchophony**

Volvulus – torsion of a loop of gut

Vomiting – oral evacuation of gastric contents

Warts – cutaneous circumscribed lesions, usually of viral origin, e.g., on hands, soles (verruca); **perianal** – of venereal origin

Weber's test – auditory test

Wegener's granuloma – destructive granulomatous disease of soft tissue

Whispering pectoriloquy – prominence of whispering over diseased lung, heard through a stethoscope

Wilson disease – degenerative cerebral disease due to abnormal copper metabolism

Xanthoma (xanthelasma) – yellowish-brown cutaneous nodules, frequently periorbital, and usually associated with raised lipids

Zollinger-Ellison syndrome – association of peptic ulceration with a secreting pancreatic adenoma

Index